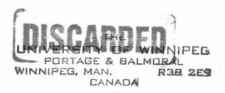

The Psychiatric Society

European Perspectives: A Series of the Columbia University Press

THE PSYCHIATRIC SOCIETY

Robert Castel, Françoise Castel, and Anne Lovell
Translated by Arthur Goldhammer

COLUMBIA UNIVERSITY PRESS
New York   1982

First published in French as *La Société psychiatrique avancée,*
© Éditions Grasset et Fasquelle, 1979

Columbia University Press
New York   Guildford, Surrey

Copyright © 1982 Columbia University Press
All rights reserved
Printed in the United States of America

Library of Congress Cataloging in Publication Data
Castel, Françoise.
The psychiatric society.

(European perspectives)
Translation of: La société psychiatrique
avancée / Françoise Castel, Robert Castel,
Anne Lovell.
Includes bibliographical references and
index.
1. Mental health services—United States.
2. Psychiatry—United States.   I. Castel,
Robert.   II. Lovell, Anne.   III. Title.
IV. Series.   [DNLM: 1. Mental health services—
History—United States.   2. Psychiatry—Histo-
ry—United States.   WM 11 AA1 C4s]
RA790.6.C3713   362.2′0973   81-15504
ISBN 0-231-05244-8   AACR2

*Clothbound editions of Columbia University Press books are
Smyth-sewn and printed on permanent and durable acid-free paper.*

Contents

Translator's Note

A book like this one, which relies so heavily on English-language source material, presents its translator with special problems. The authors have been kind in helping me to retrace their steps through the many and various texts they consulted. Robert and Françoise Castel literally emptied their closets to unearth documents available nowhere else. And closer to home, Anne Lovell interrupted her current work to find needed citations. It has still proved impossible to find a few of the documents consulted by the authors in the course of their original research. In these cases, indicated in the notes, I have retranslated from Robert Castel's French translations. I apologize to the reader for any distortions that may have crept in in the process.

Preface to the English Edition

The American reader may ask why a book such as this one, which examines the development of mental medicine and the relationship of its practices to power and structures of the state, should choose as its laboratory the United States. Or, more surprisingly, why would a sociologist and a psychiatrist, both French, and a third American author with some European background, turn to the American psychiatric system? One answer, of course, is that the United States is the most advanced psychiatric society today, whose techniques—ranging from neuroleptics and methadone maintenance to behavioral therapies to the latest California group experience—are imported and implemented at the very least by European and Latin American countries, if not the world. But there is another answer which emerged as the pieces of this book began to fall into place. An analysis of psychiatry in the United States has enabled us to break with the concept, too long prevalent in social control theories and even in some sociologies of mental health, that behind the array of mental health laws, techniques, and institutions lies one unitary system, the purpose of which is to carry out explicit political goals of the state. Before elaborating on this central idea, though, it might be useful to provide the reader with a few "European" keys to contextualize, so to speak, this study and its method.

The European interest in a social analysis of psychiatry grew out of a larger concern, first with institutions, later with minor forms of power (that institutional analyses had first brought to light), and with the expressions of power in everyday life. To backtrack: already in the 1960s, a current in French intellectual thought had begun moving away from the concept of institutions as instances of reproduction of the social structure or of ideological reflection, toward a view of the institution as a locus of *production*—of certain kinds of individuals, specific forms of submission, special relationships to a social-political order. In the explosion of the 1968 May events, this current converged with a political tendency. French students began to examine the university as an institution that dominated them and produced a certain culture.

Thus intellectuals began perceiving power where they had never looked before. On the one hand, they gave a new legitimacy to epistemological subjects that had previously been considered unworthy of reflection. On the other, intellectuals began to surpass the Marxist concepts of state and dominant ideology that had constituted power analyses. Instead of analyzing the sociological functioning of institutions, intellectuals reconstructed the discourses that institutions produced—and that in turn legitimated them—as well as the populations dominated by such discourses and the everyday social relations reflected in them. By zeroing in on a microsocial space, we may perceive the subtle forms of power that are the main focus of our book.

In France, the concern with institutions soon led to the study of medicine, psychiatry, the prison, and the police—to name a few. Of course, Michel Foucault was the ground-breaker here. And while he would never use his archaeological approach to examine a contemporary situation, his work (and that of other intellectuals) has been read, applied, and incorporated by Europeans into a process of understanding present-day psychiatry. In France, this happened in groups—themselves products of 1968— that maintained a political dimension in their critique of psychiatry: GIA (Information Group on Asylums), Marge, collectives around such journals as *Gardes-Fou* and *Cahiers pour la Folie*, all of which can be roughly characterized as comprising part of the antipsychiatry* movement. In Italy, the crucible of such activity

---

* Antipsychiatry is used here to refer to a broad movement that denounced the mental hospital as a total institution and saw a political (repressive) function to psychiatric practices and techniques. We are not referring to the original, narrower meaning developed by R. D. Laing and David Cooper.

was Psichiatria Democratica, the culmination of a fifteen-year-old anti-institutional movement among mental health workers and professionals. Practical experiences (such as the closing of psychiatric hospitals in Italy) and the groping for an alternative that was neither purely psychiatric nor institutional, demanded constant theoretical elaboration. (Perhaps the most influential work that lent itself to this task was Foucault's *Madness and Civilization*.)[1]

Unfortunately, the French antipsychiatry movement remained theoretical and ideological—basically at the level of verbal denunciations of the most blatant practices in institutions, moral proclamations, and a romanticization of madness. And meanwhile the "psy" sector (psychoanalysis, psychology) continued to expand, developing more liberalized and elaborate forms of their practices, such as institutional psychotherapy and leftist Lacanian psychoanalytical groups. It is not surprising, though, that a sometimes archaic bureaucratic and centralized mental health system should have been the target of antipsychiatry in France and democratic psychiatry in Italy. After all, French psychiatry is the first public medicine, regulated and administered from one central point, according to a single legislation. The law of June 30, 1838 provides for "special establishments" (asylums) for its practice, psychiatrists who are accountable to local prefects, and a single commitment procedure to handle persons deemed dangerous. In Italy, a 1904 law until recently similarly regulated private and public asylums alike, under the Minister of the Interior and local prefectures. (Italy recently passed a radical law known as 180, which, while abolishing involuntary commitment and the perpetuation of long-term care psychiatric facilities, does so with a similar central statute equally applicable to every region of the country.) It is only recently that both French antipsychiatry and European sociology of mental health shifted their analysis to new realms, primarily to the community (*secteur* in French, *territorio* in Italian), and to different practices (e.g., psychoanalysis) and their effects.

The French and Italian situations are now moving toward a collaboration between the old public sector and new, private initiatives; toward a multiplicity of techniques and therapies including family, behavioral, bioenergetics, transactional analysis—in short the gamut; toward the creation of newer categories of people to treat (delinquents, the handicapped, etc.). "Psychiatry as an arm of the state" is no longer an adequate heuristic device for understanding a new situation.

Instead we can look to a model—the United States—where every category of deviance and normality has its treatment modality. The *differences* (of populations to manage, of models for treatment, of strategies for implementation) comprise one unified psy sector in this model. And its very fragmentation allows a penetration into interstices that a centralized system might not reach. It is the loosening of the boundaries that define a concept of health that renders normality a legitimate concern for treatment and manipulation. Thus the American psychiatric system no longer simply censures or represses. It actually *produces* a form of relations delineating a geography of everyday life.

This book was first published in 1979. Since then we have witnessed in the United States both a turning back to the medical model and a dismantling of social psychiatry and experimental programs mentioned in later chapters. A few of the major developments may be worth pointing to.

The deinstitutionalization efforts set in motion in the sixties have developed unevenly, as can be expected in a country where multiple factors, differing from state to state, contribute to this policy. What is changing since the time we wrote this book (see chapter 4 and the conclusion) is the official discourse, which now recognizes a failure of this policy, the inadequacy and in some cases the nonexistence of community care, even the intensifying of *trans*institutionalization, whereby former patients are channeled into new institutions—nursing homes, board-and-care homes (California), private proprietary homes for adults (the East coast), even jails. The National Institute of Mental Health responded to a penury of programs by establishing, in 1978, the Community Support Systems programs to meet the needs of patients "dumped" into increasingly hostile and ghettoizing communities. New York State, appalled by a growing, unmanageable pool of "deinstitutionalized" individuals, many homeless, has declared a halt to its deinstitutionalization policy,[2] while its hospital rooms, shelters, and neighborhoods overflow with former psychiatric patients. Their situation is aggravated by the gentrification of the neighborhoods they cluster in, such as by the closing of low-income hotels and consequent displacement of its residents. Nationwide, hospitals have not been closing at a rapid pace;[3] in fact, they continue to be filled with acute care and chronic patients.

The psychiatric profession, meanwhile, continues to update itself, turning increasingly to genetic and biological models to explain a range of psychiatric disorders. Just as prison officials are calling for more cells, psychiatrists call for more treatment, turning the legal victories of the sixties and seventies (see chapters 4 and 7) into a call for *right* to treatment, asking for more facilities in which to carry it out. The psychiatric journals are replete with articles on how to work around recently established consent and due process procedures so as to administer electroconvulsive therapy or medication to unwilling patients. But just as inpatient practices strengthen, the outpatient practices expand for the range of persons with few or no psychiatric disturbances. And with them expand the new categories: the young chronic, the violent and assaultive patient, hand in hand with the multiplication of new diagnoses in the latest *Diagnostic and Statistical Manual*.[4]

With Reaganism and the return to a pre-Keynesian economic policy, we move into an era of budgetary cutbacks, which directly and indirectly affect the mental health system. First, the reduction in federal grants to such programs as Medicaid is equivalent to withdrawing incentives for community care. Second, proposed block grants will put the future of community mental health centers (still the only major federal program in mental health, see chapter 5) into the hands of local decision makers. It is doubtful that federal money will support the lively experimentation (minority-controlled clinics, rape crisis centers, to name a few) that proliferated earlier.

One may be tempted to see in the era of Reaganism an end to all liberal initiative, as the state rids itself of expensive programs (welfare, health, mental health) no longer profitable to it, in social control terms or otherwise. However, it would be a mistake to think that the control of deviancy and production of a certain type of normality should end here.

First, as has always happened in the United States, a combination of private, semiprivate, volunteer, and local, initiatives always stands ready to take up some of the slack. Witness the current tendency to make the private sector responsible for the management of psychiatric patients (growth of the nursing home industry, adult homes, private hospital beds, and even such explicit policies as the recent Massachusetts moves to contract outcare of patients entirely to the private sector). In fact, the Mental Health Systems Act of 1980, like the Presidential Commission report that preceded it, attempted to rally these varied, often contradictory programs, to respond to the many new categories of the psy sector.

Second, as the division between normal and pathological has eroded (a tendency for which the mechanisms were already in place in the beginning of this century—see Part One), so too is the social microcosm—in the form of self-help techniques, the small group, the psychological management of workplace relations, the preventive management of children as they develop— firmly implanted in our daily lives. Thus even a return to neoliberal economics (as the Europeans call it), without the direct mechanisms of state intervention in people's lives, leaves intact what is more deeply rooted: the production of certain behaviors, the technicalization of what is most "spontaneous," the transformation of needs from public to private issues, from political to individual problems.

We have attempted to trace historically how such a seemingly contradictory system of separate initiatives, of hard and soft technologies, of repressive and liberal institutions came about. The American model raises questions for the future: how do horizontal social forces at the microlevel and vertical lines to the state interact with one another in the psy sector as well as in what remains independently everyday life?

Anne Lovell
New York, 1981

Preface

The three of us have taken the chance of writing this book in the hope that we might succeed in unifying standpoints usually kept apart from one another, owing to the social division of labor, the hazards of history, and the constraints of geography: we hoped, that is, to combine theory and practice, polemic and objective research, personal familiarity and cultural distantiation. To that end we have sought to employ methods modeled on those of ethnology, or, rather, on a reversal of the traditional relationship between the ethnologist and the object of his research.

What does it mean to be an ethnologist? To familiarize oneself with another culture, we should say, while at the same time holding fast to the capacity for surprise that being an outsider affords. In the case of the traditional ethnologist, however, distance is increased still further by the fact that his or her own society is on a level very different from that of the society under investigation, the observer being a member of the dominant culture and consequently in possession of a more powerful interpretive code. Anyone who undertakes "field work" in the United States must find himself in a paradoxical situation, as his informants will seldom fail to point out: usually it is the natives who occupy the dominant position, and the observer who, in one way or another, figures as a primitive. Of course this general observation applies to the particular case of American psychiatry and, more generally, to the broad range of techniques for manipulating human behavior. Let us begin at once with a frank avowal: for more than half a century now, most of the major innovations in this area have come from the United States or been most fully developed there; it is in the United States today that we find the most abundant and comprehensive set of techniques for controlling psychic disorders, deviance, and antisocial behavior. Can one who hopes to evaluate these techniques act both as an interpreter and as a representative of the "underdeveloped" world? To judge by the attempts that have been made, it would seem to be difficult to play both these roles at once. Those who have tried have either come away with a shamefaced awareness of their own "cultural backwardness" and hastened to import the latest recipes stamped "made in U.S.A." (witness the recent burgeoning of group therapy in France, in which the appeal of California-style spontaneity has masked the other side of what is today a very profitable line of business); or else they have turned inward upon their own parochial intellectual traditions, looking upon all American imports as inferior byproducts of their own country's marvelous creations. (French psychoanalysts, for example, have adopted this latter attitude, interpreting any differences in matters of theory and practice between themselves and their far-off colleagues as so many signs of the Americans' intellectual deficiencies and willingness to compromise politically.) On the one hand awe-struck admiration, slavish imitation, and unconditional surrender, on the other hand haughty contempt, self-satisfied ethnocentrism, and intellectual arrogance. It is easier to denounce such attitudes than to move beyond them in practice, however. Having been tempted by some of them ourselves, we have thought it necessary to take certain precautions.

This book might have been entitled *Travels in America*, for in one respect it is a report of a journey. Two of us toured the United States for more than a year, working out of three main centers: San Francisco, New York, and Boston. Among our activities during this period of time, we compiled an inventory, hopefully impartial, of the whole range of psychiatric and parapsychiatric institutions, both official and alternative; we held long discussions with administrators, both responsible and not so responsible; with professionals, both orthodox and not so orthodox; and with opponents of the system, both radical and not so radical; we taped many, many interviews; we personally experimented with certain new techniques; and we gathered a fairly substantial body of statistical data and bibliographical material at the source, as it were. Our predominant feeling upon returning to France was one of perplexity. All our data, all our impressions, all the hypotheses we submitted to test and modified from one day to the next added up to a good deal, and at the same time to very little. A travel diary? Memoir writing has never tempted either of us as a pastime. Had we had it in mind to undertake a more systematic evalution of what we had seen, no brief stay, no matter how rich in experience, could possibly justify such presumptuousness with regard to a system whose surface we had only barely scratched. Even the most interesting experiences, moreover, need not make good books: of the "back from China" genre and the like, we have seen more than enough. We were ready, then, to resign ourselves to using this long detour solely as a way of gaining a better understanding of the contemporary situation in France, if only by mounting an attack on the astonishing gallocentrism of French views on American psychiatry.

That matters took a different course owes entirely to the fortunate circumstance that enabled us to combine our outsiders' point of view with the intimate familiarity brought by an insider's involvement in the social structure we were studying. One of us is an American. Anne Lovell founded a free clinic in 1970, and later took part, as a board member of the Louisiana American Civil Liberties Union and of various community organizations, in the efforts to reform mental hospitals and prisons that grew out of the civil rights struggles of the nineteen-sixties throughout the United States. Having spent a year working with Franco Basaglia at Parma, she was well acquainted with the problems on the European side as well and was planning a comparative study of Italian and American experiments in "alternative" psychiatry. The complementary features of our respective situations allowed us, we felt, to aim for a combination of involvement and aloofness, objectivity and criticism, impartiality and commitment. By looking first from one angle and then from the other we could be detached yet not uncaring, familiar yet not hampered by ethnocentricity. At least this was the ideal for which we aimed; the reader will be the judge of how close we came to achieving it.

Our work, then, has clear limits and a specific intention. It does not pretend to be an exhaustive evaluation of all the achievements of American psychiatry. But we do hope to lay out an interpretive schema useful for sorting out the specific characteristics of mental health care in the United States: the diversity of its organizational forms, the variety of services available, the mutual reinforcement of its component units, and the coordination of the system's overall operation.

Diversity of Organization

This is first of all a result of the decentralized power structure in the United States, which affords local authorities a large measure of autonomy; another factor is the existence of very special kinds of relationships between public institutions and private agencies providing mental health care. It would be an endless task to take note of the special features peculiar to each locality. There is no common measure, for example, by which to compare an East Coast city with a rural area in the South, or a solidly middle-class suburb with a sub-proletarian ghetto in a major city, in regard to quality of care or number of patients provided for. But, as we shall see, selecting one or two central themes will help us find our way through this confusing thicket: the dominant trends in the evolution of thinking about the provision of care will be one such theme, and the administrative and political scaffolding that gives structure to this highly diversified organization will be another. One possible shortcoming of our work results from the fact that except for Louisiana our most personal contacts were in the states that offered more "advanced" psychiatric services (California, New York, Massachusetts), states that are not exactly representative—far from it—of the United States as a whole. But these states offered us the best opportunities to ponder the latest developments in the field. Care has been taken at all stages of our work, moreover, to compare our data with the information compiled nationwide by the National Institute of Mental Health, as well as with the general literature on the subject.

Variety of Services

Beyond this geographical diversity, the mental health care system in America is distinguished by the variety of services that it offers. We find the broadest imaginable range of institutions and techniques, owing to which the system is able to draw into its orbit a larger and more diverse clientele than in any other country. In one place a hospital still operating under the most repressive of nineteenth-century regimes may be found. Nearby, sometimes even within the same institution, a surprisingly liberal experiment will be in progress. Constant innovation, as exemplified by the recent proliferation of groups that stress the development of the individual's human potential, coexists side by side with increasing reliance on methods of quite another sort, such as the use of patients for biological research or of knock-out doses of drugs to keep patients under control.

Our first obligation: to do justice to this variety by depicting the entire range of services, from the most standard forms of psychiatric care (hospitalization and "hard" technologies) to the most subtle techniques of control (*in vivo* regulatory mechanisms operating within the fabric of society itself in the realm of "pure" psychology). This concern is reflected in the plan of the book, which describes in the order of their emergence the major components of the system, from the asylum to the very latest therapies, ostensibly emancipated from the old prescriptive imperatives.

Mutual Reinforcement of the System's Component Units

Despite the diversity of organizational forms and the broad range of experiments, each unit has a place in an encompassing system and derives its significance from its relations with all the other units. Rather than speak of archaic practices on the one hand, and up-to-date innovations on the other (important though the relative timing of their appearance on the scene may be), we should speak instead of a range of measures *feasible at any given moment,* each of which corresponds to a specific therapeutic slot. Thus, contrary to what is commonly believed, the psychiatric hospital is hardly obsolete in the United States. To be sure, the number of such hospitals has declined, and they can no longer boast of the near monopoly in the mental health care field that was once theirs. In loosening their hold on a once captive population, however, the psychiatric hospitals have discovered their real mission, in which role they are irreplaceable. They still have their place and their function, even though some of the jobs once done more or less indiscriminately in the hospitals are now performed elsewhere (in community mental health centers, for example). Still farther removed from the hospitals' old bailiwick, new areas for mental health care have opened up in answer to "symptoms" unheard of in the golden age of alienism. What we are witnessing, however, is not so much the creation of new forms of care incorporating the latest innovations, but rather the broadening of the spectrum of available therapies, each novelty overlapping the last and all working together in the present as parts of the overall system of mental health care.

Functional Operation of the System as a Whole

As the central theme of our study, we have chosen to examine the social groups involved in the mental health care system in order to understand the system's operation as a complex whole. Despite a steady stream of innovations on the system's fringes, there is, within the constantly changing borders, a carefully laid-out market in which clients are shifted from one stall to the next. These shifts are determined by the social problems supposedly posed by each client group. Changes in institutional structures, methodologies, and theoretical models are governed by the growing demands for services. All the current efforts to redefine problems, redistribute skills, and cope with "crises of adjustment" in the American mental health care system came to the fore, as we shall see, with the advent of new client groups that had previously lain beyond the system's reach. This development gave rise to changes both in therapeutic practice and in the theory of health care. During the mid-sixties, for example, thousands of youthful dropouts descended upon the United States with no resources but their dreams and their confusions, catching the traditional institutions off guard. This led to the creation of a new type of facility (the "free clinic"), as well as to increased reliance on techniques such as counseling and group discussions instead of standard medical treatment. Nonprofessionals supplied these new services, and often, thanks to their less technical training and to the less hierarchical structure of treatment, they were able to establish much warmer relations with their clients than traditionally-trained medical personnel had been able to manage. In the end this brought about definite modifications in the relationship between the "normal" and the "pathological": coping with the problems of daily life and even individual "growth" replaced the mere restoration of sanity as the object of psychiatry. In certain respects these changes are reminiscent of those wrought by psychoanalysis, but the techniques involved were totally different, as was the patient population.

These changes, then, were fundamental, and should be judged in their own right. But they should also be seen as establishing new categories in the range of available services. Groups within the population having no other place to go (not being sufficiently disturbed or socially deprived to qualify for treatment in a mental hospital, nor sufficiently wealthy to go into psychoanalysis, nor sufficiently integrated to choose a private "encounter group") now found a place in the system. Of course once drawn into the system they could very well be shifted along the scale from one to another of the institutional programs available at any given moment. The wider the range of available programs—and it is constantly expanding—the greater the likelihood that any problem identified as being of concern to society will match up with some program ready to take charge of a new segment of the population. It is this constantly shifting clientele that constitutes the jurisdiction of the mental health system. The unity of the system really lies in the diversity of the services it undertakes to provide. There are many different forms of care, but the system as a whole has but a single function, which we shall try to illuminate as our study proceeds by analyzing each unit of the system not only as an entity in itself but also in the light of its contribution to the overall function of the system.

These, then, are the assumptions underlying our analyses; we have also described the framework within which our results will be presented. Our objective is twofold: not only to explain what is happening in the United States, but also to warn against what might happen in Europe. As we were saying a moment ago, objectivity must be coupled with commitment, for the stakes are high.

There can be no doubt that the United States is the country in which the mental health system, together with its allied activities—psychoanalysis, mental hygiene, group therapy, behavior modification, counseling, and so forth—has penetrated most deeply into the social fabric. It is idle to assume that what has taken place in the United States foreshadows what will inevitably come to pass in France. On the other hand, it is unquestionably true that all modern societies are searching for new ways and specific technologies to combat deviant and antisocial behavior. Social consensus can no longer be achieved spontaneously (if indeed it ever could). More and more the achievement of consensus is becoming an explicitly assigned task, i.e., a political undertaking requiring the assistance of planners, administrators, researchers, and troops in the field to carry out their orders. In the effort to turn the problem of social integration into a merely technical matter, i.e., into a problem capable of being dealt with by appropriate technologies, designed and perfected by specialists in human behavior, the United States has played a pioneering role from the beginning of this century right up to the present day. American technicians have opened up new frontiers in the control and standardization of human beings. It is therefore less important to decide whether one technique or another will be imported "as is" from the U.S. than to discover the logic of the process by which men and women are being transformed into targets of manipulative technologies in "advanced industrial societies" everywhere. This is true both for those who want to have such technologies around and for those interested in learning how to protect themselves against them.

Thus the American dream of mental health is not just a curiosity, a strange and marvelous fantasy from a far-off place. If we can learn to see it as in some ways a model of what is in store for us in Europe, perhaps we can keep it from becoming the nightmare of our tomorrows.

We are indebted to so many people—officials, professionals, and friends who shared with us both information and the pleasure of their company—that we can only express our gratitude to them as a group. We make one exception, however, for Mony El Kaïm, who generously placed at our disposal both his experience of two years' practice in the South Bronx and his personal files. Special thanks are due also to Professors John Clausen, Bogdan Denitch, and Stanley Hoffmann, who provided us with essential institutional support in the departments of sociology at Berkeley, Columbia, and Harvard.

The Psychiatric Society

PART ONE

——————◆•◆——————

A Resistible Rise

——————◆•◆——————

At first glance, it would seem that the project of establishing a system of care for the mentally ill proceeded at about the same pace in America as in Europe. First there was the work of a founding father, Benjamin Rush, who shared in the role that legend attributes to Pinel and Tuke; then, beginning in 1820, this was followed by systematic efforts to build a series of "special hospitals" or asylums, inaugurating a golden age of "moral treatment" and philanthropic humanism. As the nineteenth century progressed, however, the situation deteriorated, owing to severe overuse of the available facilities, pessimistic ideas about the possibility of curing mental illness, and so forth. The twentieth century is said to have witnessed two major revolutions in mental health care, first with the rage for psychoanalysis that followed Freud's visit to the United States in 1909, and later with the development of community-based psychiatric care in the nineteen-sixties, thanks to an alliance between an enlightened administration (with President Kennedy himself pushing for reform) and a mature psychiatric profession.

Doubtless this panoramic résumé of the history of American psychiatry as seen by the members of the profession and their spokesmen is not entirely false. But a closer look at the question is surely necessary: professions, like individuals, have selective memories, and their choice of what to retain from the past is not made innocently when it comes to the present. The history of American psychiatry is neither a duplicate of its European counterpart nor a foreshadowing of Europe's future. In the American case distinctive relationships were slowly built up between medicine and politics; between the public and private spheres; and between local and national authorities, which differ significantly from corresponding relationships in Europe generally and in France in particular. What is the significance of those features of the American situation that are not found elsewhere?

In the first place, if the public mental health care systems of Europe and the United States seem to have been established at roughly the same pace, the American system nevertheless came into prominence at a later date (as an imported phenomenon) and, more importantly, never attained a position of total monopoly (owing to stronger resistance to the unifying policies of the state on the part of local authorities and private institutions—see chapter 1).

Having said this, we can more readily understand the spate of other early initiatives that paralleled the growth of the public system and led to the development of flexible and multifaceted ties with the private sector, with nonpsychiatric institutions, and with groups having nonmedical aims. Although in a schematic sense the United States did tend to imitate the European asylum model during the nineteenth century, from the beginning of the next century onward a series of innovative steps were taken which gave the United States a pilot role in the ensuing years (chapter 2).

The variety of these developments raised problems of coordination and overall control. After the Second World War the Federal government took some steps in the mental health domain. But this attempt to restore control did not altogether do away with the situation that had existed previously. The organization of mental health care in America has at least in part moved beyond some of the conflicts that have hampered the development of psychiatry in the past (public–private, bureaucratic–alternative, centralized planning–experimental pilot projects, technocratization–innovation, etc.). Ever since the nineteen-sixties, the United States has been moving toward the establishment of a full spectrum of procedures for psychiatric intervention, which marks the beginning of a turn away from mental medicine and toward collective forms of social control (chapter 3).

CHAPTER 1

The Success of the Worst

As late as 1820 only one state, Virginia, had a public lunatic asylum, founded in 1773. In such large East Coast cities as New York and Boston, however, there were a few private establishments set aside for psychiatric patients, most of them based on the Quaker model of the York Retreat in England. The Pennsylvania Hospital in Philadelphia, though it had been and still remained a general hospital, was the first to admit psychiatric patients for treatment, beginning in 1752. It was there that Benjamin Rush, a very important physician, a signer of the Declaration of Independence, and the "founding father" of American psychiatry, began in 1783 a special practice devoted to these patients, which would serve as the basis for his *Medical Inquiries and Observations upon the Diseases of the Mind* (1812), the first, and until 1883 the only, American treatise on mental pathology.

Beginning in 1820 we witness a relatively rapid development of a system of publicly-supported state mental hospitals responsible for treating indigent psychiatric patients. At the same time a number of small private hospitals were established, especially devoted to the care of mental patients. In 1844 the first thirteen directors of public and private hospitals for the mentally ill formed the Association of Medical Superintendents of American Institutions for the Insane, which would become the American Medico-Psychological Association in 1893 and in 1923 the American Psychiatric Association, which now numbers nearly twenty thousand members. The association immediately began publishing the *American Journal of Insanity*, which is still in existence today (since 1921 under the name *American Journal of Psychiatry*). Thus by the mid-nineteenth century the psychiatric establishment was in place. It could claim its own specialized personnel, its own publications, and above all a specific place to practice its particular methods, the asylum. It relied on moral treatment and a firm belief in the possibility of cure: directors of the various hospitals rivaled one another in optimism, with cure rates often in the neighborhood of 90 percent.

This period was also witness to the heroic efforts of Dorothea Dix, a typical American philanthropist, who figures between Benjamin Rush and Clifford Beers (see below, chapter 2) in the psychiatric hagiography of the New World. A former schoolteacher living a quiet life of retirement (forced on her at age forty for health reasons), Dorothea Dix owed it to her good reputation and Protestant piety that she was asked in 1841 to give a Sunday school course in a woman's prison. There she was horrified to discover that psychiatric patients were being treated as common criminals. Worse still, large numbers of them were living in almshouses crammed full with the homeless poor, the blind, the sick, the aged, orphans, abandoned children, and madmen.

Dorothea Dix immediately launched a veritable crusade, going tirelessly from prison to prison and almshouse to almshouse, first in her own state of Massachusetts and then in other states, everywhere attacking the scandalous mingling of the mentally ill with other inmates, and mobilizing public opinion in favor of the creation of special hospitals for the insane. By the time she gave up her philanthropic activities in 1881 at more than eighty years of age, she had set in motion the construction and renovation of asylums in some twenty-odd states, to say nothing of her work in Scotland, Italy, and Germany.

Despite the enthusiasm with which some American historians have described this golden age of American alienism in the mid-nineteenth century, the system of mental health care in the United States was not yet established on a very firm footing. The capacity of the asylums, numerous though they doubtless were in comparison with earlier periods, was still ridiculously small for the size of the population. Moreover, the Association of Superintendents imposed a strict limit of 250 beds per hospital. In 1860 twenty-eight of the thirty-three states of the union had at least one asylum, but for a population of 31,443,322 and an estimated 24,042 insane, there were only 8,500 hospital places, even counting those reserved for psychiatric cases in ordinary hospitals.[1] A report of the New York State Senate in 1856 observed that, out of 2,123 estimated insane in the state, only 293 were treated at Utica State Asylum. Most of the rest were in the prisons, the reform schools or, more frequently, the almshouses (when Dorothea Dix visited New York in 1845, she counted 1,345 in the almshouses alone). No doubt an even larger number escaped institutional treatment altogether. Yet the state of New York was, along with Massachusetts, the most advanced of all in putting the new policy into practice.

Approximately one mentally ill person in an asylum (public or private) for every ten in the population: this state of affairs may be compared, for example, with the situation in France during the same period, where for a population of approximately the same size there were more than 30,000 places available in the public hospitals, and where psychiatrists complained bitterly that one psychiatric case out of two (compared with nine out of ten in the United States) remained beyond their reach.

The mid-nineteenth-century conquest of madness by medicine, which in psychiatric hagiography is recounted as a heroic saga, was in reality no more than a thin patina of modern innovations laid over the surface of very different methods for dealing with deviance, poverty, and illness, methods that were organized along quite different lines. But it is seldom meaningful to interpret a situation of this kind in terms of simple lags or archaic methods. Rather, the modest results achieved in the establishment of public psychiatric care in the mid-nineteenth century should be seen as the effect of an administrative and political structure peculiar to the United States, which conditioned, and in large measure is still conditioning, the organization of public welfare in all its aspects.

THE PLACE OF PSYCHIATRY IN THE PUBLIC WELFARE SYSTEM

Under the American federal system, the states occupy an intermediate position in the power hierarchy. In New England, for example, the states gradually developed out of cities and counties that were originally independent, and were not, as in France, administrative units of the central government superior to the local authorities. Only much later and after a hard-fought struggle did the federal government acquire the right to act independently.[2] These basic characteristics of American society have influenced psychiatry in the United States and, beyond that, the organization of the welfare system in general.

The Primacy of Local Government

The "special hospital" especially devoted to the treatment of mental patients was commonplace in Europe and particularly in France as early as the time of Pinel and was enshrined in official doctrine in the law of 1838. In the United States, on the other hand, the separation of asylums from almshouses proved difficult. Almshouses—lodgings for the indigent and for those incapable of taking care of themselves (abandoned children, homeless old people, the handicapped, and so forth)—were not yet a thing of the past in early nineteenth-century America, as they were on the verge of becoming in Europe. In the Old World wholesale confinement of the poor had been tried as a solution to the problem of poor relief from the seventeenth century on. But criticism from Enlightenment philosophers and those faithful to the Revolution had made such measures symbols of royal absolutism, and as such detested. By the beginning of the nineteenth century, philanthropists and social reformers were seeking new ways to deal with the poor relief problem, such as public poorhouses, which would allow indigent individuals to continue to function in society.[3]

By contrast, almshouses in the United States were seen as a new and progressive solution to the relief problem, since they represented a move away from the colonial system under which the poor were supposed to be cared for directly within and by the community. "Cared for," in actuality, meant being eliminated from the community or whisked out of sight. In most cases indigent individuals were taken to the town limits and sent on their way, or else auctioned off at public sales as farm laborers. The best they could hope for was to receive meager assistance at home, assistance provided at the discretion of well-to-do members of the community and supervised by ministers of the various religious denominations.[4]

Compared with these traditional expedients, the idea of setting up a completely new system of poor relief was thought to be the last word in philanthropy, and philanthropists set about the task enthusiastically. By the end of the colonial era there were a few almshouses in large eastern cities. Systematic efforts to open almshouses began after 1820 (thus at the same time as the asylums). By 1855, fifty-one of the fifty-five counties in New York state had at least 1, and in Massachusetts there were 180. They absorbed two-thirds of the funds allocated to poor relief in this period.[5]

Why were the almshouses so successful? Because they embodied two of the leading characteristics of the American welfare system: moralistic philosophy and local determination of the manner in which aid was distributed. The rationale behind this moralism went something like this: In our country, with its many advantages, where labor is so much in demand and so well paid, and where the needs of subsistence are so easily obtained and so inexpensive to buy, poverty need not and ought not to exist.[6] Under these conditions, if there were paupers—and the paradox was that they did exist, and even existed in large numbers—it could only be their own fault: "Official data show, though imperfectly, how large a part of the pauperism of the city and State is occasioned by indolence, intemperance, and other vices."[7]

That the almshouses should have commanded universal assent owes mainly to the fact that, as advocates claimed, this marvelous institution offered both correction for the depraved and relief for the poor.[8] Segregated from the rest of society, the indigent were stigmatized by receiving assistance. Doubtless the failure of the system was apparent from the moment it was instituted. Horrible, overcrowded jails—this is all the almshouses ever amounted to. By the middle of the nineteenth century a staggering weight of testimony had accumulated about the defects of an institution which, rather than eliminate poverty and vice, concentrated their effects.[9] So great, however, was suspicion of the poor and so widespread the fear that they would use relief to perpetuate their vices rather than be forced to discipline themselves, that even the patent failure of the almshouses failed to bring about a search for a different system before the end of the nineteenth century. As late as 1891 a welfare official was able to state to the National Conference of Charity and Correction that it was the weak, the lazy, and the slackers who were asking for relief at home. For those people the hospital, the workhouse, and the prison had been provided.[10]

The almshouses also satisfied a second requirement in that they insured that local communities would retain control over the distribution of relief. Although the construction of almshouses was encouraged by state charity boards, the houses were planned and financed by individual counties or municipalities. Some local authorities refused to build them on the grounds that communities were free to do as they pleased in this area.[11] Even after almshouses were commonplace, local authorities continued to exercise control wherever possible. The system was in fact the result of a compromise between the old idea of private "charitable" assistance (which was clearly too disorganized a system to survive the nineteenth century intact, though it continued to be viewed as an ideal) and the new idea of public assistance, an idea that carried with it the inherent danger that the poor might come to think that they had a right to relief, a right that was vehemently denied: the poor man who has been taught to beg by the state will turn against the state for its refusal to recognize his natural right to relief. This danger is not inherent in personal, voluntary charity, which is a favor and not a legal obligation and can always be cut off.[12]

No doubt this ideal of personalized dependence, in which the grant of aid was supposed to match the moral pliability of the person receiving it, was unrealistic. An increasing share of poor relief, in the United States as elsewhere, has been distributed through public agencies, while the traditional role of local and private agencies has decreased in importance. In the United States, however, this trend developed later than in other countries and was never fully carried through, so that there was never recognition of a *right to assistance*, as there was in European social legislation at the end of the nineteenth century. When, in the nineteen-thirties, the Great Depression made massive intervention by the federal government necessary, the welfare situation turned out to be extraordinarily complex and confused. Each state had its own welfare system, with public and private relief agencies distributing assistance through channels affected by neighborhood relations, membership in certain ethnic and religious groups, and affiliation with philanthropic organizations, community groups, and local political organizations.[13] Again, these were not merely remnants of an outmoded system. Although the federal government did try to bypass this hodgepodge in dealing with the two great crises of the twentieth century, in the thirties and the sixties (see chapter 3), the results were ambiguous, to say the least. In some cases federal intervention ended once the crisis was over; in others the federal effort itself became ensnared in the complexities of the local systems and their paternalistic policies. Individualize cases, isolate the poor, multiply the agencies distributing aid: this has been the persistent pattern of American welfare policy, denying that poverty is a social and political problem, instead approaching welfare recipients as cases for psychological and moral examination.[14] To take just one example, even today the United States, the first "advanced industrial society," is without a system of national health insurance.

It was no mean feat, then, to make madness "a matter of state." Given the prevailing system of relief, such an attempt was to swim against the tide. Yet the insane were the first group of "dependents" to be granted official welfare status. This was possible because madness was identified as an illness, which weakened the influence of the moralistic notions that lay behind earlier relief policies. As people suffering from a malady, these individuals were different from other indigents, who were supposed to be in the grip of vice or indolence. Since the mentally ill were regarded, whether rightly or wrongly, as posing a threat to the life and property of others, they could not be left to wander about on the loose.

Still, it took a long while before the responsibility of the states in the treatment of the mentally ill was fully recognized, and not before a long series of battles had been fought with local authorities. In New York the principle of state responsibility was not fully accepted until the Care Act of 1890. Under the law, treatment of the insane in public hospitals (to which they were to be transferred from the almshouses) was made compulsory. Twenty-two state mental hospital districts covered the entire state. More or less reluctantly, the other states followed suit.[15] Again our remarks apply more to what was enacted into law than to actual practice. A 1908 investigation revealed that 18 percent of the patients in New York asylums had spent time in prison before being admitted to the hospital. As late as 1937, Albert Deutsch found large numbers of the mentally ill in prisons, almshouses, and state farms, and the practice of chaining patients to trees was not unheard of.

A second prominent characteristic of the American welfare system has been the exclusion of the federal authorities from its operation. The public system of mental health care has never enjoyed an unchallenged monopoly in the United States because state governments have been unable to protect the system against encroachment by powerful local interests. The disparate health policies of the various states bear witness to this fact: while the eastern states and, later, California were able to carry out fairly coherent policies in the area of mental health, this has not been true in the conservative states, particularly in the South, where politics is often still under the thumb of powerful local interests. This disparity is also reflected in case statistics, which show considerable variation in hospitalization rates (relative to total population) from state to state. Conservative states had a hard time establishing state hospital systems and succeeded in doing so only recently, having been content previously to offer the insane more traditional and less costly forms of care. Accordingly, it has only been in recent years that blacks have come to be treated as a group with specific psychiatric problems; they first had to migrate in large numbers out of the South. By contrast, immigrants have long been recognized as a distinctive group, since they constituted a community of uprooted individuals concentrated in the big cities.

There are other signs, too, of differences in mental health policy from one state to the next. A large body of American professional literature deals with the effects of local politics on hospital personnel. In 1893, for example, the superintendent of Illinois Eastern Hospital at Kankakee was forced to resign because of political differences with the governor. The situation was serious enough for the American Medico-Psychological Association, in 1894, to set up a committee on relations between state institutions and the political authorities and to attack the corruption and lack of principle that was dragging public institutions into the whirlpool of political conflict, so that supervisory, medical, and other staff posts were being handed out as rewards for political services.[16] No doubt these conditions reflected widespread corruption in the American political process. But they were also an indication of how fragile the mental health care system was, for its status as a public service was never fully accepted.

Dorothea Dix, a philanthropist but not a naive one, understood that the success of her program could be insured only by establishing clear ties between psychiatric institutions and the federal government, and she therefore turned to Washington for help. After protracted discussions she persuaded Congress to set aside federal land for the foundation of public asylums. At the last minute, however, President Pierce vetoed the measure (1854). In his veto message, he stressed the conflict between two divergent views of relief policy:

> If the Congress have the power to make provision for the indigent insane without the limits of this District [of Columbia], it has the same power to provide for the indigent who are not insane, and thus to transfer to the federal government the charge of all the poor in all the states.

Pierce felt that if Congress made this choice, the fountains of charity would dry up at the source, and many states, rather than make the effort to meet the needs of their own citizens, might yield to the temptation to become humble supplicants of the federal treasury, thereby reversing their true relationship to the Union.[17] In the name of states' rights, Pierce was in fact defending the idea that relief should be locally controlled and, if possible, privately financed.

The question was thus a political one in the full sense of the word. Some American historians deplore Pierce's veto as a missed opportunity to unify the mental health care system as early as the mid-nineteenth century. But the President's decision was consistent with the whole tenor of American relief policy. The proof: not until 1963, more than a century later, when President Kennedy spoke in favor of the Community Mental Health Center program, would the federal government reconsider any part of the position laid out in the Pierce veto message and take direct responsibility for the care of a portion of the mentally ill population. In the interim there had been many major upheavals, both in psychiatry and in the society at large. The use of psychiatry, almost from its inception, as an instrument of governmental power, as was done in Europe, is one thing. It is quite another thing to establish relations between psychiatry and the federal authorities at a much later date, after psychiatry had developed in a pattern peculiar to the American situation, forging specific alliances with other social forces along the way.

THE IMPOSSIBILITY OF AUTONOMY

The strength of a psychiatric care system depends on its capacity to organize apparently heterogeneous elements into a coherent structure, which in turn defines a comprehensive policy. Among the elements constituting the system are institutions (such as hospitals), treatment technologies (such as "moral treatment"), a codified theory (such as the standard nosologies), and specialized personnel (such as medical chiefs of staff experienced in the management of mental hospitals). Once this complex system has been unifed, it finds its expression in legislation according special legal and civil status to the mentally ill. Clear lines of division are laid down between the psychiatric apparatus and other departments of government, particularly the courts and the bureaucracy. A mental health care system organized along these lines achieved its most polished form in France in the nineteenth century (it is not, we trust, because we are speaking from a French point of view that we make this judgment). French law (particularly the law of June 30, 1838) served as a model for most other European legislation in this respect. Psychiatric practices developed from the time of Pinel on were thereby linked up with the government's centralized administration. The system of psychiatric care obtained official status as a public agency charged with the administration of the mentally ill, alongside other agencies shouldering other responsibilities. Psychiatrists became government officials of a sort, reporting to the prefects and sharing in the power of the state.[18]

Nothing of the sort took place in the United States, at least not in so clear-cut a way. As we have seen, American psychiatry was caught up in the complexities of a power struggle among the many echelons peculiar to the federal system. The end result was that mental health care came to be viewed as a function of state government. But the freedom of action of the state authorities was limited by the influence of local forces. Psychiatry, moreover, could not be unified at the national level because of the diversity of state policies. The lack of a systematic approach to the problems of mental illness in the United States is reflected in the confused legislation on the subject (and above all in the lack of any definitive single body of legislation).

In the land of habeas corpus it was not until 1867 that any state (Illinois was the first) adopted special laws regulating the procedure for admission to the asylums. In theory, liberty for all was guaranteed by habeas corpus, but in fact it was not, as can be seen in an 1845 precedent-setting decision of the Supreme Court of Massachusetts, which stated that:

> the right to restrain an insane person of his liberty is found in that great law of humanity, which makes it necessary to confine those whose going at large would be dangerous to themselves or others. . . . And

the necessity which creates the law creates the limitation of the law. . . .
The restraint can continue as long as the necessity continues.[19]

The situation in the United States was quite different from the situation in Europe, and particularly in France, where political issues overdetermined the outcome: in Europe the whole question was shot through with overtones of the long struggle against absolute monarchy, so that the law of 1838 stands as an extraordinary monument to legalism and pettifoggery. America made do with a mixture of grandiose principles such as habeas corpus and outright cynicism, whereas in Europe a ponderous legacy of political theory and jurisprudence resulted in granting full official status to the mentally ill. It was therefore surprisingly easy to commit someone to an American asylum in the early days. To take one example, papers exist bearing the signature of Benjamin Rush stating that "James Sproul is a proper patient for the Pennsylvania Hospital." No more than this was needed to commit the man.[20] No one seems to have agonized unduly over such practices, except in occasional habeas corpus proceedings before the courts. The 1867 "personal liberty bill" of the state of Illinois was the work of a woman patient confined, in her view wrongly, from 1860–63 upon request of her husband, countersigned by a physician. After her release she launched a virgorous campaign that led to passage of the bill, the first special legislation concerning the insane, which laid it down that no patient may be forcibly committed except by due process before a jury. Unlike the French law of 1838, this bill was not a recognition of the power of the psychiatric profession but rather a limitation on that power.

The passage of the Illinois law in 1867 inaugurated a process that led ultimately to the passage of similar though not identical laws in many other states. Voluntary admissions became important only rather late in the twentieth century. For a long time the number of patients entering mental hospitals voluntarily remained quite small: only 5 percent of those hospitalized in 1933 and about 20 percent in 1960. Until quite recently, then, the vast majority of patients had no choice but to enter the hospital by way of proceedings leading to involuntary commitment. Today a distinction is made between emergency and nonemergency commitments. Emergency commitments require only certification by a physician; depending on the state, an individual committed on an emergency basis may be hospitalized for periods of up to thirty days. Nonemergency commitments require special proceedings, as do extensions of the term of hospitalization of patients committed under emergency procedures. The nature of these proceedings varies from state to state: some states require a court order, to be issued by a judge upon the advice of an ad hoc committee, the composition of which depends on the state but usually includes a majority of doctors; others require a specially appointed commission (with doctors again in the majority) to rule on each case; still others require a jury trial or judicial hearing.[21]

Criteria for commitment also vary from state to state. As of 1974, in twenty-nine states a person could be committed only if he was; "a danger to himself or others"; fifteen states required that he be "incapable of providing for his own physical needs"; twenty-nine states provided for commitment of patients "in need of treatment or hospitalization," half of these states stipulating further that the individual must be adjudged mentally incompetent to decide himself on the best course of treatment; and seven states required "commitment for the well-being of the patient or others."[22]

Much pettifoggery results from the complexity of these laws, which have given rise to endless litigation that has had an important impact on the transformation of the system of psychiatric care in the United States (see chapter 4). The important question, however, is not whether American laws are better or worse than their European counterparts, nor is it whether or not they provide more or fewer safeguards. There may well be advantages to having a diversity of laws and taking a case-by-case approach. Still, since the matter is one with important human rights implications, it is significant that the responsibilities of the various authorities in a position to infringe upon individual rights (government agencies, courts, medical personnel) have not been clearly delineated. Like other countries, the United States has had to deal with legal problems associated with mental illness. In an empirical way these problems have been resolved more or (usually) less satisfactorily.

Unlike France, however, the United States has never seen fit to grant true legal status to the mentally ill, thereby removing cases involving mental illness from the jurisdiction of ordinary courts. The psychiatric profession has never been granted clear legal authority. If it is true that the law only codifies actual social practice, then the ambiguous status of the mentally ill in American law is a good indication of the difficulties psychiatry has had in staking out a claim to autonomy in the United States.

THE KEY COMPONENTS OF THE MENTAL HEALTH CARE SYSTEM

It is not difficult to explain why the public system of psychiatric care was established at a later date in the United States than in France, and on a somewhat less secure footing. The reason is that in America various obstacles connected chiefly with the relative weakness of the federal government had first to be overcome. The same observation also accounts for a paradox in the history of American psychiatry: namely, that psychiatry made its greatest inroads into society just when it seemed discredited from a medical standpoint.

As we have seen, enthusiasm for psychiatry waned quickly after the middle of the nineteenth century, and the high point of that enthusiasm coincided with a period when psychiatry was in fact little practiced. The deterioration set in quite rapidly. To begin with, the Civil War upset the nation's social equilibrium, plunged local communities into crisis, particularly in the South, and stimulated migration to the big cities. The pace of change was further accelerated by foreign immigration, which eventually reached a level that exceeded the "melting pot's" capacities of assimilation. Between 1860 and 1900, 14 million immigrants came to seek their fortunes in the United States, an average influx of 350,000 immigrants per year. In the eighth decade of the last century the economy sank into depression, throwing 3 million people out of work. In the face of rumblings of worker revolt, the militia and even federal troops were called out to quell the riots. From Europe alien morals and subversive ideas flowed into the United States and threatened the cohesiveness of American society, which responded by mythifying its early years.

Social Darwinism, a synthesis of economic liberalism and the Darwinian theory of the survival of the fittest, was the philosophy of the age. Society might be a jungle, but the strongest could take care of themselves. Wide-ranging efforts were made to purge American society of its unhealthy elements. Psychiatry's role in these efforts was at first only minor. Of greater importance were merciless repression of revolutionary tendencies in the workers' movement; a witch hunt for subversives, particularly anarchists, among the immigrants; confinement of society's most rootless and wayward members in the almshouses; and the birth of the Organized Charity Movement, which developed systematic methods for surveillance of the poorer classes and inaugurated social work in the United States (see chapter 2).

A single example will suffice to show how this heavy-handed charity operated. In 1853 a hard-working young pastor founded the New York Children's Aid Society. He quickly realized that the real problem was, as he put it, to "drain the city" of its homeless children, who were seen as a threat to law and order. A veritable system of deportation was put in place, a system that over a period of twenty-five years transported some 50,000 children from New York city alone westward, where they were left to the tender mercies of farmers and industrialists. American historians view this movement as the seed from which the child welfare system grew.

What happened in psychiatry was similar but on a smaller scale. The capacity of existing asylums was limited and they were quickly overwhelmed by the flood of immigrants from rural areas and Europe into the cities. An even more serious problem was the breakdown of the consensus on which "moral treatment" had been based. The assumption underlying moral treatment was that illness temporarily removed the insane from the social order, but that they could be taught to abide by society's values once again and thereby made fit to return to normal life. Now, however, the sharp new edge to social conflict, and above all the massive influx of immigrants who had been brought up in cultures held to be "inferior" to those of earlier settlers and who were indifferent to middle-class values, triggered a veritable wave of racism in American society. Psychiatrists were not exempt from these feelings of racist hostility. No longer was the patient viewed as a symbol of suffering humanity; now he stood for all that was disturbing about alien cultures. The director of the Worcester asylum, for example, did not bother to conceal his attitude toward the Irish:

> The indulgence of their appetite for stimulating drinks . . . and their strong love of their native land . . . are the fruitful causes of insanity among them. As a class, we are not as successful in our treatment of them as with the native population of New England. It is difficult to obtain their confidence, for they seem to be jealous of our motives.[23]

This negative attitude was heightened still further as the source of new immigrants shifted from northern Europe toward central and southern Europe, bringing in fresh waves of aliens even more foreign to the "American way of life" than were the Irish.

The barrier of class, as well as that of nationality, undermined the cultural endogamy on which psychotherapeutic relations had been based. In this quarter the prognosis was equally somber:

> When . . . the patients, instead of being partly drawn according to the original purpose from an intelligent and educated yeomanry, are drawn mainly from a class which has no refinement, no culture, and not even much civilization even—that hospital must certainly degenerate.[24]

In actuality, of course, the handicaps of nationality and class often went hand in hand, and poor immigrants came to account for a majority of asylum inmates in the second half of the nineteenth century. It is not surprising, then, that as early as the eighth decade of that century we come across disillusioned judgments of "the inadequacy of the hospital to accomplish the desired end."[25] The same period witnessed an increasing tendency to diagnose mental illness as due to organic causes, which did not encourage optimism in formulating prognoses.

Following the Civil War cure rates fell dramatically. It was not long before the very principle of isolation, the basic axiom of alienist therapy, was called into question. The sudden rupture of ties to family and society was especially traumatic at that time. Families of the mentally ill were advised to keep them at home as long as this could be done without danger.[26] One of the first neurologists held that by the ninth decade of the last century medicine was quite capable of treating madness like any other malady, and that in many cases confinement was not merely useless but downright harmful.[27]

Thus the hopes placed in the asylum earlier in the century were quickly dashed. The problem was that the enthusiasm of the asylum's advocates was never translated into action. In short order, the Association of Medical Superintendents lost interest in anything other than defense of its professional traditions and prerogatives, warding off any attempts at innovation by singing the praises of the golden age. American asylums seem to have surpassed their European counterparts in routine cruelty. The scandal reached such proportions that one English alienist offered his American colleagues a critique of their practices in the respectable *Lancet* (November 13, 1875):

> It is scarcely believable, but we are almost forced to the conclusion, that our friends across the Atlantic have not yet mastered the fundamental principles of the remedial system. They adhere to the old terrorism tempered by petty tyranny. They resort to contrivances of compulsion; they use, at least, the hideous torture of the shower bath as a punishment in their asylums, although it has been eliminated from the discipline of their gaols. And worse than all, if the reports that reach us may be trusted, their medical superintendents leave the care of patients, practically, to mere attendants, while devoting their own energies principally to the beautifying of their colossal establishments.

The psychiatrists, who were isolated along with their patients (most of whom belonged to the lower strata of society), and who lacked funds, prestige, and contact with ongoing medical research, had virtually no professional standing. This was noticed rather early. With blunt candor one of the leading figures in the new and dynamic specialty of neurology, Weir S. Mitchell, told the members of the profession as much at their annual congress in 1894:

> You were the first specialists, but you were never really involved in what was going on. It is not hard to understand how that happened. You began living in a world of your own and you go on doing so even today. Your hospital is not our hospital. Your way is not our way. You are never faced with unsparing criticism. Your services are not preceded or followed up by skillful rivals or observed by knowledgeable students just out of medical school.[28]

It was in these rather discouraging circumstances, however, that the principle of state responsibility for mental health care gained currency, thereby encouraging strong and steady growth of the asylum system. When the golden age ended in 1860, there were only about 8,500 patients in American mental hospitals. Already by 1870 this figure had risen to 17,735; to 40,942 in 1880; to 74,028 in 1890; 187,791 in 1910; 267,617 in 1923; 337,573 in 1931; and 480,741 in 1941.[29] The peak came in 1955, when the patient population reached 558,000. There is no point trying to explain this progression by looking for signs of a substantial increase in psychiatry's scientific capabilities. A recent in-depth study has shown that hospitalization rates for mental illness correlate only with the fluctuations of the economy.[30] The shape of the American mental health system was molded chiefly by the ups and downs of the business cycle and by government policy on immigration. Here is confirmation, if confirmation were needed, of the impact of so-called external social and political factors on mental health care, these factors in fact being responsible for the internal structure of the system.

The asylum, it thus appears, fulfilled its social function while placing less and less emphasis on its presumed therapeutic virtues as a justification for its existence. Administrators continued to push for new mental hospitals even after it became increasingly apparent that their purpose was not to provide "care." Overcrowding grew worse (in some states the number of patients was nearly double the available capacity). Huge new institutions (of up to 10,000 beds) were built at some distance from the communities they were intended to serve, and both size and remoteness made it clear that these were not so much hospitals as lockups whose purpose was to segregate the mentally ill from the rest of society. Local politicians bargained cynically over the benefits to be obtained in return for allowing mental institutions to be built in the areas they represented. These issues took precedence over the therapeutic role of the hospital. Staff members were undersupervised and underqualified, doctors were overwhelmed with administrative chores, and while there were psychiatric nurses available to do the jobs that required special skills, the bulk of the staff consisted of attendants or untrained guards whose job was to insure discipline and keep costs down.

The truth of the matter is surely that American alienists were the least medical of doctors and the asylums in which they practiced the least therapeutic of hospitals. Today, more than a few traces of this legacy remain. One striking feature of the state hospitals is the high·proportion of foreign physicians on the staff. Often they have not even mastered the language spoken by their patients—though, to be sure, there is precious little communication between doctors and patients anyway. These doctors fill positions that require some modicum of medical training, positions that native-born members of the august American Medical Association would not deign to hold, owing to their low pay and lack of prestige. The mental hospitals have been and still are ghettos for the medical staff as well as the patients. Physicians will work in these institutions in most cases only as a last resort, when all other doors have been closed. As we shall see in the next chapter, the major innovations in mental medicine have been introduced outside the hospital system and (in contrast to what has often happened in, say, France) have been the work of individuals trained outside the public mental health institutions.

The main features of the public system have often been described. The hospitals are bleak "jails" in which few are cured and many die (40,000 deaths per year during the fifties). Patients are segregated according to their relative docility, independence, and availability for work in the institution. Superintendents have dictatorial powers over the internal life of the institution and the release of patients. And so on. As recently as 1970, the conditions to which 5,000 patients in one Alabama mental hospital were subjected every day were described by an eyewitness:

> The dormitories are barn-like structures with no privacy for the patients. . . . The toilets in restrooms seldom . . . have partitions between them. These are dehumanizing factors which degenerate the patient's self-esteem. . . . Contributing to the poor psychological environment are the shoddy wearing apparel furnished the patients, the nontherapeutic work assigned . . . and the degrading and humiliating admissions procedures which creates [sic] in the patient an impression of the hospital as a prison or as a "crazy house."[31]

One unmistakable sign of the fact that these institutions function as prisons: the ratio of voluntary admissions to involuntary admissions is much lower than in Europe.[32]

In some respects this picture is no doubt out of date (see chapter 4). Then, too, the situation in America is not unique. Hospitalization rates, which peaked in 1955 at one inpatient for every 300 Americans (a total of 558,000 patients in mental institutions), were on the rise elsewhere as well. The organization of mental hospitals in other countries is similar: when Erving Goffman hit upon the concept of "total institution" to describe the organizational structure of the mental hospital in 1961, his analysis, but for a few minor differences, held good for European mental hospitals as well.[33] There is nothing peculiarly distinctive, then, in the way American hospitals are run or in their primary social function: to provide a medical excuse for the exclusion from society of certain categories of undesirables. Statistics (of which a fuller discussion may be found in chapter 4) show that in the United States as in other countries mental hospitals are populated mainly by those who are suffering not just from illness (which is often difficult to define in any case) but also from one or more social handicaps, such as loneliness, poverty, lack of education, old age, etc.

Although American society has therefore added nothing new to the asylum system as such, it has carried the logic of that system to its extreme conclusions. Furthermore, a widespread prejudice against federal intervention in the administration of welfare has made it difficult for psychiatry to establish hegemony over the mental health care system. As a result, psychiatrists have for many years been forced to accede to the development of other forms of mental health care, owing to which new subgroups of the population have been brought into the orbit of the system. As we shall see shortly, the United States was the first country to see the emergence of novel types of institutions, unheard of elsewhere, aimed at treating newly specific classes of clients. These various mental health services sometimes support and sometimes clash with one another, but together they constitute a complex and comprehensive system. It is this pattern of contemporary American psychiatry that we shall next try to elucidate.

CHAPTER 2

———◆◆◆———

The Progressive Era

In France, the asylum system came very early (1838 at the latest) to dominate older forms of treatment of mental illness (religious methods, family care, assistance in the village, etc.) and also took precedence over other medical approaches such as outpatient services, whose development was for a long time impeded by the presence of the asylum. Even criticism of the asylum came mainly from within. Most French reformers were staff physicians in mental hospitals. Last but not least, the major modern-day institutional reform in French mental health care, the so-called *politique de secteur,* was conceived, carried through, and brought to fruition essentially by a dynamic group of such insiders.

As we have seen, the situation in the United States was quite different. This fundamental difference makes sense of reams of data that would otherwise remain incomprehensible. Innovation in psychiatry came mainly from outside the state hospital system, both from more prestigious institutions, such as medical schools, and, at the other end of the spectrum, from such marginal experiments as the therapy groups that are such a common feature of the contemporary scene. Whereas in France the power of the public psychiatric establishment stymied most initiatives and mobilized the energies even of its opponents, in the United States the relative weakness of the public system allowed other forms of care to develop early in the game and independent of the asylums. Generally speaking, these initiatives were begun with virtually no institutional support and little or no coordination, but for that very reason their influence was extensive and flexible. Usually connected with government only loosely if at all, they nonetheless managed to meet the needs of large segments of the society.

We have no wish to attribute mythical significance to any supposed discontinuity in the development of the system, nor do we place much store in the idea of locating an absolute zero on the scale of historical time. Having said this, we must nevertheless record our initial surprise at discovering that fundamental changes took place in the United States in the first two decades of the twentieth century—more precisely, around 1910. Hitherto more or less content to imitate Europe, American society, it seems, then set its mind to innovation, at any rate in the area of human manipulation. A fresh start was made during this period in a number of areas apparently without relation to one another—and yet we find the same individuals in back of all of them. The actions these people took, at first blurred in their outlines, eventually established new methods for the management of human beings.

A NEW MEDICAL CLIMATE

As we have seen, the first systematic attack on alienism came from the neurologists. Neurology was a new specialty, dating back no farther than the post–Civil War years, but its development had been very rapid, particularly in the larger eastern cities. Publication of the *Journal of Nervous and Mental Diseases* began in 1874, and the American Neurological Association was founded in 1875. From the start, neurologists took a very aggressive attitude toward their colleagues, the psychiatrists. The New York Neurological Society even went so far as to establish a "commission on abuses in the asylums." We can follow the violence of the polemic by comparing the circulation of the *Journal of Insanity* in the eighties and nineties of the last century with that of the *Journal of Nervous and Mental Diseases*.

The bone of contention between the two disciplines lay first of all in their two very different conceptions of mental illness, as may be seen in the titles of the rival journals: "insanity," for one, was madness, and the proper techniques for treating it revolved around custodial care in the asylum; "mental disease," on the other hand, was conceived as a brain disorder, and the proper methods for treating it were said to be "scientific" and medical. A second difference between the two specialties had to do with their clientele and the places in which they practiced. The neurologists were concentrated in large cities, practiced in general hospitals and medical schools, and in addition saw private patients. For example, Mitchell, who led the attack on the alienists (see the preceding chapter), practiced in Philadelphia, where he treated wealthy hysterics who came to him from all over the United States (hysteria was at this time becoming fashionable in America as well as in Europe). Neurologists, then, lived in the cities, belonged to the upper classes, were trained in prestigious eastern schools, practiced in the most dynamic institutions, and saw private patients, whereas alienists were in most cases born in smaller towns, were not as well trained medically, and were left to treat the uneducated masses in overcrowded hospitals relegated to remote rural settings.[1]

At the end of the last century, however, the somatic style in mental medicine fell into crisis and neurologists were thereby prevented from capitalizing fully on their gains. The results of research on brain lesions proved disappointing, and disease classifications based on the structure of the nervous system were widely viewed as abstract and arbitrary, incapable of providing an adequate account of complex mental pathology. At the same time, interest in one form or another of psychotherapy was on the increase. A number of different schools of thought competed for supremacy in the early part of this century. Some came out of the academy. Janet, for example, enjoyed a wide audience in the United States, where he was invited to lecture three years before Freud.[2] Other schools had a religious tinge and displayed hostility to professional psychologists. One such was the Emmanuel Movement led by the Reverend E. Worcester, whose popularity reached a peak in 1908–9, only to be dethroned by psychoanalysis. Various forms of hypnotism, counseling, and "help" were commonly practiced. Questions of childhood, sexuality, and the family were coming to preoccupy psychology.

These were matters of interest, for example, to Stanley Hall, a professor at Clark University. It was no accident, then, that he soon issued an invitation to Sigmund Freud.

If we examine the relative frequency with which mental disorders were diagnosed as being due to somatic causes on the one hand and psychic causes on the other, we find that the trend toward organic explanations of mental illness was reversed in the first decade of the twentieth century: the new century turned away from the somatic view to become the era of "feelings" and "relationships."[3] Not only scholarly journals were affected by the shift. Already there were magazines especially devoted to psychotherapy, such as *Psychotherapy: A Course of Reading in Sound Psychology, Sound Medicine, and Sound Religion*, which commenced publication in 1908: its title is a whole program in itself. Women's publications were particularly susceptible to the new influences: for example, an article in the August 1907 issue of *Good Housekeeping* was entitled "Become Beautiful by Thought."[4] Thus, even before 1910, alienism had lost its dominance in the field of psychopathology. And the groundwork was being laid for the appearance of certain innovations.

First of all, a new type of medical institution appeared: the psychopathic hospitals. These hospitals not only conducted treatment but combined it with research and teaching. Growing numbers of the mentally ill could, in consequence, be cared for outside the asylum setting. In hospitals in a few cities (such as New York's Bellevue as early as 1879), mental patients had been kept in special wards for observation before being transferred to asylums. By the turn of the century some of these special wards (such as Ward F of the Albany Hospital in 1902) were offering treatment. Somewhat later, psychopathic hospitals began offering intensive care as well as facilities for research and teaching (e.g., the University of Michigan in Ann Arbor as of 1906) and outpatient consultations (Boston, 1912).

Another innovation was the opening of psychiatric institutes. Some mental hospitals had responded to the late-nineteenth-century challenge of neurology by opening laboratories, which at first did little more than perform autopsies. Research-oriented clinical departments were, however, organized in some hospitals, particularly in New York, as early as 1902. Case studies replaced autopsies, and the new departments attracted a type of medical student whose background was different from that of the typical alienist.

A third innovation was the opening of psychiatric wards in a number of general hospitals, such as Mount Sinai in New York. These private hospitals accepted patients suffering from milder forms of mental illness than the typical asylum patient; they also offered intensive treatment. Cases in which these methods proved unsuccessful were dispatched to the state mental hospitals. These new departments attracted doctors who would have been loath to practice in the asylums, where the pay was low and scientific stimulation lacking. Young doctors accepted posts in these departments in order to round out their training in intellectually stimulating environments while awaiting teaching posts or preparing for private practice.

Independent of the asylum system, the new institutions were at first few in number and treated only small numbers of patients. They were centers of dynamic activity, however, in this respect standing in sharp contrast to the mental hospitals, where chronic cases predominated. Out of the new institutions came innovative treatment ideas (such as outpatient and follow-up services and special wards for children), new teaching methods, and a stream of research papers. Rather than give statistics about the growth of these institutions (which, in any case, we are not equipped to do), we shall next try to explain how all these developments were related by taking a brief look at the career of Adolf Meyer, who was destined to become one of the leading figures in American psychiatry during the nineteen-thirties.

Adolf Meyer, a Swiss doctor schooled in the German tradition and trained at the Burghölzli Clinic in Zurich, emigrated to the United States in 1892, when he was twenty-five. Thanks to his thorough European training, he was the first pathologist to obtain a laboratory post in a mental hospital, first in Illinois and later in

Worcester, Massachusetts, in the thick of New England's active medical community. He offered a free course at Clark University and established ties with the progressive intelligentsia, whose leaders included psychologists Stanley Hall and William James and philosophers John Dewey, Charles Peirce, and George Mead, among others. In 1902 Meyer became director of the Pathological Institute of New York (which became the Psychiatric Institute in 1908). He was responsible for its reorganization as a teaching clinic. In 1913 he became the first director of the newly-created Henry Phipps Psychiatric Clinic of the Johns Hopkins Medical School of Baltimore, which was destined to become the most dynamic mental hospital in the United States. He developed a teaching and research program that was to serve as a model for other medical schools for twenty-five years to come.

Adolf Meyer was not responsible for all the new developments, but he had a hand in most of the major ones. Consider three examples. Psychoanalysis: we find Meyer's face in the photograph commemorating Freud's visit to Clark University in 1909, where he stood in the front row to Jung's left, and he was a founding member of the American Psychoanalytic Association, which was formed in 1911. Social work: Meyer's wife was the first psychiatric social worker, one of the founders of the specialty that was to build a bridge between psychiatry as it was traditionally practiced and work in the community. The mental hygiene movement: it was Meyer who, in 1909, suggested the name of the movement to former patient Clifford Beers, its organizer, whose activities focussed on the prevention of mental illness and soon drew a considerable following.

We shall encounter Adolf Meyer's name at other key points in the history of American psychiatry. Our purpose in mentioning him here, however, is not to retrace the steps of his career (which, among other things, included the distinction of being Zelda Fitzgerald's therapist). Rather, his example is one clue that a new mental health care system was already forming alongside the existing one; furthermore, it is no mere happenstance that one of the pivotal figures of that new system should have been a man who was not an alienist but a little of many things: psychiatrist, psychoanalyst, social worker, mental hygienist—a figure of a new type, harbinger of a rich future.

THE PSYCHOANALYTIC DELUGE

A well-known anecdote has it that Freud turned to Jung in 1909 as their ship approached the shores of the New World and told him that they were bringing a plague to America. An epidemic did indeed ensue, but it was not the one Freud envisioned. By 1911 there were already two American psychoanalytic organizations, the New York Psychoanalytic Society and the American Psychoanalytic Association, based in Baltimore. Morton Prince, reflecting on these exciting early days in 1929, epitomized the significance of the new developments in an image: "Freudian psychology had flooded the field like a full rising tide, and the rest of us were left submerged like clams buried at low water."[5] What was it that Freud had sold so successfully? Essentially two things: one affected the balance of power within the medical profession, while the other altered the relationship between the profession and the larger society.

1. *Psychoanalysis helped to resolve an internal crisis in mental medicine,* or at least suggested an elitist response to that crisis. In the early years of this century, as we have seen, the situation in mental medicine was confused: alienism had been discredited, neurology had lost its forward momentum, and several different forms of psychotherapy were competing for dominance in the field. None, however, offered a comprehensive vision, an integrated view of the problems of childhood and adulthood, individual and family, mind and body (sexuality). None had both the sanction of the medical profession and answers to the most pressing questions of the day. All authorities agree that psychoanalysis was and remains highly "medicalized" in the United States. But what sort of doctors were involved? To answer this question, we must look at early converts to the "cause."

Two of the three most prestigious early converts served chiefly to provide a cover for the movement, for they never actually practiced psychoanalysis. We have already encountered their names: Adolf Meyer, then on his way to becoming the dominant figure in American psychiatry, and Stanley Hall, professor of psychology at Clark University and a pioneer in American research on child psychology. Hall's attitude toward Freud seems to have been ambivalent, perhaps because he felt that Freud's work unfairly overshadowed his own. The third major convert was a Harvard Medical School professor by the name of James Jackson Putmann, one of America's best known neurologists. Of the three, his was the only total conversion: he became the only American analyst to win the genuine respect of Freud, and his high standing reflected great credit on the rather heterogeneous group of early analysts.[6]

The rest of the group was in fact made up almost entirely of young doctors, most of whom had no permanent positions and practiced in the medical schools or general hospital clinics. The first fifteen members of the New York Psychoanalytic Society were all doctors: ten were practicing or had practiced at the Psychopathic Institute of New York, upon which Meyer had impressed his stamp. They were graduates of the leading schools in America or had been trained abroad (nine had been born outside the United States, and seven of these were Jews). Most would hold teaching positions, go into private practice, or, at a somewhat later date, run such prestigious clinics as the Meninger Foundation at Topeka or Chestnuts Lodge near Washington.[7]

This, then, was an avant-garde of a very distinctive type, at first utterly cut off from the sort of psychiatry practiced in the mental hospitals. There was one exception: William A. White, who from the first ranked as one of the leaders of the movement, was the medical director of the 6,000-bed Saint Elizabeth's Hospital in Washington, the only federally-run mental institution. As early as 1917 White foresaw the possibility of using psychoanalysis on a wide scale in the hospitals.[8] The practical import of such foresight should not be overestimated: bear in mind the fact that, even though the head of Saint Elizabeth's had been won over to psychoanalysis as early as 1912, it was this very institution that was studied by Erving Goffman in 1959 for his book *Asylums,* the strongest indictment to date of what has come to be known as the "total institution."[9]

Not until the thirties, when the emigration of many European psychoanalysts to the United States gave the movement a second wind, did psychoanalysis cease to be peripheral to the bulk of psychiatric practice and become the basis for the training of the new generations of psychiatrists who were to gain prominence in the years after World War II.

Until then psychoanalysis had not by any means won over a majority of professionals. In fact, most neurologists and psychiatrists steadfastly persisted in denying that the new discipline had any scientific validity whatsoever. Psychoanalysis made its inroads on the periphery of the system, though it is true that it often won followers in very prestigious places: courses in psychoanalysis were offered in the leading medical schools—Harvard, Johns Hopkins, Cornell. Among doctors, then, psychoanalysis enjoyed limited and circumscribed success among a rather elitist audience.

2. More than just a response to a crisis in medicine, *psychoanalysis was a response to a crisis in American values,* particularly in regard to the rigid traditional sexual morality inherited from colonial days. This aspect of the movement was responsible for its success in "high society." From the first, the new doctrine seduced the intelligentsia, which was then in rebellion against New England puritanism and moral conformity. Members of this intelligentsia controlled the enlightened press: *The New York Times,* the *New Republic, Vanity Fair,* etc. Writing in the latter, a journalist gave an apt definition of the new symptoms that psychoanalysis was designed to treat, and showed how far the expectations of the cultivated middle-class minority that flocked to analysts' couches differed from the needs of the patients traditionally cared for by psychiatrists. Psychoanalyis was needed as a remedy for "the inability to achieve results in one's work commensurate with the efforts put forth; infelicity in personal relationships, and a sense of not being able really to get at grips with the realities of life."[10] The circle of Friends of Psychotherapy, to borrow Charles Kadushin's phrase (see chapter 8), was clearly already gathering.[11] In this circle, psychoanalysis found not only a class base but above all a vehicle to help spread its renown as the very paradigm of psychological reductionism.

From the outset, the champions of the new doctrine worked hard to "psychologize" American life in all aspects, imposing a crude and one-sided interpretation on political and social events. On March 24, 1912, *The New York Times* Sunday magazine published an article by Morton Prince, editor-in-chief of the *Journal of Abnormal Psychology* and future founder of the famous Boston school of psychology, entitled "Roosevelt as Analyzed by the New Psychology." It described the leader of the Progressive Party and candidate for the presidency as a case of "the distortion of conscious mental processes through the force of subconscious wishes."[12] Advertising was quick to find work for psychoanalysis when Freud was asked to help in an advertising company's campaign to get women to smoke. He referred the company to Brill, who suggested ways in which ads might appeal to a woman's unconscious desires. Psychoanalysis also worked its way into the media, literature, and film. In 1925 Metro-Goldwyn-Mayer contacted Karl Abraham about undertaking a major production on Freud and the unconscious. Abraham was quite tempted, but the discussions came to nought.

Chiefly by such apparently "unmedical" means, psychoanalyis stamped the American social fabric with interpretive and manipulative patterns that drew attention away from more traditional forms of psychiatric intervention. Thus the conclusion that American psychoanalyis was "colonized" by the medical profession, thereby sealing its fate, is a hasty one, not altogether supported by the evidence.

What sort of psychoanalysis did come to prominence in America? Was it a betrayal of the movement's true principles, a psychoanalysis coopted by conservative forces? Or was it a psychoanalysis lucidly aware of its true social functions? We shall here sidestep this question, whose answer, perhaps, is more ideological than sociological.[13] One thing is certain. At a crucial moment in the development of American society, phychoanalysis was tapped to play a key role as a new technology of human relations. As we shall see shortly, psychoanalysts cooperated with other outside innovators (involved in such activities as the mental hygiene movement, social work, child welfare, scientific management, and so on) in forging sophisticated tools for the psychological manipulation of human beings. These tools have since come to be seen as distinctive characteristics of American society.

THE MENTAL HYGIENE MOVEMENT

In 1908 Clifford Beers published *A Mind That Found Itself,* a book that enjoyed extraordinary popular success.[14] A former mental patient, Beers told of spending years being treated first in a private clinic, then in a charity hospital, and finally in a state mental institution. His, however, was not just one more story of capricious commitment. Beers acknowledged that he had been seriously ill. But he modeled his book after *Uncle Tom's Cabin,* deliberately seeking to draw attention to the inhumanity of psychiatric treatment and hoping to stir up a movement of popular protest. Rather than dwell on his own misfortunes and attack conditions in the asylums, Beers, in a stroke of genius, emphasized the *avoidance* of hospitalization. As far as possible, this was to be the goal, which he proposed to achieve by developing a program of public education and new and less debilitating forms of treatment.

Beers immediately won the support of dynamic psychologists and psychiatrists led by William James and Adolf Meyer. On Meyer's advice, he founded the National Committee for Mental Hygiene in 1909. The group's bylaws stressed the idea of prevention through research, as well as education of the public in regard to mental disorders of all sorts. They also called for coordination of all existing public and private institutions:

> To work for the protection of the mental health of the public; to help raise the standard of care for those in danger of developing mental disorder or actually insane; to promote the study of mental disorders in all their forms and relations, and to disseminate knowledge concerning their causes, treatment, and prevention; to obtain from every source reliable data regarding conditions and methods of dealing with mental disorders; to enlist the aid of the Federal Government so far as may seem desirable; to coordinate existing agencies and help organize in each State in the Union an allied, but independent, Society for Mental Hygiene, similar to the existing Connecticut Society for Mental Hygiene.[15]

After early difficulties, the committee, which had no connection with the government, secured the aid of private charities and foundations, including the Rockefeller Foundation. From the outset, it sponsored studies that looked beyond a narrowly defined notion of insanity. Thus the first such study, carried out in a Baltimore school in 1913, purported to show that 10 percent of the school children were in need of psychiatric assistance. Pilot programs were also begun at Sing Sing prison. The upshot of this research was that psychiatric departments were established in the juvenile courts and the prisons.

The war gave new impetus to the movement. A neuropsychiatric unit was set up to select recruits to take care of psychiatric problems at the front (ultimately, 72,000 troops were to be discharged for mental problems), and to help demobilized soldiers readjust to life at home. Named medical director of the movement in 1912, Dr. Salmon later became chief psychiatrist of the American Expeditionary Force in Europe. "War neuroses" provided new material for observation and highlighted the relationship between psychic disorders and everyday living conditions.

The usefulness of the mental hygiene movement emerged most clearly, however, in the treatment of the problems of returning soldiers. There were no institutions or specialists prepared to cope with these postwar difficulties, so the movement mobilized all its resources. Special training courses were offered to "social workers." To that end, Smith College, the first school of social work, was opened in Boston, soon to be followed by the New York School of Social Work. It was not long before these schools broadened their objectives and began training hundreds of new specialists in psychiatry with a particular orientation to "social" problems. Most important, they provided social work with the ideological basis it was lacking (see below).

Thus the differences between the mental hygiene movement and traditional psychiatry grew more pronounced in the postwar years. The movement took a particular interest in children's problems and played a leading role in the child guidance movement, which first flourished in the twenties (see below). This opened the way to important future developments, both in new institutions (diagnostic centers and treatment clinics for children) and new methods; as one official of the movement put it, "the [children's] clinic treats these problems by treating not only the child through whom they become manifest, but as well the family, schools, recreational and other involved factors and persons which contribute to the problem, and whose disorder the problem may reflect."[16]

The courts, the military, the schools, the family—what about industry? It too played a part. As far as business was concerned, the problem was not so much to diagnose and treat illness per se as it was to measure the "personality potential" of an individual, or the likelihood that he would perform satisfactorily in a particular job. The new psychological discoveries could be put to good use in personnel selection, enabling people to be assigned to jobs so as to maximize job satisfaction without compromising efficiency. This development marks the beginning of interest in "human factors" in industry. For the present we need not consider what functions were fulfilled by manipulation of these factors. As one early specialist in the field put it,

> As our work progressed, it became more and more clear to us that the largest issues involved in this failure [of workers] were personal and constitutional in nature; were to be found in the makeup of the workers themselves rather than "in the slings and arrows of outrageous fortune," or terrible working conditions, or general economic situations and the like.[17]

Increasingly, then, the mental hygiene movement fostered a shift away from the traditional institutions and methods of psychiatry. In every important area of social life, these were replaced by new methods under the auspices of new kinds of specialists. The change marks the transition from a focus on mental *illness* to a focus on mental *health*, which opened the door to the introduction of manipulative methods inspired by psychological medicine. Once again, we may cite Adolf Meyer as witness; he summed up his considerable ambitions as follows: "Mental hygiene as a philosophy of prevention is an ideal and a guiding principle working wherever possible with the assets of life before the differentiation into the 'normal' and the 'pathological'."[18]

The combination of mental hygiene and psychoanalysis thus had one important consequence: medicine was freed of its dependence on disease and fired with a new ambition to intervene in the lives of the healthy. The movement aimed beyond prevention at the *improvement* of health by medical and psychological means. Probably the first person to state clearly that this was the aim of the program was William A. White, who, like Meyer, was a psychiatrist, psychoanalyst, and hygienist. It is worth citing at length from his inaugural address to the First International Congress of Mental Hygiene, which he chaired:

Mental hygiene is on this account alone more important than ever before, and its significance can be seen to be gradually changing from one of the simple prevention of mental disease, which is a negative program, to the positive attitude of finding ways and means for people to live their lives at their best. Medicine has long enough maintained as ideals freedom from disease and the putting off of death. It is time that these were replaced by ideals of living, of actual creative accomplishment. The art of living must replace the avoidance of death as a prime objective, and if it ever does succeed in replacing it in any marked degree, it will be found that it has succeeded better in avoiding death than the old methods that had that particular objective as their principal goal. Health is a positive, not a negative concept.[19]

THE PSYCHIATRIZATION OF CHILDHOOD

The simultaneous success of psychoanalysis and mental hygiene led to a spectacular increase in the number of children treated. The change came not because new techniques flooded the marketplace, but rather because a problem already existed, waiting for appropriate means to deal with it. In fact, a White House conference on the problems of childhood—a conference described by historians of welfare assistance as "historic"—was held at the behest of President Roosevelt in 1909, that is, in the year when both psychoanalysis and mental hygiene first burst into public attention. This led, two years later, to the creation of the U.S. Office of Children, charged with coordinating and encouraging assistance, especially medical assistance, to children throughout the United States.

Not only was psychiatry involved in the general trend toward medicalization of childhood, it was the driving force in the whole process. Also founded in 1909 was the Juvenile Psychopathic Institute of Chicago, a private foundation connected with the Chicago juvenile courts. William Healey, its director and a pioneer in the field, had found in a 1908 study that there were no satisfactory sources of assistance to children in need.[20] During the nineteenth century, abnormality in children was still lumped together with the problem of idiocy. The only special facilities that existed were devoted to the provision of some modicum of education to children classed as idiots or imbeciles.

Psychiatric concern with childhood originated, not accidentally, with interest in juvenile delinquency: the young offender was thought to exemplify a new dimension of pathology, of a kind irreducible to idiocy or retardation.[21] The Psychopathic Hospital of Boston soon had a section of its outpatient department devoted to young female parolees (1912).[22] At the same time the mental hygiene movement was sponsoring research into the related problems of delinquency, psychiatry, and childhood. In 1917 William Healey founded the important Judge Baker Foundation for delinquent children in Boston. This later expanded through branch agencies known as the Judge Baker Guidance Centers. In his theoretical work, Healey stressed the influence of mental factors in delinquent behavior.[23]

The movement gathered momentum after the war with the creation of the child guidance clinics. In 1919 a Massachusetts law was passed requiring examination of any child who fell more than three years behind in school. Thus the question of emotional disturbances in children was separated from the problem of delinquency without being reduced to a matter of retardation, as had been done in the past. The "problem child" was discovered, and new methods, mainly relying on outpatient clinics, were developed to deal with the personality "disorders" of such children. These methods involved such new services as family counseling. The clinics "deal not so much with definite psychiatric entities as they do with the socially maladjusted who are personally within reasonably normal limits."[24] Stevenson listed the following "behavioral disorders," all calling for intervention: "tantrums, stealing, seclusiveness, truancy, cruelty, sensitiveness, restlessness, and fears."[25] Later, the vocabulary took on an increasingly psychoanalytic cast.

Some of these institutions came into being in ways that prefigured the type of relationship with the community that was later to be systematized in the community mental health centers (see chapter 5). Governmental agencies and private organizations such as the Judge Baker Foundation sponsored "demonstration clinics"

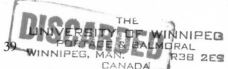
as part of their programs: teams of skilled practitioners would be sent to spend several months in a city, where they would open a clinic and train local people to carry on after they had gone. Once the experiment was successfully launched, the team would move on to another city, leaving behind a working community center. Other programs revolved around training. At the Institute for Child Guidance in New York, for example, not only were 3,600 cases treated between 1926 and 1932 but, even more important, special training courses devoted to children's problems were given to 366 psychiatrists, psychologists, and social workers.

In 1939 there were 776 centers offering ambulatory psychiatric care to children throughout the United States, with such diverse designations as "child guidance clinics," "child guidance bureaus," "institutes for juvenile research," and the like. Some of these were public and some private, and organizational structure and methods of financing varied from one facility to the next. Fewer than one-third served children exclusively. Together, these facilities accounted for between one-third and one-half of the ambulatory psychiatric care services in the United States. Though no real central policy was ever promulgated, these facilities amounted to a highly developed system of mental health care services for children, which was already in place on a nationwide scale before the outbreak of World War II.

THE PSYCHOLOGIZATION OF SOCIAL WORK

The psychoanalytic and mental hygiene movements together also led to professionalization of workers in the field of welfare: "social work" became a new specialty. Social work is perhaps best thought of as a reinterpretation of the problems of welfare assistance in psychological terms. Once again, the new methods in psychology did not by themselves create a social function to which they could be applied, but rather contributed to bringing about important quantitative and qualitative changes in the way a previously existing need was met.

Social work is rooted in the philanthropic tradition. Given the pervasive influence of religion in the United States, together with the constant refusal to see the problem of poverty in social and political terms, it is not surprising that we persistently find paternalistic and moralistic attitudes among social workers. But professionalization and, increasingly, politicization were the dominant trends in social work in the late nineteenth and early twentieth centuries.

Professionalization grew out of efforts to coordinate the charitable activities of a host of philanthropic organizations. Although public assistance continued to revolve chiefly around the almshouses, the private religious organizations that oversaw most household relief were beginning to regroup and rationalize their methods. "Scientific charity," as the new outlook was known, placed great store in research to develop new techniques for evaluating the indigent. As one of the organizers of the scientific charity movement put it: "The fundamental law of its operation is expressed in one word. 'INVESTIGATE.' Its motto is 'No relief (except in extreme cases of despair or imminent death) without previous and searching examination.'"[26] The technique devised to meet this imperative was case work: relief was not to be handed out until a thorough investigation of each individual case had been made. The case work method required trained personnel to implement it. Accordingly, paternalistic charities declined in importance beginning in the late nineteenth century. Officials of the old philanthropic organizations were relegated to honorific roles, and the real responsibility for dispensing relief was taken over by the new professionals. In the field of mental health, the years 1904–6 saw the first assignments of social workers to follow up on mental patients after their release from the hospital. Further changes followed with the establishment of new institutions distinct from the asylums, such as the Boston Psychopathic Hospital and the Phipps Clinic of Baltimore. In 1913, one social worker, Mary Jarrett, set up a training program in psychiatric social work. By 1915, according to one author, the services of at least one social worker were available to every mental hospital in Massachusetts.[27]

Professionalization went hand in hand with a reaction against the outmoded moralistic ideology of charity. The new professionals still spoke of "preventive charity," but their attention was focused on the need to change the social environment rather than to assess the "moral deficiencies" or "merits" of the relief recipient. In 1909, a committee that was an outgrowth of the National Committee for Social Work proposed a program that anticipated the key planks of the Progressive Party platform on which Theodore Roosevelt was to run (unsuccessfully) for President in 1912: minimum wage, health insurance, the eight-hour day, decent housing, etc. The Settlement House Movement also rose to prominence during this period: middle-class youth groups went to live in slum neighborhoods and worked to improve housing, help the poor, and defend the dignity of the individual (among these groups were the first civil rights activists and many feminists). These new methods broke sharply with the tradition of "friendly visitors." By 1910 there were as many as four hundred settlement houses.[28] These, however, were by no means the dominant force in the social work profession. The professionals were torn in two directions, which are described in Mary Richmond's *Social Diagnosis*, published in 1917, a fine overview of the social work profession and its main concerns of the day. The aim of social work, according to Richmond, was to develop the personality by helping man adjust consciously to his surroundings, stressing "the idea of the sympathetic study of the individual in his social environment."[29] This clearly points up the ambiguity in the term "case work," the social workers' preferred method. On the one hand there was a proclivity to interpret all problems in terms of the individual, though interpretation now could no longer rely on traditional forms of religion and morality. On the other hand the influence of the social environment on the relief recipient, the way in which social conditions could reduce an individual to a state of helpless dependency, was just beginning to be perceived. Just prior to the First World War, the results of such major investigations as Paul Kellog's *Pittsburgh Survey* were published, revealing the conditions in which poor people in industrial areas were living (suffering from unemployment, lack of hygiene, wretched housing, low wages, etc.).

At this point, the ambiguity was swept away in what Kathleen

Woodroofe has called the "psychiatric deluge," the result of the simultaneous triumph of psychoanalysis and social hygiene.[30] Buffeted between broad "environmental" explanations and moralistic paternalism, social work had lacked a methodology of its own. The "new psychology" was to provide it with one and was therefore welcomed by social workers with open arms. "Social case work was starving for practical human psychology, and had been fed for the most part on academic husks. The doctrines of mental hygiene and the new psychology [psychoanalysis] came as the fulfilment of a long-felt conscious need."[31] Thus "moral deficiency" became "psychological maladjustment" or "emotional instability": in any case, the idea was that psycho-medical techniques could be applied directly to the treatment of moral deficiencies. To do so, however, the social and political causes of poverty had to be neglected. Somewhat later, the medical director of the Mental Hygiene Movement, Dr. Thomas Salmon, declared that attention must be focused exclusively on the individual, "first, last, and all the time."[32] In 1930, with the Great Depression already under way, Miriam Van Waters, president of the National Conference of Social Work, stated that "The true springs of action are in the internal nature of man. Hence the uselessness of programs, particularly those dependent upon state action, or force."[33] In short, the problem was not to help the unemployed worker to find a job, but rather to explain psychologically why he had lost his old job and why he could not find a new one.

It is impossible not to notice correspondences between these declarations and those made by spokesmen for triumphant capitalism and partisans of unfettered individualism in the same period. In the same depression year, for instance, the president of the National Association of Manufacturers offered his opinion that to seek to abolish unemployment or poverty was "neither a legitimate nor proper function of government" because poverty is the result of "voluntary unemployment, thriftlessness, sin in various forms, disease, and other misfortunes."[34] Of course, confidence in the virtues of capitalism was de rigueur during the so-called Progressive Era. Herbert Hoover was swept into office in 1928, before the onset of the depression, in the wake of a presidential campaign that he ended with the following words: "Our American experiment in human welfare has yielded a degree of well-being unparalleled in all the world. It has come nearer to the abolition of poverty, to the abolition of fear of want, than humanity has ever reached before."[35]

There is a clear relationship between this political ideology and the ideology of "professionalism" that accompanied the general medicalization of social ills. Just as social workers expanded their services to include "case work above the poverty line," as one social worker aptly put it in 1918,[36] so psychiatrists expanded their services to include intervention in cases falling "above the line" of outright mental illness. Psychiatrists and their associates now treated more than just cases of unmistakable pathology, and welfare officials thought of themselves as performing a function broader than just providing material assistance to the poor in hard times. Both psychiatrists and social workers became specialists in "psychological maladjustment." There were many forms of maladjustment, but in describing them the specialists invariably neglected the social and political dimensions of want and mental anguish. The rising tide of professionalism swamped the other trend to emerge in the late nineteenth century, the trend toward increased politicization in social work. The fact is inescapable: psychology and psychopathology equipped the social work profession with new analytic tools and methods of intervention. Thus psychology provided the means to put the treatment of poverty on a "scientific" basis. This, at least, was the view of apologists for the wealthy, who argued that poverty did not exist as a social and political phenomenon. Only "the poor" existed, i.e., individuals who bore within themselves the seeds of their own failure. The new outlook has a somewhat different focus from the old moralistic and religious view of poverty, but the basic position is similar. The strategy is once again one of blaming the victim.[37]

Thus the psychiatric deluge merely flowed into familiar moralistic channels. By the time the crisis hit in the thirties, the transition was complete; the public welfare system was staffed by professionals who had been trained (whether for good or ill) in an atmosphere permeated by the ideas of mental hygiene and psychoanalysis for fifteen years. The truth of the matter is that welfare in America has never really recovered from this deluge. Bureaucracy and psychology still dominate the welfare system— a system for dealing with poverty that is unique to America.[38] Not until the late fifties do we witness the emergence of a new type of social worker, a worker trained more in civil rights agitation than in schools of psychotherapy. Even at this late date, these new members of the profession accounted for no more than a small minority of all social workers.

EUGENICS

As we have seen, confidence in the virtues of the asylum began to collapse around 1850. In the latter part of the century, organic theories of debility and emphasis on hereditary causes of mental illness seemed to lend scientific backing to growing feelings of pessimism, which the deteriorating conditions in the asylums only reinforced. When Mendel's laws were rediscovered in 1900, work on heredity seemed at last to be established on firm foundations. Thus belief in the hereditary and incurable nature of mental deficiencies grew increasingly firm in the latter half of the nineteenth century. Families were studied in order to trace the persistence of symptoms from generation to generation and to understand why they sometimes became aggravated. On a more practical level, too, anxieties emerged with regard to the treatment of hereditary disease, now a fashionable topic because of the influence of Social Darwinism: not only nature but also society harbored unfit individuals. In society, however, natural selection did not insure that unfit individuals would be eliminated in the struggle for social survival. How were they to be gotten rid of? By the end of the century the first institutions for the feeble-minded were in operation, "feeble-mindedness" being used as a generic term to cover idiocy, imbecility, and retardation.

The introduction of intelligence tests into the arsenal of psychological techniques raised the question of feeble-mindedness to the status of a national problem, to the point where the feeble-minded came to be seen as Public Enemy Number One.[39] A translation of Binet and Simon's book appeared in 1908 (three years after its publication in France—uncommonly soon). Its conclusions, adapted by Terman, were universally accepted. The mechanical conception of the mind advocated by utilitarian psychologists was now joined by an instrument capable of indicating when the brain-machine failed to operate up to specifications (derived from the one-dimensional utilitarian notion of rationality). The results were disastrous. The most conservative initial estimates placed the number of feeble-minded at between one-fifteenth and one-tenth of the population. When the tests were administered to wartime recruits, 47 percent turned out to be below average. Extrapolating these figures to the entire population of the United States yielded a figure of some 50 million mentally defective citizens!

Though these estimates were quickly revised downward, the implications of the problem remained tragic, because "stupidity" was viewed so pejoratively, connoting far more than mere intellectual deficiency. "The feeble-minded menace" became a universal obsession, shared by the press and scientists alike. To give some feeling for what this hysteria involved, we cite the following:

> The feeble-minded are a parasitic, predatory class, never capable of self-support or of managing their own affairs. . . . They cause unutterable sorrow at home and are a menace to the community. Feeble-minded women are almost invariably immoral, and if at large usually become carriers of venereal disease or give birth to children who are as defective as themselves. . . . Every feeble-minded person, especially the high-grade imbecile, is a potential criminal, needing only the proper environment and opportunity for the development and expression of his criminal tendencies.[40]

Investigation after investigation found that more than 50 percent of criminals, tramps, prostitutes, and the like were mentally deficient. How were they to be eliminated from society?

The first solution proposed was institutional: confinement for life. In 1904, 14,347 persons of deficient intelligence resided in custodial institutions. By 1920 this figure had risen to 20,731, by 1923 to 42,954, and by 1935 to around 80,000. Since, however, the most conservative estimates put the size of the handicapped population at several hundred thousand, this solution was clearly incapable of coming to grips with the magnitude of the problem. Even the "asylum farms" then under consideration as a backup for the asylums themselves could not begin to meet the enormous "need." One preventive measure was proposed, however, that did hold out the promise of reducing the figures to reasonable proportions within the space of two or three generations: prevent the handicapped from reproducing—eugenics, or rather sterilization, was held out as a panacea. In 1883 Darwin's cousin Francis Galton had defined eugenics as "research carried out under the auspices of society to improve or alter the racial, physical, or mental characteristics of future generations." Mutilation was not in principle a necessary part of eugenics, which also envisioned other sorts of measures, such as improvements to the environment. Still, the extremes to which eugenic ideas were carried by the Nazis are not at variance with, but rather a logical extension of, the principles and practices of the eugenics movement. Eugenics has always been associated first and foremost with the elimination of hereditary "defects," a program of clearly racist inspiration. It was no different in the United States. Sterilization of the feeble-minded, as well as incurable mental patients, murderers, rapists, and even ordinary thieves was seen as the most rational and economical solution to the problem. The annals of America psychiatry record that the president of the American Medico-Psychological Association (the professional organization representing the psychiatric profession in the United States), speaking in his official capacity, recommended the following solution.

> That a radical cure of the evils incident to the dependent mentally defective classes would be effected if every feeble-minded person, every imbecile, every habitual criminal, every manifestly weak-minded person, and every confirmed inebriate were sterilized, is a self-evident proposition. By this means we could practically, if not absolutely, arrest, in a decade or two, the reproduction of mentally defective per-

sons, as surely as we could stamp out smallpox absolutely if every person in the world could be vaccinated.[41]

With such unimpeachable advocates, it is not surprising that sterilization became the officially sanctioned method of restoring law and order. The state of Michigan was the first to pass a law in 1907 mandating compulsory sterilization of "confirmed criminals, idiots, imbeciles, and rapists." The finest example of repressive legislation in this area is doubtless House Bill 290 of the Missouri State Legislature (1923). To paraphrase this bill:

> When a person is convicted of murder (except in the throes of passion), rape, highway robbery, theft of chickens, use of explosives, or automobile theft, the judge trying the case shall immediately designate a competent physician residing in the area in which the offense was committed to perform upon said individual the operation known as vasectomy or salpingectomy for the purpose of sterilizing that individual and depriving him or her forever of the power to procreate.[42]

Tender America!

These laws were attacked as unconstitutional and in particular for violating the Eighth Amendment prohibition of "cruel and unusual punishment," provoking protracted legal battles. In 1927, however, the United States Supreme Court handed down a celebrated opinion on the matter. This decision held that it was legal to sterilize a woman in whose family three successive generations had produced feeble-minded offspring. The Chief Justice justified so strenuous a measure on the grounds that the principle according to which compulsory vaccination is justified was broad enough to cover removal of the Fallopian tubes. Presumably he felt that three generations of imbeciles was enough.[43]

This decision opened the door to compulsory sterilization on a very broad scale. It is only fair to say that in spite of this, the actual practice of sterilization remained relatively limited. While almost all the states passed laws concerning sterilization, only two or three made systematic use of the practice for any length of time. As of 1944, 41,928 *official* sterilizations had been performed in the entire United States.[44] (Only a third of the cases involved feeble-minded individuals, while more than half suffered from allegedly incurable mental illness.) Of these operations 16,332 were performed in California alone.[45] The spread of the procedure was surely impeded by public reluctance (particularly in the face of Catholic opposition to the practice) and growing doubts as to its "scientific" justification.[46] Other counterarguments were based on quite different considerations: it was feared, for example, that sterilization, by eliminating the risk of pregnancy from sexual intercourse, might provoke widespread immorality and lead to an increase in venereal disease. Regardless of the reasons, the great hope that feeble-mindedness might be prevented ended in failure; while the laws are still on the books, recent attempts to enforce them have run into stiffer and stiffer opposition.[47] This kind of preventive intervention, however, is hardly to be thought of as a barbaric legacy of a remote past. As we shall see when we come to discuss the relation of psychiatry to the courts (chapter 6), the dream of using technological manipulation to stamp out "moral disease" is still alive in contemporary American Psychiatry.

MODERN TIMES

Why were there so many changes in the related areas of psychology, welfare, hygiene, psychiatry, industrial relations, and so forth in the period around 1910, which American historians have dubbed the "Progressive Era"? An answer to this question would require a sweeping analysis of American politics and society, which is beyond the scope of the present essay. The best we can do is to venture a hypothetical response, drawing together two or three of the dominant trends in American society during this period.

This was a time of extraordinary growth in production, wealth, technology, and so on, during which a capitalist notion of rationality came to dominate all areas of life. Quantitative measurement was applied across the board, and all performance was rated numerically to determine success or failure. Taylorism (Taylor's *Principles of Scientific Management* was published in 1911) is an extreme example of the trend, an ideal-type, if you will: the minutes and seconds of human existence were significant only for their value within the productive process.

Within American society, however, there remained dark corners into which the supertechnologists could not see, much as they wished to believe that psyches were completely malleable and that human lives must be subordinated to the objective needs of technology. In particular, there came to the shores of the promised land hordes of near brutes, afflicted with all the maladies of the Old World. These people had to be reshaped to fit the American mold—they were given the choice of fitting in or being crushed: there were no alternatives. What is commonly referred to as the "melting pot" functioned more like a sieve, allowing only the most malleable individuals to pass and rejecting the rest.

But what did rejection mean in this context? For those whose differences proved fundamental, who were utterly incapable of meeting the requirements of American society, there were the foul ghettos in which poverty and delinquency pullulated, the prisons, the almshouses, and the asylums—to say nothing of the "preventive"alternative, sterilization. Misfits were thus liable to be dealt with harshly: crude methods temporarily or permanently "took care" of anyone who openly repudiated the new system of values.

Alongside such crude, segregative methods, more subtle methods came to assume increasing importance, methods that were aimed at patients still functioning within society, who were manipulated into obeying social norms. Such techniques are of course used by all societies, but during this period Americans were developing full-blown technologies for orchestrating the new techniques in a coordinated, rational way: in other words, technological, industrial rationality was being applied instrumentally to man himself. With increasing sophistication, the various institutions we have discussed above learned how to exercise this new "psy-function" (the French refer to anything psychiatric, psychological, or psychoanalytical as "psy"), relying on ever more adaptable human technologies. A broad range of new teaching programs and rehabilitative methods was made available to more and more specific subgroups within the population: services were now offered not only to those who were clearly ill or unmistakably delinquent, but more and more to people who found it "difficult" to adjust to the one-dimensional rationality prevalent in American society. Among the malajusted were workers who fell short of productivity goals, children who misbehaved, adults whose social efficiency was impaired by dissatisfaction, and so on.

What is striking is that, from 1910 on, these new technologies to a large extent functioned as an ensemble, one substituting for, backing up, or being used in conjunction with another. We wish neither to be unfair nor to exaggerate. But the coincidence in the dates, the multiple affinities of the institutions, and the constant flow of personnel from one to another indicate that what was happening was not a chance coincidence of independent developments. There is a certain consistent pattern in the multifaceted careers of an Adolf Meyer or a William A. White, for example, as we noted briefly above. Another name that might be mentioned is that of Dr. E. E. Southard, director of the Psychopathic Institute of Boston, where clinical treatment was combined with teaching and research and a new type of service was offered to children. Southard was the first president of the American Medico-Psychological Association who was not an asylum superintendent. He helped to popularize mental hygiene in industry and, with a social worker, coauthored a manual of social work that was widely regarded during the twenties as authoritative in the field, to mention only a few of his outside activities. Others with similar backgrounds include Thomas W. Salmon, James Jackson Puttman, A. A. Brill, etc. Other encounters between different traditions were even more astonishing, such as the early flirtation between psychoanalysis and behaviorism. The vogue for behaviorism, like the vogue for Taylorism and social psychology,[48] dates from 1910— the crossroads years, the date when the various manipulative techniques for dealing with human problems encountered one another. In that year John Watson was initiated into psychoanalysis by Meyer at Baltimore's Johns Hopkins University. He was immediately "convinced of the truth of Freud's work" and undertook to reinterpret what he believed to be the fundamental findings of psychoanalysis within the framework of his own system (which shows that recent attempts to synthesize psychoanalysis and behaviorism are far from being the first).[49] What is more, it was none other than the father of behaviorism who suggested that any man in a position to serve in high public office should be obliged to submit to psychoanalysis![50] Among our contemporaries, many psychoanalysts are fond of using the metaphor of "cooptation" to describe this sort of relationship between the disciplines, but to our mind the real point of the flirtation is so obvious that we cannot but be astonished by the continuing resistance to acknowledging it: yet it seems that we must spell it out.

The point is this: psychoanalysis and behaviorism connived and collaborated because both assume that man is to some degree malleable (behaviorism believes in total malleability, while psychoanalysis believes only in a relative degree of malleability—though it is no accident that psychoanalysis came to be seen in the United States primarily as an ego psychology rather than a technique for exploring the primary processes).[51] Psychoanalysis and behaviorism joined the mental hygiene movement and preventive methods of one sort or another in offering an alternative to somatic theories of mental illness, to innatism, and to heredity-based policies of confinement and sterilization. Both offered similar ways out of the impasse that older methods threatened to create by requiring that larger and larger populations of "uneducables" be permanently segregated or completely incapacitated. The new technologies offered more flexible solutions to the same problems, solutions that promised to be less costly and to lend themselves to an infinite variety of applications. This was because henceforth one could hope to correct asocial tendencies and undesirable behavior without isolating the patient from his ordinary environment. Hence treatment revolved less and less around the "special hospitals," the old fortresses of segregation. At the same time, control over that treatment was taken out of the hands of the courts, as in the case of sterilization. Now the skilled specialist, with his "neutral" technical training, could hasten to the scene of trouble—to the family, the school, the factory, and so on—to nip disturbances in the bud.

In making this interpretation, we are not assuming that the various methods were strictly equivalent or interchangeable, independent of the special circumstances of each particular case. William White, psychiatrist, psychoanalyst, and propagandist on behalf of mental hygiene, opposed sterilization of the feeble-minded, for example, basing his opposition on arguments drawn largely from psychoanalysis: violating the body's integrity, he maintained, risked provoking reactions in the unconscious. In this we see a sign of conflict between two kinds of control technology: one set of "hard" technologies, including asylum-style psychiatry, Taylorism, eugenics, and, later, psychosurgery, knockout drugs, and the like, and another set of "soft" technologies, including mental hygiene, psychoanalysis, psychotherapy of one sort or another, encounter groups, and other more or less amiable "human potential" techniques. We have watched this antagonism begin to take shape, and in subsequent chapters we shall follow the development of the associated tensions into the present era. It is important to underscore, however, that we are dealing with two divergent tendencies within a single, unified system, which systematically responds in specific (differential) ways to problems of a given type. The nature of the response is determined by the urgency of the problem, by its social and institutional setting, by the characteristics of the population in need of care, and so on.

The earliest recognition that such a system exists, so far as we have been able to determine, dates from 1919. It occurs in the presidential address to the annual congress of the American Medico-Psychological Association made in that year by E. E. Southard, whose strategic position in the field at this period has already been mentioned. In that address, Southard applauded the fact that a new man like himself, trained in novel ways and expert in novel techniques, could have been called upon to head the old guild of asylum superintendents, founded in 1844:

> Do you not agree with me that in all the *pot-pourri* of the years this great problem of the place of the individual stands out? That American thought, trans-illuminated as always by the softened European lights, contains within itself immortal fundaments of the mental hygiene of nation, race, and person? And may we not rejoice, as psychiatrists, that

we, if any, are to be equipped by education, training, and experience better than perhaps any other men to see through the apparent terrors of anarchism, of violence, of destructiveness, of paranoia—whether these tendencies are shown in capitalists or in labor-leaders, in universities or in tenements, in Congress or under deserted culverts? It is in one sense all a matter of the One and the Many. Psychiatrists must carry their analytic powers, their integrated optimism, and their tried strength of purpose into not merely the narrow circles of frank disease, but like Séguin of old into education, like William James into the sphere of morals, like Isaac Ray into jurisprudence, and above all into economics and industry. I salute the coming years as high years for psychiatrists![52]

CHAPTER 3

The Third Psychiatric Revolution

Contrary to popular opinion, psychiatry's mass exodus from the asylum is not a recent occurrence. It happened before World War II. Since the thirties there have been hundreds upon hundreds of private institutions available to care for tens of thousands of adults and children outside the hospital setting. More than that, psychiatry itself has come to be conceived in a new way, focussing more on preventing mental disorders than on curing them after they have occurred. The mental health worker no longer waits for patients who have nowhere else to turn to come to him or her. Rather, the worker has set up shop in the center of the community and moved into other institutions in the role of counselor, personnel specialist, educational adviser, and so on. As early as 1934, an impressive inventory of all these new methods was compiled in the book *Mental Hygiene in the Community*.[1]

Schematically speaking, two parallel systems exist: one official, the other alternative; one public, associated with state governments, the other private, supported by the efforts of local citizens. But this dichotomy is overly rigid, and one of the objects of the present analysis is to take a closer look at how things really work. For example, the mental hygiene movement, due originally to private initiative, enjoyed a national audience that state agencies lacked. Services in child psychiatry were sometimes provided by private local groups or charitable organizations, sometimes by city agencies or hospitals or by state medical officials. Personnel costs—regardless of whether the personnel involved were full-time or, more commonly, part-time, tenured or consulting—were met in a variety of ways, sometimes out of public, sometimes out of private funds. The bewildering variety of organizational arrangements has not prevented some rather surprising collaborations. Consider the following typically American example. When World War II broke out, there were not enough army psychiatrists to examine all draftees. A private agency, the New York Mental Health Committee, suggested using its social workers to survey families, employers, schools, hospitals, courts, and so on, in order to prepare a report on each recruit, informing the military authorities if there was anything in the man's "life history" to render him unfit for military service. Before long, seven hundred social workers were examining 19,000 "cases" per month in New York state. The service was deemed so effective that it was broadened to national scope in October 1943.[2]

Care should be taken, therefore, to avoid over-dramatizing the consequences of pluralism in the mental health system. The absence of comprehensive planning has partially been compensated by the willingness of the various agencies to cooperate, or, in other words, by their common adherence to the values of American society. The system was held together by widespread conformity, which also insured its flexibility: wherever government officials were unwelcome or inappropriate, employees of private agencies could take over, in the finest philanthropic tradition. Such a system of organization was not without weaknesses, however. In certain circumstances the lack of a single chain of command directly responsible to the federal government and immediately obedient to its orders made itself felt. Before the war the need for federal intervention had arisen in only two or three limited areas. After the war, however, the need became more and more urgent, as a new federal welfare strategy emerged, a strategy that represented a sharp break with the earlier policy of laissez-faire with respect to local agencies. From this time on, the willingness of the federal government to intervene must be seen as an essential element in American psychiatry. Far more than the evolution of psychiatric knowledge, it is this change in the government's attitude toward intervention that has brought about a restructuring of the American mental health care system over the last thirty years.

PSYCHIATRIC EVANGELISM

There is no better way to counter the false image of American psychiatric policy as a policy designed to meet the "needs of the consumers" than to examine its successive goals. The first federal intervention in psychiatric matters involved immigrants. In 1905 Dr. Thomas Salmon (who in 1912 became medical director of the Mental Hygiene Movement) set up a psychiatric department on Ellis Island under the auspices of the Public Health Service. The purpose was clear: to detect immigrants afflicted with mental disorders before allowing them to mingle in the American melting pot.[3] Because of the importance of the job, it was felt that the examination ought to be entrusted to public officials, who, like police officers or customs agents, would represent the interests of the United States.

A second "national need" for psychiatry emerged during the First World War. In 1918 General Pershing, commander-in-chief of the American Expeditionary Force in Europe, sent the following telegram to Washington:

> Prevalence of mental disorders in replacement troops received suggests urgent importance of intensive efforts in eliminating the mentally unfit from organizations in new draft prior to departure from the United States.[4]

Once again, a leading role was played by Dr. Salmon, who had in the meantime become chief of psychiatry in the AEF. He assigned a psychiatrist to each division, with orders to treat mental health problems at the front as far as it was possible to do so, so that soldiers could be sent immediately back into combat. Resources for a systematic application of this policy were lacking, however, both at the front and back in the United States. Psychiatry scored its first real success in helping to cope with the problems of demobilization. In this it was assisted by the mental hygiene movement. With the return to normalcy, however, the interest in psychiatry waned, and in the end the First World War had little effect on the overall structure of the American mental health system.[5]

A third significant episode involved drugs. In 1929 a federal law was passed concerning the "confinement and treatment of drug addicts." A special narcotics division was set up within the D٠partment of Public Health to administer two hospitals for addicts (one in Lexington, Kentucky, opened in 1935, and another in Fort Worth, Texas, opened in 1938), which also carried out drug-related research. Medical science being what it is, the claim was soon made that the major causes of drug addiction were emotional, and so the Drug Division became the Mental Hygiene Division in 1930. The latter was concerned not only with drug problems but also with criminality, delinquency, and immigration. From this seed emerged the National Institute of Mental Health, which was to play a fundamental role in the postwar period. In 1936, the director of the division (a psychiatrist) conceived the idea of setting up a national neuropsychiatric institute with research and treatment facilities. The project had reached a fairly advanced stage of planning when it was interrupted by the war. Nevertheless, an embryonic agency had been created whose task was to administer on a national scale certain issues relating to mental illness and deviant behavior.

A fourth major event, quantitatively the most important of all, was the Second World War. The same problems that had cropped up in 1917 had to be faced again, but now on a much vaster scale: there were 15 million recruits to be examined, and 1,875,000 were rejected for neuropsychiatric reasons (accounting for 12 percent of all inductees and 39 percent of all rejections). Of the recruits actually inducted, 387,000 were later discharged for neuropsychiatric reasons, accounting for 37 percent of all discharges. Nearly a quarter of the men evacuated from the combat zone were suffering from mental problems.[6] The war not only brought new awareness of the magnitude of the mental health problem but also showed that new forms of treatment, based on on-the-spot diagnoses and carried out in the field, could be more effective than long-term treatment in an institutional setting. Of course the means for implementing such measures were again lacking and day-to-day solutions had to be improvised. But this time the lesson was not forgotten. During the Korean War the rate of evacuations from combat zones for mental health problems dropped to 6 percent, and was as low as 1 percent in the Marines, with its more selective recruitment policies. Between World War II and the Korean conflict the military had trained psychiatrists to treat most mental disorders in the field and send the soldiers immediately back into combat.

Psychiatry, then, turned out to be useful and effective, provided one was willing to pay the price. It was ready to perform a service in the national interest, for which organization would be needed on a permanent, nationwide basis rather than just in the military under wartime conditions. Extrapolated to the entire population, the above figures indicate that one American in ten was suffering from a mental disorder serious enough to impair his or her performance, at least in critical conditions. Given the magnitude of these requirements, which if not new were at least being looked at in a new light, the system of state mental hospitals seemed inadequate and obsolete. The alternate system, while more flexible, was still uncertain in its operations and poorly coordinated. What was needed was a comprehensive reform to establish a public service capable of meeting these new needs.

At the end of the war a group known as the Group for the Advancement of Psychiatry was formed. Its members were young, reform-minded psychiatrists, many of whom had served in the army and now wanted to put their wartime experience to use in civilian life. As its leader the group chose psychoanalyst William Menninger, codirector with his brother Karl of the celebrated Menninger Foundation, one of the chief agencies in the spread of psychoanalysis in the United States. During the war William Menninger had been the army's chief psychiatrist. The group also included Francis Braceland, formerly chief psychiatrist for the Marine Corps and future president of the American Psychiatric Association, as well as future editor-in-chief of the American Journal of Psychiatry; Jack Eswalt, a consultant to the Air Force during the war, who would become chairman of the Joint Commission on Mental Illness, the importance of which we shall see later on; Robert Felix, trained before the war by the federal Division of Mental Health and future director of the National

Institute of Mental Health as well as the man who coordinated the establishment of community psychiatry under the auspices of the federal government. Around this core group gathered a number of young, modern-minded psychiatrists, trained in psychoanalysis and eager to sponsor in the United States the new idea that psychiatry could be designed to serve the public interest. This group soon forged alliances with enlightened bureaucrats and politicians in Washington, as well as with certain active philanthropists with good political connections. They set up what their enemies ironically dubbed the "Washington health syndicate," an effective, unified pressure group whose efforts were to culminate in 1963 in the passage of the Community Mental Health Centers Act.[7]

As a first step in this strategy, Robert Felix, head of the Division of Mental Hygiene (the only federal mental health agency) since 1944, arranged for two Democratic legislators, Senator Hill and Representative Fogarty, to file the National Mental Health Bill, which in 1946 was passed without opposition. The act left intact the main elements in the public mental health care system (the state mental hospitals), but appropriated federal funds for research, training of a new breed of psychiatrists, and financing of new services, in almost all cases clinics designed to provide diagnostic and preventive services and intensive treatment in a nonhospital setting. The spirit of the project is summed up in Albert Deutsch's testimony before the Senate committee: "The institutional care of psychotics has been traditionally mainly a state responsibility. It should remain so. But the job of getting preventive devices and using them is a national responsibility."[8]

The National Mental Health Act established the National Institute of Mental Health as the agency responsible for implementing the new policy. This was a crucial development: under Felix's leadership, the NIMH became the driving force behind nearly all the innovations that were to have a profound impact on contemporary American psychiatry, at least in its publicly-financed aspects. By 1963 the very modest initial budget of $8 million had grown to $144 million. The Institute financed clinics and experimental programs associated with universities and private hospitals (the state mental hospitals played almost no role). The primary focus of its policy was on training and retraining specialists and on a broad research effort ranging from perfection of new drugs to investigations of the social components of mental illness. Plentiful funding was available to anyone who wished to specialize in the study of mental illness. Many students availed themselves of the opportunity, sometimes out of genuine conviction, sometimes for opportunistic reasons, and often with a mixture of the two. It is worth mentioning in passing that this was one of the reasons for the fact that the sociology of mental health was early to be established as a discipline in the United States.[9] Though still a matter for ostracism at the end of World War II, by 1960 mental illness had become a subject of great interest to the general public, to judge by the number of publications, investigations, debates, and newspaper articles devoted to it. Meanwhile, the National Institute of Mental Health had financed more than three thousand research projects.

It had also supported more than fifteen hundred teaching programs. Accordingly, the number of psychiatrists in the United States rose from around three thousand at the time of the Second World War to seventeen thousand in 1964 (while the number of health professionals in general increased only 30 percent in the same period). In addition to training psychiatrists and to a lesser extent auxiliary mental health workers, NIMH also sponsored refresher courses in psychiatry for several thousand general practitioners. These efforts, carried out on a large scale and frequently hastily organized, helped to insure the ascendancy of psychoanalysis: psychoanalysis seemed to provide a technology of social relations as the basis for specific forms of psychiatric intervention, giving psychiatry a distinctive role within the field of medicine.

A new phase of this strategy began in 1955 with the passage of the Mental Health Act. Once again, the changes appeared to be modest and of limited scope. A national investigative commission, the Joint Commission on Mental Illness and Health, was established to report to Congress on the status of American psychiatry and to suggest comprehensive reforms. As the law states, its purpose was to give "an objective, thorough, and nationwide analysis and reevaluation of the human and economic problems of mental illness."[10] In theory, the commission was to include representatives of thirty-six different organizations concerned with mental health problems. In fact, official spokesmen for associations of health professionals and for the various welfare bureaucracies played a clearly preponderant role, joined by members drawn from a few more or less typical consumer organizations, whose presence lent credence to the fiction that all sectors of public opinion had been consulted.[11] Based on a wide-ranging series of investigations, the commission's report was completed in 1960. Entitled "Action for Mental Health," it was intended to be at once a diagnosis of the existing situation and a proposal of ways to remedy the system's deficiencies. The actions recommended were not without ambiguity (see below). A consensus emerged, however, around the need to reexamine the state hospital system, which was deemed outmoded, and to develop services of a new type with ties to the community.

The third phase began after Kennedy's election to the presidency with the appointment of a committee responsible for working out comprehensive new legislation based on the commission's proposals. At the same time a group led by the President's sister, Eunice Shriver, was working on a program of prevention and aid in the area of mental retardation. On February 5, 1963, Kennedy addressed Congress specifically on these two problems (the first time in the history of the United States that a President had made a major speech on matters of mental health).

Kennedy proposed a national mental health program that would take a completely new approach to the problem of treating the mentally ill. Central to the new program was the concept of a broad range of community health care services.

> To use federal grants only to perpetuate the existence of outmoded institutions will make no great difference. We need a new type of health facility, one which will return mental health care to the main stream of American medicine, and at the same time upgrade mental health services. I recommend, therefore, that the Congress authorize grants

to the States for the construction of comprehensive community mental health centers.[12]

The Congress immediately went to work and within a few months had passed the Community Mental Health Center and Retardation Act. Opposition from both the American Medical Association and congressional Republicans succeeded in limiting federal aid to the construction of centers, whereas the original proposal had called for payment of federal funds to cover staff salaries as well. Not until collective guilt over the assassination of President Kennedy had altered the national mood and a new Congress with an overwhelming Democratic majority had been elected was the Johnson administration able to amend the act in 1965 to include staff costs.

As early as 1963, however, the community mental health center (CMHC) idea had clearly come into its own as the centerpiece of the whole project. CMHCs were to provide at least five types of service: hospitalization, ambulatory care, emergency care, partial hospitalization services, and so-called community consultation and education services.[13] In signing the act on October 31, 1963, President Kennedy gave voice to the implicit hope that it would result in a profound transformation of the mental health care system:

> Under this legislation, custodial mental institutions will be replaced by therapeutic centers. It should be possible, within a decade or two, to reduce the number of patients in mental institutions by 50% or more. The new law provides the tools with which we can accomplish this objective.[14]

In rough outline, the foregoing paragraphs provide a summary of one version of the main events in the "third psychiatric revolution" (the first two being those associated with the names Pinel and Freud). Thanks to this third revolution, we are told, the insane were freed from confinement to become first-class patients, cared for in and by the community. As a general rule, American commentators have extolled these various acts and programs as humanitarian, even in works written quite recently. These writers see the reforms as a consequence of the growth of psychiatric knowledge, of increased tolerance of mental illness by society, and of the openhanded generosity of an enlightened administration under the leadership of a President "not like the rest," John F. Kennedy.[15] The transformation of the mental health care system was indeed orchestrated by a group of dynamic and hard-working individuals. Their success can be explained in psychological and sociological terms, as has been done on more than one occasion by some of those involved in designing and executing the new policy. Among other things, such analyses make the point that a leading role was played by a group of liberal and cultivated Bostonians, of which Kennedy was himself a member (as the former chairman of the commission recalled nostalgically when we interviewed him during the Nixon years, Kennedy was "a President who actually read the reports submitted to him"). For personal reasons, moreover, mental health issues were a particular concern of Kennedy's. Another decisive factor was the charismatic personality of Robert Felix, an effective leader and dedicated champion of this particular cause.

Beyond these special circumstances, however, what was the balance of forces that made success possible? There are troubling analogies between the American reforms and the so-called *politique de secteur* instituted in France, even though the circumstances and the individuals involved were, of course, different. In both cases dynamic professionals forged an alliance with forward-looking bureaucrats. In both cases the state sanctioned and assumed responsibility for the compromise that was struck. Although the process involved twists and turns peculiar to each country, and the differences between the two should not be neglected, still what we see is that the logic of the transformation of the issues taken to be central to modern psychiatry was the same in both places. This raises certain questions. What interests and forces on the part of both health professionals and bureaucrats resulted in the eventual political decision? What social and historical circumstances made the new policy desirable in the eyes of those invested with the decision-making power (i.e., in the American case, the Democratic administration)?

DYNAMIC PROFESSIONALS

At first sight, it seems anomalous that a group of American psychiatrists with an interest in public service should have managed to carry out their reform. In American society, probably to an even greater extent than elsewhere, the medical profession has been a powerful conservative force. Time and again, the American Medical Association has aligned itself with the most conservative forces whenever the threat of federal intervention has reared its head. The best proof of the AMA's unconditional support for the free enterprise system has been its unwavering, fierce opposition to national health insurance. Whether the target was Teddy Roosevelt's Progressive Party in 1908, the New Deal, or the Truman Administration, the AMA has consistently met its opponents by launching a campaign of hysteria financed by "war checks" contributed by its members. By raising the specter of "socialized medicine" or "communist plots" (a strategy that worked particularly well during the McCarthy era), the AMA has been largely responsible for the fact that of all the advanced industrial countries, the United States has the worst system of health insurance. As recently as 1965, i.e., after the passage of the Kennedy Act, the medical guild mobilized all its resources to oppose the passage of even such limited programs as Medicare (which provides partial coverage of medical costs for persons older than sixty-five) and Medicaid (which provides medical coverage for the needy). To this day the AMA has not significantly modified its opposition to the leading proposals for national health insurance, an issue that has bedeviled American domestic politics for years.[16]

The AMA's ultraconservatism has always gone hand in hand with its Malthusian attitudes toward the structure of the medical profession itself. In 1970, 70 percent of health service workers were women, but only 7 percent of doctors were, doubtless the lowest figure of any "developed" country. Nonwhite doctors accounted for only 2 to 3 percent of American physicians. Medical school admissions standards are such that many American students go abroad to study medicine. Conversely, as we have seen, some public institutions are forced to recruit foreign doctors to fill posts held in relatively low esteem by native physicians.

To be sure, the power of the American Medical Association has been on the decline since World War II, as more and more doctors choose to practice in a hospital setting (in 1970, only half of all doctors were engaged in private practice,[17] accounting for only 29 percent of medical care costs). But this has only meant that to some extent the AMA has been replaced by other powerful pressure groups, such as the American Hospital Association and the American Association of Medical Schools. These are dominated by the major hospital complexes and university medical centers, whose concern is to enhance their own profits and prestige through advanced research and elitist instruction. It is not because they are powerful that these groups are free to operate outside the free enterprise system as quasi public services. On the contrary, the way the system is organized accounts for the central paradox of American health care: on the one hand, there are vast material resources, highly skilled professionals, and technology that is undoubtedly the most advanced in the world, while, on the other hand, services are so unequally and inhumanely distributed that illness is a nightmare for tens of millions of Americans—and not only the poorest.

> Every day three million Americans go out in search of medical care. Some find it; others do not. Some are helped by it; others are not. Another twenty million Americans probably ought to enter the daily search for medical help, but are not healthy enough, rich enough, or enterprising enough to try. The obstacles are enormous. Health care is scarce and expensive to begin with. It is dangerously fragmented, and usually offered in an atmosphere of mystery and unaccountability. For many it is obtained only at the price of humiliation, dependence, or bodily insult. The stakes are high—health, beauty, sanity—and getting higher all the time. But the odds of winning are low and getting lower.[18]

Policy in these "empires" is set by the powers-that-be in the world of medicine, by representatives of insurance companies and of industries supplying the hospital market, and by officials of charitable organizations, which helped to found many of the system's institutions. These groups have gone the old medical guilds one better in establishing a more dynamic and effective hegemony over the health care system, but with similar effects on society. In particular, their policy has always been hostile to the idea of organizing medicine around the client and offering services accessible to all. Accordingly, it came into conflict with federal efforts in the sixties to relocate mental health services in the community and to encourage extension of the benefits of medical discoveries to the entire population (see below). Recent attempts at national health planning—such as the Comprehensive Health Planning Act, as well as the Regional Medical Program Act, designed to define new priorities in teaching, research, and practice, and the Professional Standards Review Organization, intended to supervise and set standards for professional practice, and Health Systems Agencies—have all ended in failure or been reinterpreted in a manner in keeping with the interests of the medical profession and its affiliates.

Astonishingly enough, however, this very same medical establishment was apparently in favor of a would-be progressive reorganization of the mental health care system. In fact, matters are more complex than appearances suggest. Doctors initially entered into alliances to protect their own professional interests and, later, policies inspired by the Democratic administration attempted to move beyond those professional interests toward a more comprehensive approach.

Psychiatry has always been the weak link in the medical system. Mental hospital superintendents, who had long languished far from the centers of power owing to their role in the system and their lack of scientific credibility, took almost no part in the debate during the fifties, though its outcome was first and foremost of concern to them. By the time they woke up, it was too late.

Similarly, private psychiatric practice was not very widely developed when the reform process got under way in the fifties. So private practitioners were not much of a pressure group, either. The real prestige and power in psychiatry belonged to doctors at universities, general hospitals, and major private psychoanalytic clinics such as the Menninger Foundation, Chestnut Lodge outside Washington, McLean's outside Boston, and Hillside near New York. French experience, too, shows that a dynamic group of individuals can take the lead in a profession during a period of transition, particularly if that group can make profitable use of political capital amassed during wartime (or, as in France, during the Resistance). In France progressive hospital psychiatrists took control of the union apparatus and of the journal *Information psychiatrique* in 1945. In the United States the Group for the Advancement of Psychiatry rose to prominence within the American Psyciatric Association, a section of the American Medical Association, and took over the *American Journal of Psychiatry* after forcing out the traditionalists, who had formed a Committee for the Safeguard of Medical Standards in Psychiatry.[19]

The success of groups such as these, however, depends in large part on the fact that they serve the interests of the profession quite effectively: in the present case, the reform group proposed a program that made it possible for psychiatrists to overcome their isolation and enjoy some of the benefits of technical progress. As we have seen, this became the policy of the National Institute of Mental Health. The NIMH mobilized all available resources to train specialists, to create new technologies, and to experiment with more flexible institutional structures. As a result, a discipline that had become estranged from "scientific" medicine over the years—if it had ever really had anything to do with science at all—was able to return to the fold. Felix pointed to "the developments of the past two decades which have made psychiatry not only a part of medicine but have placed it at the very heart of it."[20]

If the Joint Commission achieved a consensus, it was built around an outlook centered on the profession. Its proposed objectives for psychiatric reform were therefore to move away from an outmoded idea of the profession's role, which was bound up with the asylum, and to lay the foundations for a genuinely medical approach to mental illness, an approach that had been made possible by the development of a new kind of knowledge, propagated by modern institutions and highly trained teachers. The hope was to create a sort of utopia for professionals, helping them to establish their practice on a firm new footing, thereby legitimating their privileges and increasing their power—a program that could hardly fail to attract the support of many specialists.

In fact, the apparent unanimity concealed differences over how the desired *aggiornaménto*, or bringing up to date, was to be achieved, differences that existed even before the onset of crisis (see chapter 5). The Joint Commission recommended that state hospitals be modernized and made more humane, and that community centers be established to provide the mentally ill with treatment close to where they lived. At this point the community clinics were still quite narrowly defined:

> Community mental health clinics serving both children and adults, operated as out-patient departments of general or mental hospitals, as part of State or regional systems for mental patient care, or as independent agencies, are a main line of defense in reducing the need of many persons with major mental illness for prolonged or repeated hospitalization. Therefore, a national mental health program should set as an objective one fully staffed, full-time mental health clinic available to each 50,000 of population. Greater efforts should be made to induce more psychiatrists in private practice to devote a substantial part of their working hours to community clinic services, both as consultants and as therapists.[21]

These proposals, as is evident, were thoroughly eclectic. The same thing happened in France: eclecticism was the price that had to be paid in order to rally the various segments of the profession, with the exception of the fundamentalists. In the *politique de secteur* the hospital remained the centerpiece of the system, ostensibly modernized and humanized. To it were added outpatient services, clinics, and consultations. Support was solicited from the private sector. And so on. Everyone was likely to support reform, because everybody benefitted from it in one way or another. "Psychiatric revolutions" are in many cases no more than judicious compromises for avoiding difficult choices and structural change.

Between the time the Joint Commission issued its report and the passage of the Community Mental Health Center Act, however, there was a basic shift in policy. The new policy was more radical: to establish as an alternative to the old system a new, independent community system—the long-term objective being to supplant the state mental hospitals altogether. The reformers' thoughts turned from community mental health *clinics* to community mental health *centers* (CMHC). The operation of the clinic still required a symbiotic relationship with a hospital: in a word, the clinic served as the hospital's outpatient department. The center, on the other hand, was conceived as an autonomous organization offering a full range of services. At the same time, the plan to reform the state mental hospitals via a direct infusion of federal funds was abandoned. Under the new policy, all resources were devoted to the establishment of community mental health centers. The thinking was that two thousand CMHCs, each serving a so-called catchment area comprising 75,000 to 200,000 people, would ultimately replace the asylum system.

The reasons for this change of orientation were not merely technical, however. The groundwork was laid by the cabinet committee appointed by Kennedy. The President's men reinterpreted the proposals of the NIMH bureaucrats in accordance with their own strategy,[22] and thereby destroyed the consensus within the profession. Why? Because in the meantime the problem had become a political issue. In July 1960 the community plan for the reorganization of mental health services was incorporated into the platform of the Democratic Party at its convention in Los Angeles.[23] In his February 1963 speech, Kennedy himself came down clearly in favor of one of the two options proposed in the Joint Commission report. Speaking on the President's behalf, a special assistant from the Department of Health, Education, and Welfare put it this way in testimony before the House committee holding hearings on the bill: "The basic purpose of the President's program is to redirect the locus of treatment of the mentally ill from State mental hospitals into community mental health centers."[24]

How did it happen that the choice of a medical model coincided with a political strategy? The proponents of bold reforms in psychiatry had come up with a medical technology for mental health care. This was now seen as a way of combatting social instability, as one element in a new policy designed to control marginal groups within the population, a policy on which the Democratic administration was just then putting the final touches. To understand the importance of the issue, however, it must be viewed against the background of American welfare policy in general, which in the early sixties was undergoing a fundamental change.

A NEW FEDERAL STRATEGY

For a long time what was distinctive about American welfare policy was that the bulk of the aid was handed out by local and private agencies rather than by the federal government (see chapter 2). During the twenties social work was dominated by interpretive models based on psychiatry and psychoanalysis, which further accentuated the tendency to treat individual cases one by one. In general, American welfare policy was directed toward dealing with defects in individual personalities rather than with the social causes of mental illness, the association of insanity with poverty. It was natural, therefore, that this policy should have relied upon ideologies that revolved around the individual case, ideologies that were at first of moralistic and later of psychological derivation.

When economic crisis hit in the thirties, however, the central issues in the formulation of welfare policy had to be redefined. For the first time, the federal authorities intervened on a broad scale to cope with the social instability brought on by the crisis and to counter the threat of political subversion. Typical of the New Deal were such projects as the Federal Emergency Relief Act, which distributed direct aid, and the Works Progress Administration Act, which provided funding for major public works projects. These were spectacular measures, which brought relief to 20 million people and absorbed a tenth of the national income. What is more, they were effective, in one way or another helping the United States to recover from the crisis and starting the country down the road to imperialism. Recovery was given a decisive lift by the onset of World War II, but even before then the decline had been arrested. And yet, when we look closely at the New Deal programs, we find that they were both tentative and limited in scope. They dealt only with those who were "poor by accident," chiefly people who had previously played productive roles in the society but who had been plunged into difficulties by the economic collapse. Once the crisis was over, these emergency programs were allowed to lapse and things once again followed their normal course in the best of all possible capitalist worlds.

There had never been any question, then, of really attacking the structural causes of poverty and racial inequality. Other measures were, however, aimed at different groups within the population, groups cut off from the benefits of the affluent society by some handicap. These measures were embodied in the Social Security Act of 1935. At best, however, these efforts were extremely modest. The Democratic administration was unable to enact free medical coverage, even for the elderly. Except for a 1942 amendment providing unemployment insurance and old-age benefits (both of which applied only to people already integrated into the labor market), the Social Security Act offered public assistance only to the blind, to certain of the elderly and handicapped, and to dependent children. For thirty years these provisions would remain the backbone of the entire welfare program. All welfare policy was built around the aid to dependent children program. Needy families, particularly those in which the father had either died or disappeared, received aid that varied from state to state. Thus only a small segment of the poor population received welfare assistance: namely, broken families with no resources, provided they were able to prove their poverty and neediness to the welfare bureaucracies, which developed a most humiliating array of techniques for checking, controlling, and manipulating needs.[25]

For the most part, the picture of the welfare situation sketched above remained true until the early sixties, except for a few amendments to the 1935 Social Security Act that it would be tedious to analyze here, and a slight increase in the number of welfare recipients and the amount of aid paid out. In the sixties, however, a new federal offensive began to take shape. The new policy was influenced by awareness of the political importance of ethnic minorities, particularly blacks, and of their subversive potential. The latter was made evident by riots that shook American society to its foundations, riots that exploded one after another in nearly every major city in the United States. Driven from the South by modernization of agricultural methods, blacks settled in big-city ghettos, where they gained political power thanks to their ability to swing elections in several eastern and midwestern states as well as California. Kennedy, it will be recalled, only barely beat Nixon in 1960. In several states, such as Ohio, he won by only a few thousand votes, thanks to having run up a large majority in the ghettos.[26]

An "other America," forgotten amid the self-congratulatory affluence of the preceding period, suddenly forced itself on the attention of the nation.[27] Politicians, journalists, and social scientists set out in search of new solutions to the newly discovered problems. No longer treated merely as an afterthought in the affluent society, poverty became a central social issue and elimination of the threat it represented became a political imperative.[28] Poverty now came to mean not merely lack of resources, but rather a condition of deprivation, in which unemployment, poor housing, racial segregation, juvenile delinquency, physical illness, and psychic imbalance took a terrible toll in a large number of cases. These conditions were not only destructive for those who had to endure them but dangerous for the government and society at large, which might have to deal with the rebellion that widespread social misery could easily produce.

Immediately upon taking office, the Democratic administration took a series of steps directed toward accomplishing two goals: first, to help groups within the population that did not share in the benefits or values of American society and therefore represented a subversive potential; and second, to enable the government to exert more effective control over the behavior of such groups. The redistributive effects of the measures taken were modest at best: at the height of Johnson's War on Poverty, in 1965, an average of ninety-five dollars in supplemental benefits was added to each welfare check. But federal intervention was carried out in such a way as to insure the presence of federal officials in the heart of areas that had previously been neglected, for the most part in the cities.

The measures taken were impressively far-reaching, beginning with the Juvenile Delinquency and Youth Offense Control Act of 1961 and the many acts that followed throughout the sixties. More remarkable, however, than the number and variety of different programs is the unified strategy that was the basis for them. The main targets were chronic poverty and despair in the ghettos, scenes of daily violence and smoldering rebellion. To attack these targets, new institutions were established within the areas to be controlled. The work was carried out by a new type of professional, aided by volunteer workers. The aim was to enlist the participation of the community itself, relying on minority group leaders to gain access and attract the attention of community activists to the reform programs promoted by the government. The money and the initiative behind these efforts came from Washington, the intention being to bypass the traditional welfare agencies and municipal bureaucracies, which were suspected of wanting to maintain the status quo.

Among the various measures taken, those concerned with health and juvenile delinquency stand out: Juvenile Delinquency and Youth Offense Control Act, 1961; Community Mental Health Center Act, 1963; Medicare and Medicaid, amendments to the Social Security Act of 1935, 1965; Regional Medical Program Act and Comprehensive Health Planning Act, 1966; Safe Streets and Omnibus Crime Act, 1968. It will not be possible to go into detail here about the methods used in each of these programs and the way they interacted with one another. It should not be assumed that the effects of all the programs were similar. There can be no doubt, however, that behind all of them lay a coherent political strategy, a strategy that was pluralist in orientation yet centrally orchestrated in execution. All the programs were designed to deal with the same population subgroups, and all worked together toward a single goal. Two of the best observers of this period, who also happen to have been involved as actors, put it this way: "It made little difference whether the funds were appropriated under delinquency-prevention, mental-health, antipoverty, or model-cities legislation: in the streets of the ghettoes, many aspects of these programs looked very much alike."[29]

Thus the community mental health centers were but one element in a multifaceted strategy. Like the other new social services inspired and financed directly by Washington, they were established mainly in disadvantaged urban areas. Regulations issued under the 1963 act regarding submission of step-by-step plans by the states for the construction of CMHCs required that "the frequency of mental illness and emotional disorders" and "the proportion of low-income individuals, the unemployment rate, and the prevalence of substandard housing" all be taken into account.[30] Accordingly, more than half the new centers were built in the ghettos, and the only reason the proportion was not even higher was that some local officials managed to take advantage of the new laws to undertake programs in less deprived areas.[31]

In this context, not all practices labeled "medical" were strictly medical in content—nor could they possibly have been. Many so-called medical practices were in fact based on theories of prevention and went far beyond what Goffman has called the "servicing" model, long standard in psychiatry: that is, a model in which treatment is limited to manifest disorders of undeniably pathological origin.[32] Since the twenties, much has been made of "prevention," which has generally been touted in connection with programs designed to maintain or improve the health of the American people, programs that are as vague as they are ambitious. The prevention ideology had one major defect: it lacked specific technologies, institutions, and personnel to inervene on a large scale. The community mental health center may be seen as one institution designed to fill this gap. In fact, the supporters of the CMHC movement within the medical profession were proponents of prevention:

> The main focus of this unit is on extramural services to the community which concentrate upon the primary prevention of mental disorders.[33] The staff of the centre will be deployed within the framework of a variety of non-psychiatric community educational, social, and medical agencies, where they will be available for preventive intervention in crisis situations.[34]

Plainly, the new frontiers of medical intervention have become indistinguishable from the new frontiers of social action. The implementation of a primary prevention program requires effective control over the decision-making process, so that intervention takes on a political dimension. This was explicitly noted by another leading theorist of prevention: "The psychiatrist must truly be a political personage in the best sense of the word. He must play a role in controlling the environment which man has created."[35]

The community mental health centers enabled psychiatrists to plunge into the thick of the community so that they could actually play this sort of political role, especially among marginal social groups, where there is so much to "control." Consider the issues: The urban crisis?

> If we can reach the mayors and the people concerned by the cities in their crisis with assistance in the acute problems they are facing, they will begin to use us and we can help bring about change. I suggest that we begin to take them on as clients. We cannot wait for them to request our services, because they are not going to ask us. We must begin right now to fill in and be of assistance to them with the issues they are facing.[36]

The immorality of the poor, resulting in increased welfare costs?

> In some states the regulation of these grants in the case of children of unmarried mothers is currently being modified to dissuade the mothers from further illegitimate pregnancies. Mental health specialists are being consulted to help the legislators and welfare authorities improve the moral atmosphere in the homes where the children are being brought up and to influence their mothers to marry and provide them with stable fathers.[37]

Further examples could easily be adduced. Perhaps the most comprehensive statement of this conception of politics coupled with medicine has been given by Caplan:

> The mental health specialist offers consultation to legislators and administrators and collaborates with other citizens in influencing gov-

ernmental agencies to change laws and regulations. Social action includes efforts to modify general attitudes and behavior of community
members by communication through the educational system, the mass
media, and through interaction between the professional and lay communities.[38]

This statement is a succinct summary of the ideology that underlies community mental health. The professionals who took
part in the movement were agitating for more than just the right
to provide standard types of medical care to those who had been
deprived of it. Of course, one of their goals was to move away
from hospital-based treatment and narrowly-defined, traditional
patterns of medical and welfare assistance and toward providing
new, on-the-spot services wherever psychic and social disorders
emerged; another was to aid society's most underprivileged members and in some instances even to forge alliances with them
against the older city and state bureaucracies, which staunchly
defended the status quo; and to use Washington's desire for reform
to overcome certain entrenched local opposition. But another part
of their goal was to defuse the society's most explosive segments.
As we shall see, there was a constant danger that the movement
would get out of hand. As it happened, some psychiatrists were
tempted to switch sides, abandoning technical expertise in favor
of militant activism—inevitable mishaps in a movement of this
sort. Intervention had its limits, and these are stated below in a
paraphrase of the views of one ideologue employed by the National Institute of Mental Health:

> As individuals, professionals may or may not be political activists. But
> the field of mental medicine as such cannot be involved in radical
> changes in the power structure or drastic changes in the structure and
> function of society. It can be involved to the hilt in community plan-
> ning, of which the implementation of mental health programs is an
> important part. It cannot be involved in the overthrow of the govern-
> ment or change of the Constitution. In this country, it accepts the
> framework of a democratic society as the basis for particular contri-
> butions by mental health professionals.[39]

In general, administration-inspired social policy thrived on this ambiguity throughout the sixties. Community mental health was one element in a strategy of community participation. In other words, the program was part of a broader effort to grant some power to people at the grass roots. In some cases citizens were enlisted to participate in the supervision of community services (see chapter 5 below for a discussion of the so-called community advisory boards). Some personnel were recruited from the community, providing upward mobility for certain members of minority groups (see the discussion of paraprofessionals, also in chapter 5). In the final analysis, this policy suffered from the same ambiguity that characterized federal policy as a whole during the sixties. On the one hand, federal programs did in some areas foster a new political awareness on the part of ethnic minorities; conflicts did result that disturbed entrenched local interests; and some groups were able to obtain concessions locally that had not been planned at the federal level. On the other hand, federal policy was not without success in achieving the government's domestic objectives. It quelled the most explosive ghetto violence, if only for a while. And it drew into the system and promoted through the ranks certain local leaders, who took over functions formerly handled by city agencies and officials, though meanwhile the basic conditions of the poor remained essentially unchanged.

We are now in a position to see more clearly the nature of the alliance between the mental health professionals and the "enlightened" bureaucrats in Washington, an alliance that figured in a fundamental way in all the important changes in mental health policy. The point is not that the new psychiatry was merely an instrument of unmediated political interests. Beyond interest-group politics, the community mental health centers also represent an attempt to modernize psychiatric practice and to resolve contradictions internal to the profession. The mental health care system in the sixties was chaotic and in need of reorganization. Its rationalization placed a new instrument in the hands of the politicians and administrators whose job was to deal with mental illness and, more broadly, to control "problem groups" in the society. Invariably, this is how new psychiatric methods come to be "recognized," i.e., given a social mandate. For example, the methods perfected by Pinel and his successors were used by legislators as a basis for reformulating the sociopolitical issues connected with madness in nascent bourgeois society, and led in 1838 to legislation for dealing with mental health problems. In the same way, the work of the National Institute of Mental Health produced new concepts and methods for dealing with mental disturbances, and these were incorporated into a comprehensive strategy designed to enhance social stability in the United States in the areas in which it was most fragile. Everyone involved found some benefit in the new approach. The bureaucrats and politicians responsible for mental health policy acquired new resources for exerting more effective control and exercising closer surveillance of potential trouble spots. Mental health professionals developed flexible new methods of treatment and extended their jurisdiction into new domains:

> The community mental health centers established under this act reflected the expansion of the mental health world's system-conception to include non-mental illness concerns, but continued to rely upon psychiatry as the ruling discipline for the centers.[40]

One question has not yet been asked, however: How did this program of modernization and expansion of psychiatric medicine actually work? What has struck us wherever we have looked—whether at programmatic pronouncements such as those excerpted above or at the ideas of NIMH bureaucrats gleaned in Washington interviews—has been the enormous disparity between the psychiatric gospel and what is actually practiced in the field. Let us turn now to reality and look next at how old institutions were transformed and new ones established. And let us also consider, in concrete terms, the status of the mental patient in contemporary American society. Does what we see embody the utopian ideals of the reformers?

PART TWO

An American Dream

The history of mental medicine in America up through the fifties was dominated by one overwhelmingly important phenomenon: the inexorable increase in the number of mental hospital inpatients, which rose from 8,500 in 1860 to 558,000 in 1955. This increase certainly cannot be explained by the growth of the country's population: the hospitalization rate rose from 0.27 per thousand inhabitants to around 3.5 per thousand. The rise was temporarily halted by certain events, most prominently war. But as soon as the political situation returned to normal, the growth resumed.

Suddenly, however, during the fifties, the curve flattened out and then began to plummet. This downturn was not peculiar to the United States alone. Beginning in 1952 in France and in 1954 in Great Britain we see the same decrease in the rate of hospitalization. It was in the United States, however, that the drop was most marked and sudden: by 1966 there were no more than 452,000 hospitalized mental patients, and by 1975 only 193,000, or 0.9 per thousand inhabitants, a decrease of 65.5 percent in twenty years and 57.5 percent in ten years.

At the same time, discourse about mental illness shifted from nineteenth-century apologetics for "therapeutic isolation" (no cure without confinement) to the no less dogmatically asserted contention that community treatment is superior:

> Nothing succeeds like an idea whose time has come. The institution as a means of coping with the problems of specific sectors of our population seems at this point to have run its course. Whether one is aged, below par intellectually or emotionally, delinquent, alcoholic, or

drug-addicted, the source—and the remedy—of the problem lie in the communities where such people come from. By bringing them back into the community, by enlisting the good will and the desire to serve, the ability to understand which is to be found in every neighborhood, we shall meet the challenge which such groups of persons present, and at the same time ease the financial burden of their confinement in fixed institutions.[1]

Two certitudes lent each other support: first, the psychiatric hospital was believed to be dead in the United States, or at least its demise was seen as necessary; and second, the community was deemed ready to take responsibility for the mentally ill and socially deviant, ready to offer them treatment where they lived.[2]

A look at the facts, however, indicates that skepticism is called for. Some of the mental hospitals that closed down after 1960 have since reopened: in 1967 there were 307 "operational" mental hospitals, in 1973, 334, and in 1975, 313. In the state of New York no hospitals have closed down, although there have been mergers, and 80 percent of the state mental health budget is still poured into the chronic care psychiatric institutions. While the number of patients actually in the hospital at any given moment has undeniably decreased, the number of *admissions* each year remains high: 32,000 in 1978 for New York State alone. On the national level, annual admissions have increased considerably: 375,000 in 1975 compared with 178,000 in 1955, or more than double.[3]

There is some doubt, moreover, that whatever decrease there may have been in the number of patients treated in hospitals in comparison with the number treated elsewhere actually reflects a far-reaching change in attitude toward the users (or victims) of the mental health system. There are surprises in store when we come to look closely at how the number of hospitalized patients was reduced (that is, what pressures motivated the reduction, what the costs were in human and financial terms, and what actually happened to the "liberated" patients).

Then, too, as the reformers saw it during the fifties, ending the confinement of large numbers of mental patients was supposed to go hand in hand with the organization of a new system of mental health care, a system that was supposed to revolve around the community mental health centers and provide care to anyone in need. This was the essence of the new psychiatry, whose spirit Bertram S. Brown, assistant director of the National Institute of Mental Health, defined in the following terms in 1964:

All mental health services are to be available to all people of a community—the rich and the poor, the young and the old, the resident and the transient, the healthy who are merely curious or in need of education, and the ill who are mildly neurotic or severely psychotic, and the chronic cases of illness as well as the acute. They all comprise a community, and a comprehensive community health center, to deserve the name, must serve them all. . . . [It should also meet the needs of] special problem groups (for example, the alcoholics, the aged, and the juvenile delinquents) [and should take increasing interest in] the social frames of reference within which human behavior is the better understood . . . [including] such relatively new foci of attention as poverty, unemployment, substandard housing and all the echelons of economic status. . . . Consideration of the mental patient as a single individual is everywhere being complemented by a concern for the community itself.[4]

What has become of this great promise fifteen years later?

CHAPTER 4

Psychiatric Hospitals: The New Order

A CHANGE OF DIRECTION

In 1955 inmates of American mental hospitals numbered some 558,000; by 1975 the figure had fallen to only 193,000. The importance of the state mental hospitals also decreased in comparison with that of other psychiatric institutions: witness the distribution of treatment episodes[1] in 1955 as compared with 1973 (see figure 4.1). And, in 1955 half the cases calling for psychiatric treatment were handled in state hospitals, while by 1973 the corresponding proportion had fallen to 12 percent.

The governmental agencies involved were quite willing to interpret this change as a direct consequence of the "bold new approach" to mental illness called for by President Kennedy. Stanley Yolles, the successor of Robert Felix as head of the National Institute of Mental Health, stated to Congress in 1969 that

> Largely because of the impetus of community mental health centers we have seen a startling reduction of patients in mental hospitals in the United States. We are predicting now that instead of having reduced the population of mental hospitals as in the 10-year period 1963 to 1973 by one-half, we will reduce it by two-thirds because of the services thus provided.[2]

The new psychiatry had triumphed over the old policy of segregation—so runs the litany—so that patients who would formerly have been institutionalized could now be treated in the community. This is a very optimistic, or in any case a very incomplete, interpretation of the figures.

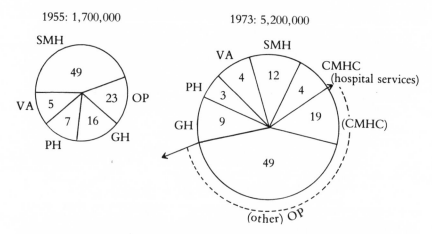

Figure 4.1: Percent distribution of inpatient and outpatient care episodes in mental health facilities, by type of facility, in the years 1955 and 1973.

ABBREVIATIONS: SMH, State and County Mental Hospitals; VA, Veterans Administration Hospitals; PH, Private Mental Hospitals; GH, General Hospital, Inpatient Psychiatric Units; OP, Ambulatory Care, Outpatient Psychiatric Services; CMHC, Community Mental Health Centers (Residential Treatment Centers for children are included in the private hospitals).

SOURCE: Based on figures given in National Institute of Mental Health Statistical Note no. 127, February 1976.

In the first place, the numbers make clear that, although the deinstitutionalization process did accelerate after 1964, it actually began more than ten years before the inception of the new federal policy.

Responsibility for the first wave of deinstitutionalization, which lasted from 1956 to 1964, can be assigned to two related factors: criticism of the psychiatric hospitals and postwar innovations in therapy.

1. As we have seen, the earliest attacks on conditions in the asylums date from the late nineteenth century (chapter 1). Such criticisms received wide publicity thanks to the efforts of Clifford Beers and the mental hygiene movement. A second phase began with the end of the Second World War. The war had breached the walls of the asylum for many conscientious objectors who had done their alternate service in asylums and later denounced the scandalous conditions they had witnessed. Albert Deutsch launched a press campaign against the outrages. In 1947 and

1948 two works destined to have a major impact on public opinion were published: *The Snake Pit* by Mary J. Ward, a former patient, and *The Shame of the States* by Albert Deutsch.[3]

These criticisms were soon broadened by others of more scholarly inspiration. The best known of these studies, Erving Goffman's *Asylums*, out of which grew a whole school of sociology, viewed the mental hospital as a "total institution" and undermined the therapeutic justifications that hid the real meaning of what went on in the asylums.[4] Many other analyses of state mental hospitals appeared, written from sociological, psychosociological, and medical standpoints, in some cases at the behest of, and financed by, the National Institute of Mental Health itself.[5] These works attacked the asylums as outmoded institutions without therapeutic effect and even inherently harmful, while arguing in favor of modern—and profitable—new ways of doing psychiatry. Ultimately, a consensus was achieved, a consensus reflected in the report of the Joint Commission. "Enlightened" professionals and social scientists took the view that the state mental hospitals, as they were then organized, were dysfunctional, ineffective, inhumane, costly, and therefore outdated institutions. Already the most energetic and forward-looking professionals were experimenting with new treatment methods, methods that were beginning to change the nature of the asylum.

2. Hesitantly, these therapeutic innovations were introduced after the war. Taking their inspiration from psychoanalysis, from group experiences (Moreno), and from English therapeutic communities (Maxwell Jones), some advanced hospitals followed certain private clinics in experimenting with new techniques. Rounding out their staff with volunteers, these hospitals instituted special programs, usually in separate buildings with patients selected on the basis of favorable prognoses; in this way it proved possible to eliminate isolation, restraint, and hydrotherapy and "packs," as well as to reduce the use of sedatives (at that time barbiturates, bromides, and paraldehydes). The involvement of staff and patients in the running of the institution was increased. Certain patients also received more individualized treatment.[6]

But these experiments never got very far, and it was not until the advent of psychotropic drugs that it became possible to combine criticism of the way things were done in the asylums with the new therapeutic methods so as to make far-reaching changes in hospital procedures. Chlorpromazine came on the market in

May 1954 under the name Thorazine. Within eight months the drug had been administered to more than 2 million patients. In 1955 New York became the first state to adopt a complete program of treatment involving neuroleptics in all of its mental hospitals. It was also the first state to see a slight decrease in the number of mental hospital patients, beginning in mid-1955.[7] In effect the potency of the neuroleptics in quelling behavioral disorders— whether for better or for worse is another matter—made it possible not only to improve conditions within the institution but also to shorten the stay of new patients considerably and even to release certain chronic patients. Inside the hospital a variety of new therapies became feasible—recreational therapy, group therapy, music therapy, occupational therapy, dance therapy. But these therapies involved only a minority of patients, and in some cases quickly degenerated into nothing more than a form of "work therapy" for chronic patients, who were assigned jobs in the hospital.

In the outside community, the fact that increased numbers of patients were being released after short stays in the hospital while still under psychiatric care called for the creation of postcure facilities, or so-called drug maintenance clinics. A minority of patients was thereby enabled to carry on with normal life while still receiving treatment. Thus by 1966 or so, when operations were just getting under way in a few community mental health centers, the patient population in the state mental hospitals had already fallen by nearly 20 percent.

THE NEW GHETTOS

The role that is so facilely attributed to the community centers in the recent trend toward deinstitutionalization deserves closer examination. The new centers did come into being just as the decline in the inmate population began to accelerate, in 1964 or thereabouts (see figure 4.2). As we shall see in the next chapter, however, the community mental health centers did not take over the job of the asylums: the centers were effective mainly in treating

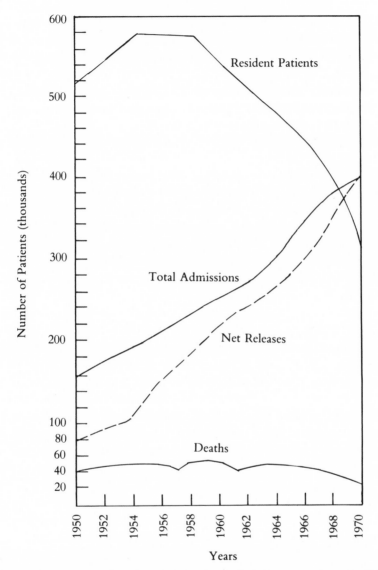

Figure 4.2: Number of resident patients, total admissions, net releases in U.S. state and county hospitals, 1950-1971.

SOURCE: NIMH Biometry Branch. Printed in Franklin D. Chu and Sharland Trotter, *The Madness Establishment* (New York: Grossman Publishers 1974), p. 36.

a different patient population. This much is today conceded even in such official documents as the Comptroller General's Report to Congress, albeit in diplomatic language:

> The CMHC program had not been fully effective in preventing unnecessary admissions to public mental hospitals, providing care and followup treatment to persons released from such facilities, or developing a coordinated system of care for the mentally ill.[8]

If the new psychiatry brought little in the way of relief to beleaguered state hospital residents, the existence or even the prospective existence of community centers provided a golden alibi to those who favored cutbacks in the state hospital budgets for reasons that had nothing altruistic or therapeutic about them. The new treatment philosphies, implemented with state or federal monies, served mainly to camouflage maneuvers motivated in fact by economic and political considerations.

The fact is that it cost states an average of twenty dollars a day to keep a patient in a public hospital at this time. This amount had to be raised out of local taxes, losing votes for local politicians. It cost far less to treat the same individual as an outpatient or in a community mental health center. Of course cost estimates are always unreliable and subject to manipulation by interested agencies. Accurate estimates are even more difficult to come by in the case of outpatient services, which are often financed from multiple sources. For the purposes of a rough calculation, however, we may rely on a California Department of Mental Hygiene document, which estimated the cost of community treatment at between five and twelve dollars per day.[9] Thus the state saved on the order of $3000 per year on each patient cared for outside the hospital setting. Cynical readers will no doubt remark that even more could have been saved had the patient not been treated at all—and, as we shall see, this is not merely armchair speculation. In any case, between 1956 and 1974 the share of the total state budget devoted to mental hospitals decreased by more than 50 percent for all states combined, despite the particularly severe impact of inflation on medical costs. In New York, for example, the share of the state budget allocated to mental hospitals dropped from 7.8 percent in 1956 to 3.2 percent in 1974, and in California from 2.56 percent to 0.86 percent.[10] Had the number of residents continued to grow at its previous rate instead of beginning to decline in 1956, moreover, there would now be more than half a million *additional* Americans confined to mental hospitals, requiring still further allocations for construction, administration, staff, and so forth. This the always financially-strapped states simply could not have afforded. The budget has weighed far more heavily than either humanitarian or scientific considerations.

And there is more: if patients released from state hospitals are pointed in the direction of private institutions for follow-up treatment, large profits stand to be made. Indeed, while the progress made in social legislation in the United States may have been modest in recent years, it has nevertheless been enough to provide indigent or once indigent patients with the means to fill the coffers of big business. Medicaid payments, for example, have poured into nursing homes and care homes, which have managed to reap huge profits by failing to comply with the minimum standards set by public agencies. Even larger sums go directly to welfare recipients, and since 1974 Supplemental Security Income payments of $150 to $200 per month have been paid to blind, handicapped, and elderly individuals. Since these funds are received by the individual rather than by the institution providing him or her with care, the institution is not accountable to the funding agency; no one is in a position to oversee the conditions in which former inmates are forced to live or the treatment that is administered to them. It is assumed that the patient has freely chosen the service he prefers from among the various institutions competing for his business when he is released from the state hospital.

Summing up, the release of large numbers of chronic patients, once confined to inhumane, disorganized, authoritarian hospitals, was motivated in part by two needs: to curtail public spending and to enhance private profits.

The situation in California is an extreme case, a clear illustration of the significance of the new policy. Always in the forefront of innovation, California had already greatly reduced the number of patients in its mental hospitals when noted conservative Ronald Reagan, now President, was elected governor on a campaign promise to cut taxes drastically. He hoped to use his election as a steppingstone to a run for the presidency in 1976. Hence he set out to show that he knew how to reduce public expenditures. Cutting the budget for mental hospitals was a key element in his strategy.

He first came up with two gimmicks to reduce the number of admissions. One was to give local authorities a stake in drying up the supply of mental patients: a target goal was calculated for each county for hospital admissions among its residents. If the number of people from the county seeking hospitalization turned out to be below the target figure, the county would receive a "bonus" of 15 percent of the per diem cost of care for each patient not admitted. Wags referred to this program as the "county-bounty." Local bureaucrats could thus increase the amount of money they received from the state by not hospitalizing patients, regardless of their symptoms and regardless of the availability of alternate treatment. The second gimmick was designed to make it easier for hospital superintendents to turn down applicants for admission. Reagan signed the Linterman–Petris–Short Act, which contained a number of liberal provisions (extending the rights of patients, for example), but which required a psychiatric examination prior to any hospitalization and increased the complexity of the procedures that had to be gone through in order to hold a patient more than seventy-two hours against his will. The superintendents (who were directly responsible to the state government) enforced these new provisions to the letter, so that few patients were admitted or kept against their will for more than the allowed seventy-two hours, regardless of their condition and whether or not help was available to them outside.

The best way to save money, though, was still to get rid of chronic patients. This was easy to do, since American law allows patients to be released at the sole discretion of the superintendent. Nor did relocating the patients released present any problems, at least for those receiving government benefits, who represented a potential source of profit. By a curious coincidence the fee for licensing nondescript buildings as "board-and-care homes" deemed suitable for housing former hospital patients was reduced to ten dollars. By another curious coincidence, the local agencies representing Medicaid, as well as those responsible for regulating the homes, suddenly became quite accommodating and approved a series of agreements with the new institutions in spite of violations of the laws governing medical facilities and failure to comply with even the minimum standards of safety and comfort required of ordinary dwellings.

The results were spectacular. In six years, the number of hospitalized patients fell by almost three-quarters, from 26,567 in 1966 to 7,011 in 1971 (the peak of 37,489 had been reached in 1956). At the same time the nursing home business received a considerable boost, which drew a critical report from the Senate in 1976.[11] Bankrupt hotels and motels and dilapidated buildings were acquired and patched up for very little money. New buildings were constructed as cheaply as possible, and even old garages, not to mention former chicken coops, were pressed into service. Patients released from the hospitals were crammed into these places, where living conditions resembled those of the hospital ghetto, and were kept in isolation, poorly fed, deprived of all comforts, and left with nothing to do, neither cared for nor supervised, and in some cases tied to their chairs or locked up with other patients in a "quiet room" if they failed to remain calm. In their new setting they cost the state nothing and represented a source of handsome profit to others. One private nursing home business, Beverly Enterprises, opened thirty-eight board-and-care homes and raised its profits 550 percent in one year. By a happy coincidence, five of the directors of this company had been prominent in the Reagan campaign and provided financial backing to the candidate.

To be sure, Reagan was unable to fully carry out his "antipsychiatric" policy. He had planned in 1973 to close all the state mental hospitals by 1977, except for two prison hospitals. The employees whose jobs were threatened moved to protect themselves, playing up scandals that they had earlier winked at. The newspapers revealed what happened to ex-inmates after they were thrown out of the hospitals, publicized crimes committed by "dangerous" patients who had been turned away from mental hospitals or released prematurely, attacked the profits being earned in the new industry of homes for former patients, and so forth. After an investigation, the state legislature refused to allow any further hospital closings without its consent. Reagan was so attached to his "liberal" policy that he vetoed this measure, but the legislature overrode his veto—the first time in twenty-three years that had happened to a California governor. Thus in the end the Reagan policy was a failure, but not a total failure: the final resolution left thousands of ex-patients formerly classified as chronically ill outside the hospital, where they were forced to live in intolerable conditions, without hope of being readmitted.

The California example is hardly unique. Many states that pursued this sort of policy aggresively for many years have recently been forced to call a halt to a process whose effects have become intolerably scandalous. States that instituted similar policies later or that proceeded more cautiously are continuing to empty out their hospitals even though no adequate replacement has been found.

New York belongs to the former group, having pursued an aggressive policy of deinstitutionalization for many years. In 1963 the state inaugurated a program whose express purpose was to replace the state mental hospitals, huge custodial facilities located far from the cities they served (with 93,000 inmates in 1955), with more centrally located institutions offering intensive treatment. Furthermore, patients who had been committed without good reason were now supposed to be cared for in more appropriate facilities (community mental health centers for those who were more seriously ill, nursing homes for those who required only daily upkeep). The newly-modified law on confinement increased the power of doctors (hence of mental hospital superintendents) to decide when to admit or hold nonconsenting patients and to change the status of present inmates to voluntary commitment. In 1965 Governor Rockefeller announced long-range plans to construct community mental health centers (there were to be 150 in all) and modern hospital centers employing medical methods.

There was explicit awareness, however, that "if we waited for all the necessary programs to develop before discharging, nothing would happen, there'd be no felt need."[12]

Patients were therefore discharged, but still there was no "felt need." By 1972 the budget had been pruned back to allow for only 28 of the planned 150 community mental health centers (another study showed that only 17.5 percent of the clients of these centers were "seriously" ill, and only 5 percent of these were elderly) and only 2,892 of the planned 7,500 beds in modern hospitals (most of which were unable to operate in 1973 owing to a personnel shortage).

Nevertheless, the mental hospitals were emptied: in 1974 there were 39,000 residents, compared with 93,000 in 1954. As in California, the—financially speaking—most "interesting" patients wound up in one of the new boarding houses that were springing up like mushrooms all over the state. Many were located in beach resorts near New York, such as Long Beach and South Beach, a choice of site not apt to foster good relations with local residents. Some patients were bussed to Manhattan and dropped off near so-called welfare hotels. These facilities quickly filled up. Some who had been left to languish in single room occupancy hotels and others who wandered homeless through the streets besieged the psychiatric wards of municipal hospitals, such as Bellevue, begging for permission—not easily granted—to stay for a few days off and on or to be sent back to their old hospitals, just to escape the intolerable state of loneliness and abandonment in which they had been forced to live.

> "Living in a welfare hotel gets to you. The place is unbelievable. You can't even call it an existence. But the worst thing is just being alone, just being ignored completely." The person speaking was a 31-year-old unmarried man who had been discharged some months earlier from a New York State mental hospital. He went on to explain that he had admitted himself to the psychiatric unit of Bellevue Hospital four times in two months since his discharge "because I just couldn't stand not having others I could reach out to. I preferred the hospital to my SRO [Single Room Occupancy] room."[13]

Former patients had to cope with hostility as well as isolation.

In Manhattan as well as Long Beach, South Beach, and other areas, the local populace had a hard time dealing with the feelings of insecurity and the loss of property values caused by the presence of the new "ghettos" and the bizarre, unsettling mental patients, by no means a boon for the neighborhoods. Once again, the state was forced to put the brakes on its policy in the wake of newspaper stories, lawsuits, and even criminal charges brought by neighborhood organizations or municipalities such as South Beach against the responsible governmental agencies, official investigations, complaints by welfare agencies and beleaguered municipal hospitals, protests by mental hospital workers threatened with dismissal, and so on. But the patients already discharged are still living in miserable holes, seeing no one and receiving no care, exploited in one way or another by their landlords, and there is little hope of seeing more adequate facilities constructed owing to the present penury of the city and state of New York.

Other states also had scandals, though they caused less of a stir. Wisconsin, for example, amended the old statute that had governed its county mental hospitals and succeeded in reducing the inpatient population by 77 percent in 1974. It is hard to see how the state could have found lodging for the 4,300 patients discharged as a result, or helped them to readjust to social life. One Wisconsin nursing home was found guilty of 136 code violations.

The National Institute of Mental Health took over the administration of the enormous St. Elizabeth's Hospital in Washington, D.C., in 1967, with the intention of making the institution into a model for the nation. Within four years the number of inpatients had been reduced by two thousand. This result was achieved, however, at the cost of transferring six hundred patients to foster homes between June 1969 and June 1970, in spite of a report submitted to the officials in charge of such placements on August 19, 1969, by a psychiatrist and a chaplain, which stated, among other things, that

> [One] problem has been the finding of several cases of undernourishment and inadequate nutrition of foster care patients. Three patients . . . have stated that they were having to spend some of their very limited weekly allowances for food since they were not getting enough

to eat at their foster homes. Another patient . . . said that the patients in his home were receiving for lunch only a small bowl of soup, two soda crackers, and a cup of cold punch . . .

[Another] problem is the inadequate protection of the patients from violence in their community. Several incidents of assaults on foster care patients were not reported to the police or to the hospital.[14]

Most of these pseudoasylums for ex-inpatients were located in the poorest sections of the ghetto, where violence was rampant. Things were not necessarily any better, however, when more suitable surroundings were chosen. Families that had scrimped and saved to buy homes in safe, respectable neighborhoods greeted the arrival of these undesirables with something akin to racist outrage.

It is hard to give a precise idea of the circumstances of these "outcasts among outcasts," because statistics are lacking. Existing documents can give us a rough idea, however. When Grafton State Hospital (in Massachusetts) finally closed after a period during which no new patients were admitted, its last 641 chronic inpatients were discharged. Official documents trace what became of them: 283 were transferred to another state mental hospital; 131 went to nursing homes; 57 to rest homes; 23 to cooperative apartment houses; 26 to collective residences; 1 to a foster family; 1 went to the Salvation Army; 59 lived on their own; 8 moved outside the state; and 52 died.[15] Thus the largest group of those discharged consisted of patients who were merely transferred to other, similar institutions. Of the 358 patients actually discharged from the hospital system, we may ask what sort of life awaited them in the places to which they headed. That as many as 14 percent died in just twenty months says a great deal . . .

In any case, there is little in the recent trend toward deinstitutionalization that corresponds to what the official liberal and humanitarian ideology describes as the "liberation of mental patients" and the integration of former inpatients into the community. "Freedom to be sick, helpless, and isolated is not freedom. It is a return to the Middle Ages, when the mentally ill roamed the streets, and little boys threw rocks at them."[16]

A new nosographic concept has made its way into the American sociomedical vocabulary: "transfer trauma." It was first observed in chronic patients who had been transferred to "mini snake pits," as the facilities set up to receive them were dubbed. Transfer trauma refers to the intense mental suffering and serious bodily injury—serious enough in some cases to cause death—that can result when the patient finds the transfer from one institution to another unbearably difficult. Injuries result when the elderly patients become disoriented because their surrounding physical structure has changed. Many of them can take bad falls and bump into things.

It is hard to say how many ex-inmates are vegetating in private homes, rotting away in welfare hotels or slum tenements, or roaming the streets, but their number should be added to the number of patients still in hospitals before the demise of the asylum is taken for granted. It seems likely that the total would turn out to be quite close to the number of inpatients in mental hospitals before deinstitutionalization began in 1960 or so. The National Institute of Mental Health itself recognizes that the number of nursing home boarders "afflicted with mental disorders" increased from 221,721 in 1963 to 426,712 in 1969, an increase of from 28 to 50 percent of all mentally ill patients in long-term facilities. In the over-sixty-five age group, the increase is especially marked: from 187,675 to 367,586,[17] or from 53 percent to 75 percent of patients with mental disorders in that age group. An official report disclosed that in 1978 there were more chronic mental patients in Medicaid-approved nursing homes than in mental hospitals.[18]

The gravity of the situation has increased to the point where even groups that have tended to take an optimistic view of deinstitutionalization have been forced to acknowledge it. In 1974, the following recommendations were published by the American Psychiatric Association in conjunction with the American Hospital Association. In veiled terms, they amount to self-criticism of current practices by members of the profession themselves:

> While we applaud the trend toward the growing adequacy of community resources and the concurrent reduction of the patient population in public mental hospitals, we now view with considerable concern the

trend toward the phasing out of the capacity for providing long-term inpatient care and treatment for the mentally ill or disabled. . . . Our reasons for our concern include: (1) *Dehumanization.* Pressure to discharge patients from the public mental hospital too often results in discharging patients without adequate planning, which in turn results in their living in substandard and dehumanizing circumstances, be it in nursing homes, boarding homes, or the streets of a ghetto. A portion of the significantly impaired psychiatric patient population will continue to lack the capability of maintaining even a marginal adjustment to the community, in spite of vigorous therapeutic efforts. (2) *Unbalanced Programs.* If the mental health center or other mental health resource attempts to meet the demands for service for people who have been inappropriately placed in the community, it finds it has neither the funds nor the staff to do so without diverting these resources from other patients who could be helped, or otherwise restricting the other services of a mental health center. The unfortunate end result can be a change in the primary mission of mental health centers.[19]

How well bureaucratic language lends itself to the discussion of matters such as these!

LEGAL BATTLES

What we see, then, is that "antipsychiatric" politics need not be left wing and that practical criticism of the asylum system has been inspired by motives other than respect for patients' rights and concern to provide them with decent living conditions. Still, these motives were not lacking, as is shown by recent efforts to change the way American mental hospitals are organized. Humanitarian and professional criticism, whose heyday was in the fifties and early sixties, has given way in recent years to legal and political battles over the way treatment is structured. In the process, the mechanisms at work behind the therapeutic rationalizations have been laid bare and the confidence of psychiatrists in their traditional methods has been shaken. One consequence of these battles has been a reduction in the number of inpatients. There is good reason, however, to ponder the limits of this type of criticism and to reflect upon the fact that it has been used by those whose motives for attacking the system are cynically economic.

To understand how the lawsuits we are going to consider next relate to other criticisms of psychiatry, it should be borne in mind that the American left has traditionally made use of the courts in protesting the status quo. In the late nineteenth century, for example, anarchists used the tribunals that were trying them as platforms from which to denounce the power of the state, inverting the logic of jurisprudence. This tradition has persisted down to the present day: antinuclear groups, for example, have frequently chosen a legalistic strategy. Think, too, of the role played by the Supreme Court in the fight against segregation in the United States.

Until the sixties, however, the courts took a "hands off" attitude toward institutions: judges felt that institutional problems were administrative matters, properly the concern of the officials responsible for running them. The first signs of a change in this attitude were connected with the prisons. In 1961 a group of Black Muslims accused the staff of a penal institution of denying them their right to practice their religion: they claimed they were not allowed to buy the Koran, to attend services, to contact ministers of their sect, and so on. Between 1961 and 1966 prisoners won other "rights" (such as the right to receive mail, consult a physician, etc.) after going to court and challenging the principles of the law and the practices of the prison administrations. Finally, in 1970, prisoners won a more far-reaching victory: a judge ruled that the way prisons were organized violated the Eighth Amendment, which forbids "cruel and unusual punishment."[20]

The legal procedure involved in this case was what is known as a class action suit. Such a suit is not brought by an individual claiming compensation for damages done to him personally. Rather, it is brought in behalf of a group of indeterminate size whose members all share a common situation. Such suits can thus be used to popularize a cause and win recognition of collective rights. In this way the class action suit is used as a political weapon. Many such suits have been brought or sponsored by activist groups: consumer movements (Nader's Raiders, for example), legal assistance collectives that grew up under the War on Poverty, and groups of liberal and radical young lawyers, such as those who fought for civil rights. Taking a case to court is a way of bringing isolated individuals together and of uniting the oppressed by raising their consciousness as to the situation they collectively share, paving the way for a counterattack. Taking the law at its word, protesters have turned the legalistic mentality that is so deeply rooted in American life against the law itself, broadening its scope and drawing out concrete consequences unforeseen by the lawmakers. These procedures were used to attack, in addition to prison-related problems, the way public services were provided, inequities in the schools, welfare cases, federal aid to private hospitals that failed to provide certain free services in return, and so forth.

The mental hospitals were among the last institutions to be challenged in this wave of lawsuits. No doubt they were protected by the mystique of medical knowledge and by the image of the mental patient as a person unable to think or act independently and therefore to be deprived of all rights. In 1966, however, two cases in the courts cast doubt on this hitherto protective ideology. The first (*Baxstrom* v. *Herald*) involved a prison inmate who had been involuntarily committed to a forensic ward. The Supreme Court declared this commitment illegal, since it had not been ordered by any civil court of competent jurisdiction. As a result of this decision, 992 inmates of the same prison hospital were transferred to ordinary hospitals.[21]

The second case also involved a person judged criminally insane, who, after four years' hospitalization (four times the maximum sentence he could have received for possession of a weapon), requested release on the grounds that, being in a hospital, he ought to have been treated and cured during this time. The judge, in delivering his opinion, enunciated the principle of a "right to treatment":

> The purpose of involuntary hospitalization is treatment, not punishment . . . the provision of commitment rests upon the supposed necessity for treatment of the mental condition . . . Absent treatment, the hospital is transformed into a penitentiary.[22]

This latter case was particularly significant because the institution found to be at fault was St. Elizabeth's hospital in Washington, D.C., which was under federal control and claimed to offer the most modern methods of treatment, such as group and milieu therapy. Accordingly, the American Psychiatric Association reacted strongly:

> Mental hospital administrations may vary in quality as do all human institutions. It is one thing, however, for outside community agencies to render constructive criticisms of the relative adequacy of a psychiatric facility and quite another for it to interpose its judgment on the professional managerial affairs of that facility.[23]

Clearly, the profession's monopoly of psychiatric questions was at stake. Were medically-trained personnel to have supreme authority over all aspects of institutional life, provided they met "scientific" standards of correct and proper treatment? More generally, could a nonmedical authority properly contradict a psychiatrist's expert judgment? The issue was stated by the judge trying the case in a way we find it difficult to improve on:

> Diffidence in the face of scientific expertise is conduct unbecoming a court. Very few judges are psychiatrists. But equally few are economists, aeronautical engineers, atomic scientists, or marine biologists. For some reason, however, many people seem to accept judicial scrutiny of, say, the effect of a proposed dam on fish life, while they reject a similar scrutiny on the effect of psychiatric treatment on human lives. It can hardly be said that we are more concerned for the salmon than [for] the schizophrenic.[24]

It is significant that in the two cases just discussed, the courts intervened in actions involving patients who had committed a crime, and who therefore could be regarded as falling within their purview. But in Alabama in 1970 a trial began (*Wyatt* v. *Stickney*) which is significant because it broadened the issues involved in legal challenges to mental institutions to regular mental hospitals and to the treatment of regular (i.e., noncriminal) patients. A state mental hospital was accused of maintaining conditions so deplorable as to preclude all possibility of treatment. In 1971 the case was broadened to include nearby mental hospitals and an institution for the mentally retarded. In other words, the whole system of state mental institutions in Alabama was brought under attack. Such national organizations as the Mental Health Law Project and the American Civil Liberties Union joined the plaintiffs, in attacking the living conditions in these institutions: racial segregation, overcrowding, understaffing, deplorable hygiene and food, brutality, etc.[25]

The court found that the main points of the accusation were justified: "To deprive any citizen of his or her liberty upon the altruistic theory that the confinement is for humane therapeutic reasons and then fail to provide adequate treatment violates the very fundamentals of due process."[26] The judge specified three conditions necessary for effective treatment: psychologically and physically humane surroundings, an adequate number of trained personnel, and a program of treatment tailored especially to each individual case. The court listed seventy-two standards to be met by an institution wishing to be regarded as therapeutic and named a special Human Rights Commission made up mainly of nonspecialists to oversee the implementation of the new standards.

In many respects this is an exemplary case. In the first place it ended the secrecy that had shrouded institutional practices in the name of therapeutic necessity. Personages from both within the institution and outside it took part in the legal arguments. This explains how it came to pass that George Wallace, well known for his segregationist politics, defended the confinement of patients—by citing none other than Erving Goffman: "The primary function of civil commitment is to relieve the burden imposed upon the families and friends of the mentally disabled . . . [who] are the 'true clients' of the institutionalization system."[27] The hospital staff defended its position and its professional independence. Most important, however, as one hospital director observed, was the fact that

one of the unintended consequences of the court order has been the disruption of the hospital's administrative channels by legitimating the use of outside pressure groups, such as the media, state legislators, and the human rights committee, to influence administrative decision-making.[28]

This case has had profound effects on the way mental hospitals are run. Patients' living conditions were made more humane, more and better qualified personnel were hired, the daily cost of hospitalization doubled, and the budget of the Alabama Health Department tripled. The number of inpatients decreased from 6,912 to 2,672 between October 1970 and October 1975, owing both to a more aggressive discharge policy and to greater strictness in admissions procedures. Many states passed new laws regarding mental patients, including clauses inspired by the standards laid down in the Wyatt case: patients were given the right to keep their own clothes, to control the spending of their own money, to refuse certain kinds of treatment, etc.[29] Undeniably positive though these changes were, they helped to perpetuate the closed institution. One Community Mental Health Center director pointed out that the decision in the case led to the bulk of Alabama's mental health budget being devoted to large traditional institutions, at the expense of community services.[30] There is also reason to wonder what fate actually lay in store for the 4,200 Alabama patients who were deinstitutionalized over a five-year period. The court made no rulings in this regard, confining its decision to specifying what constitutes genuine treatment and how it should be carried out within the institution.

But what can "genuine treatment" mean in such an institutional setting? Essentially, the point was to rationalize the institutional management of patients. One term that recurred frequently in arguments in court was "normalization." The meaning given this word is somewhat curious: for example, to keep the doors of the wards closed was declared to be "antithetical to principles of normalization."[31] In short, the goal was to "clean up" the total institution and make it over into a facility that could be run efficiently without violating the Constitutional rights of patients. The patients in these new asepticized mental hospitals were to be treated in such a way as to eliminate the most glaring differences between these and "normal" institutions. The patient was to live as "normally" as possible, though "normal" life was still not allowed to intrude upon the life of the institution. The new methods harked back to the old "moral treatment," in that they required behavior consistent with the norms of society.

Other cases led to similar outcomes. In 1973, for example, an institution for the mentally retarded was required to pay retroactive wages to residents who had been made to work without pay.[32] In many states this decision set a precedent, and in 1975 the Labor Department established a salary scale for residents working in and for mental institutions. But the same court decision that recognized the economic value of the labor also recognized its therapeutic value. All labor, whether done inside or outside the institution, was deemed therapeutic in the sense that "arguably, assignments which constitute therapy or vocational training for a patient serve the compelling purpose for which most patients were originally committed."[33]

Third, even though the courts and outside pressure groups effectively challenged the medical monopoly over the setting of treatment standards, this challenge was not as radical as it first seemed. It is significant that, after trying to resist outside interference, the American Psychiatric Association lent its support to the concept of a "right to treatment," recognizing how much it stood to gain from legal sanction for the notion of compulsory care:

> Despite the many problems it is clear for reasons of both prudence and morality that psychiatrists must try to seize the initiative in right to treatment litigation. Psychiatrists should try to lead the mental health professions in shaping the power of the court so that decrees suit the needs of patients. This can be done only by participating in litigation, learning from past mistakes, and formulating standards that are workable and realistic.[34]

Accordingly, it was not long before the American Psychiatric Association went so far as to become party to a suit against one of its own members in a case involving St. Elizabeth's Hospital.[35] Even more important, the normalization of psychiatric practices could serve as a means to normalize patients' attitudes toward psychiatry. A well-known psychiatrist argued that implicit in the recognition of patients' rights was a definition of patients' duties which, in keeping with the inherent logic of psychiatry, consisted essentially in submission to medical authority both for their own sake and for the sake of the institution:

> Perhaps the list of responsibilities of patients should include that they cooperate in treatment, that they do not lie in bed all day if they are physically able to get up, that they do not attack other patients or staff, and they do not destroy property.[36]

There are of course other lessons to be learned from the study of litigation besides those we have chosen to focus on here (see chapter 7). Still, when we consider the question of whether mental hospitals were on the way out or holding their own, two tentative conclusions do already begin to emerge.

First, although pressures stemming from litigation did contribute to some extent to deinstitutionalization, reformers seem to have been no better at controlling the consequences of their efforts than were those with more cynical economic motivations. Administrators tried to hold down rising costs by getting rid of many patients (in Alabama the number dropped by 4,200, or nearly two-thirds, in five years). Since all the criticisms and reforms were directed at the hospitals, the fate of the "liberated" patients was again left to improvisation.

More important, perhaps, the institutional reforms made necessary by these court challenges to the status quo did contribute to the modernization of mental hospitals. People had been saying for twenty years that asylums were obsolete, being irrational and nontherapeutic, not to say antitherapeutic, institutions. The unspoken assumption underlying much of the litigation was that total institutions could be reformed so as to provide genuine treatment, if only the necessary means were made available. Henceforth stress was placed on training of the staff and "normalization" of the institution. If the institution could be made to answer to the patient's right to treatment, its existence would be justified. In other words, the mental hospital emerged from these battles modernized and rationalized, thus in a sense stronger than it had been.

This conclusion is different from, but complementary to, the conclusion we drew earlier from our examination of the decrease in the number of patients for economic reasons. We saw then that the number of patients did not decrease because mental hospitals had been supplanted by new treatment facilities. Now we see too that current efforts to refurbish the mental health system in the United States invariably involve shaping and reshaping the total institution of old. Rather than lament its demise, we would do better to analyze how and why it has managed to go on living.

MODERNIZATION

Two equally illusory images of American mental hospitals are widespread, and few people even notice that the two are contradictory: sometimes the mental hospital is said to be in its death throes, merely hanging on until the last chronic patients have died off and the new psychiatry has been fully developed; while at other times it is claimed that the elimination of overcrowding and the improvement of services made possible by the criticism of humanitarians and professionals, court battles, and new techniques have transformed the hospital into a real treatment center where specialized care can be offered. In fact, even with a reduced number of inpatients, the state hospitals continue to play a role in the system, but patient care is not their only activity.

Quantitatively, the state hospitals are still the most important resource for inpatient care of mental illness: in 1974 two-thirds of the beds available for psychiatric patients were in state mental hospitals.[37] State hospitals also lead in the number of cases treated, accounting for more than a third of all cases treated in hospital (see figure 4.3). The state hospitals employ more than half of all mental health workers and 61 percent of the hospital staff,[38] and they consume more than a third of the mental health budget and more than half the hospital budget.[39] Accordingly, we may ask what functions these hospitals are performing today that might explain their longevity. In what respects are they irreplaceable?

One major role of the state mental hospitals, now as always,

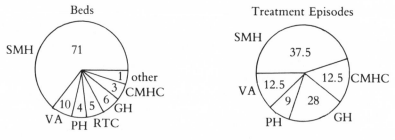

Figure 4.3: Percent of hospital beds and number of treatment episodes during the year 1973.

ABBREVIATIONS: SMH, State Mental Hospitals; VA, Veterans Administration Hospitals; PH, Private Hospitals; GH, General Hospitals; CMHC, Community Mental Health Centers; (Residential Treatment Centers are included in the private hospitals).

SOURCE: Based on National Institute of Mental Health Statistical Note no. 127, February 1976.

is custodial. More than three-quarters of the beds are still taken up by patients institutionalized for periods longer than a year—more than half have been confined for more than five years, and nearly a third for more than twenty years. The vast majority of these chronic patients are people who really could not be placed elsewhere when the hospitals were emptied.

A rough profile of the typical patient runs as follows: a man or woman over fifty years of age, single, widowed, or divorced, hospitalized for upwards of five years, of low socioeconomic status, without assets, not entitled to enough social benefits to attract the interest of private profit-making institutions (or else too disturbed to be accommodated in a private hospital), originally diagnosed as schizophrenic (which means little, given the widespread debasement of the notion of schizophrenia in the United States), maladjusted in the past and now passively dependent on the institution, having lost all contact with the outside world and all hope of returning to normal life.

The number of chronic patients has tended to decrease as patients die off and efforts are made to send as many elderly residents as possible to the less costly nursing homes. This tendency has been counteracted in part by the fact that 10 percent of incoming patients are not released within a year of their admission, becoming chronic residents of the institution just as before, though now their number is fewer. Whether kept in underequipped open wards or dispersed, as three-quarters of the patients are, in individual houses, these "old" patients, the dregs of the institution, make the state mental hospital system as a whole smack of the asylum.

Today, however, the state hospitals must play other roles as well, and we find in them a new patient population, not admitted in the same way as ten or twenty years ago and differing from the earlier population in their psychiatric history and in many other respects. Only the socioeconomic background of today's hospital users remains comparable to what it was a decade or two earlier: the state mental hospitals are for the most part reserved for the underprivileged. But the age and sex of the average patient and the most common reasons for hospitalization (as indicated in a crude way in diagnostic reports) have changed. Looking only at patients entering a mental hospital for the first time (of whom there are around 130,000 each year, a figure that has not changed much over the years), we find: far fewer elderly people, many of them being sent to nursing homes and other similar institutions for reasons of economy; far more young people (under twenty-five years of age)—three times as many in 1972 as in 1955, as measured both in absolute terms and as a percentage of all first admissions; twice as many men as women (compared with a ratio of 125 men to every 100 women in 1955), and, in the under-fifteen age group, seven times as many boys as girls; fewer cases of organic brain syndromes (the senile, in particular, are placed elsewhere) as well as fewer instances of "schizophrenia" and "other psychoses" (the latter perhaps benefitting from new outpatient facilities); but far more alcoholics, drug addicts (six times as many in 1972 as in 1955), "psychopathic personalities," depressives, mentally retarded, and cases of childhood and adolescent pathology. The majority of the cases in each of these categories except the depressives consists of men and adolescents.[40]

The total number of admissions has more than doubled since 1955 (376,000 in 1975 compared with 178,000 in 1955), the difference being accounted for by readmissions, which in 1975 made up 65 percent of all incoming patients. This is a recent development: in 1956 readmissions accounted for only 27 percent of the intake, and in 1966 for only 35 percent. All the talk about deinstitutionalization has tended to conceal its equally noteworthy counterpart, reinstitutionalization. While far more patients are now released from mental hospitals, far more enter and, above all, far more enter more than once. Similarly, while much is made of the decrease in the average term of commitment (from 211 days in 1955 to 38 days in 1974),[41] something should also be said about the many patients who enter the hospital several times a year, in each case for only a short period.

What do these figures tell us about the new patient population? There are three main points to notice.

First, there is the now well-known phenomenon of "revolving-door patients," who are quickly released from the hospital and sent back to face the hardships of the outside world, with no real place to go, no resources, no work, no care or supervision to speak of, and who immediately try to get back into the hospital, which promises greater security than the streets, the welfare hotels, or the prisons. These patients are among the victims of the hasty evacuation of the state mental hospitals and account for a sizeable portion of the 65 percent readmission rate.

The second point worthy of note is that the state mental hospitals have increasingly come to be seen as treatment centers for social deviants and misfits categorized as dangerous even though they do not fall under any recognized disease type. Usually they are labeled alcoholics, drug addicts, or psychopathic personalities. Some commit themselves voluntarily, seeking temporary refuge from a hostile world.[42] They are usually kept a short while in a wing of a regular ward. Others are involuntarily committed (in some cases after more or less deliberately trying to appear more threatening then usual, so as to gain admission to the hospital and be committed for a lengthy term), and are housed in admissions wings where violence and fear lurk constantly just below the surface, as the never-empty isolation cells attest. A not inconsiderable minority are admitted after committing a crime of some sort: the patient may be judged "not guilty by reason of insanity," or "incompetent to stand trial"—in the latter case he remains under indictment but trial is delayed for observation or treatment of the patient, sometimes for longer than the statutory punishment for the crime he is supposed to have committed. In 1972 placements of this type accounted for 1.2 percent of all admissions of whites but for 6.9 percent of admissions of nonwhites, which says a great deal about the function of the mental hospital at present.[43] Finally, some prison inmates serving time for criminal convictions are transferred from the prisons to the state mental hospitals for psychiatric treatment. Many of these patients, along with others not convicted of any crime but deemed too violent and dangerous for treatment in a regular ward, are confined to forensic hospitals or high security wards, the relative importance of which has been growing steadily. These special wards are particularly badly equipped, which leads one to believe that the method chosen to neutralize these supposedly dangerous patients is not intensive care: in a sample of sixteen such special hospitals, we find an average of only 52 staff, 14 of them professionals, per 100 patients.[44]

The third new development is a considerable increase (150 percent in ten years) in the number of young children and adolescents entering mental hospitals, while the number of adults has been on the decline. If hospitalization is deemed appropriate only for children suffering from major mental disorders, then even by the standards of medical ideology more and more children and adolescents are now being placed in hospitals who should not be there: of 26,000 children admitted in 1973, 3,000 were identified as retarded (and in the United States the retarded are supposed to be treated in special institutions), and 15,000 were classified as suffering from "personality disorders," "adaptation reactions," and "behavioral problems."[45] In chapter six we shall see what these diagnoses really signify when we come to examine other institutions for children: problems in adapting to the values of the family, school, and society having little to do with pathology, psychiatry being used to camouflage the way these problems are actually being handled.

Children who are institutionalized face conditions that vary widely from one hospital to the next. The twenty state mental hospitals devoted exclusively to children, which provide facilities for 20 percent of those hospitalized among the under-eighteen age group, have the best staff–patient ratios of any hospital: 174 staff, 94 of them professionals, per 100 patients in 1974.[46]

Other young patients are distributed among special wards of regular mental hospitals, which offer very disparate services. Even within a single hospital (Creedmore, for example, outside New York City), it is possible to visit a spanking new ward equipped with a luxurious swimming pool and game rooms and practicing the latest in therapeutic techniques, while right next to it the most difficult and unwanted children are locked in an old-fashioned, prisonlike section of the hospital.

As this last example makes clear, it is impossible to give an exhaustive description of the methods and therapies used in the mental hospitals because of the disparity between one hospital and another. We shall therefore confine ourselves to making a few general remarks, based both on personal observation and on the recent literature.

To begin with, given the continued presence of a large contingent of chronic patients, the tradition of the asylum, with its own institutional life and "secondary adjustments," is being perpetuated.[47] Many wards are now as backward and underequipped as ever, and hardly less overcrowded. For reasons of economy many wards have been closed, so that the remaining patients have scarcely any more room than they had before. Accordingly, in some of these chronic wards we find scenes worthy of any nineteenth-century asylum. Some patients sit impassively in filthy rooms with hardly any furniture; others circulate aimlessly, assail visitors for cigarettes, or ask them to leave. On one side of the room some patients join in a heartrending celebration with cookies for refreshment and a few records to listen to, while on the other side an attendant tries desperately to involve a group of elderly patients in a ridiculous game of catch. Still other patients watch television without really seeing it (the fact that there are no fights over which of the twelve channels to watch attests to this). The clocks do not tell the right time, and the newspapers and magazines

lying about are several months old. Everywhere there is empti-
ness, lifelessness, timelessness, utter isolation in promiscuity, and
not the least iota of comfort or care.

The overall staffing of the state mental hospitals is far from
adequate (57 staff, 18 of them professionals, per 100 patients in
1974), but matters are even worse in the chronic wards, which
are rarely visited by the professionals. Because of the personnel
shortage,[48] not only is there no question of treatment, but jobs
must inevitably be shared between patients and staff, leading to
all the usual abuses of power, conflicts of authority, rancor, manipulation, and overt or covert brutality generally associated with
such situations. Consider testimony given recently during the
Wyatt trial at Bryce Hospital in Tuscaloosa, Alabama. All the
witnesses agreed that physical conditions in the hospital were deplorable, and one reported that

> four residents died due to understaffing, lack of supervision, and bru-
> tality. One had a garden hose inserted in his rectum for five minutes
> by a working inmate who was cleaning him; one died when a fellow
> inmate hosed him with scalding water; another died when soapy water
> was forced into his mouth; and the last died by a self-administered
> overdose of drugs which had been inadequately secured.[49]

The use of more "modern," more "medical" methods, however, has almost everywhere begun to chip away at the remnants
of asylum-style practices—all the more so where acute rather than
chronic patients are involved. For one thing, there is liberal use
of medication. Neuroleptics are administered in massive doses,
stronger than in France, though "drug cocktails" are avoided: a
common dosage is 800 mg. of chlorpromazine, administered
without any other drug (except to correct for side effects). Depot
injections of neuroleptics, antidepressants, and antianxiety drugs
are used in much the same way as elsewhere. By contrast, two
products have been in vogue longer and are prescribed for a wider
variety of symptoms than in Europe: lithium is used to treat
manic-depressive psychoses and prevent crises, as well as to calm
aggressive children and adolescents and to treat any manifestation
of depression or agitation, even in cases where the symptoms do

not fit the manic–depressive pattern; and amphetamines are used to balance children who are hyperactive or suffering from a "minimal brain dysfunction," a nosological category that is bizarre yet very much in vogue, since it ascribes an ostensible organic etiology to troublesome infantile behavior (see chapter 6).[50]

There seems to be little evidence of systematic doubt as to the wisdom of administering heavy medication, nor is there much criticism of the use of "chemical straitjackets" or of drugs for the treatment of symptoms in such a way as to mask the real problems of the disease. On the other hand, there is evidence, in recent years at any rate, of extreme caution with regard to experimentation on human subjects in the hospitals, because of widespread fear of provoking another scandal comparable to the one that surrounded the revelation of the use of prisoner "volunteers" as experimental guinea pigs. Drug experiments are strictly regulated: they are carried out by investigators who work for research laboratories not tied to the hospital in which the research is done or to the manufacturer of the drug, either administratively or financially. Only patients who have given their consent and received the approval of their families are used as experimental subjects. The doctors and staff treating the patients collaborate in the experiments, though more as subjects than investigators, not really taking an active role.

Shock therapy, including both electroconvulsive and insulin treatments, and psychosurgery, ranging from the most rudimentary kinds of lobotomy to the most refined stereotaxic methods are represented among the "medical" forms of treatment, along with chemotherapy. Statistics on the use of these methods are not particularly illuminating, and it is hard to know exactly how widely they are practiced today. Litigation and other actions by former mental patients (see chapter 7) have made doctors more cautious about resorting to these techniques. Psychosurgery in particular has been the target of vigorous attacks. An estimated forty thousand prefrontal lobotomies have been performed in the United States since the Second World War, most of them in the decade between 1946 and 1955. In the wake of a press campaign and a series of lawsuits, the average number of such operations performed each year dropped to around 400 in the early seventies. It is worth remarking, however, that an official commission has recently recognized that lobotomies may be justified in some cases, even on patients unable to give their consent, provided that legal protections are enforced.[51]

At the other end of the therapeutic spectrum, psychoanalysis and analytically-inspired psychotherapies are the oldest and most systematic "psychological" forms of treatment. In spite of proposals to "democratize" psychoanalysis made as early as 1914 by William A. White (see chapter 2), this form of treatment has played almost no role in state mental hospitals for reasons that are obvious: uneducated patients and inadequately trained personnel. Nevertheless, owing to the great influence of analytic ideas in the postwar era and to the importance of psychoanalytic training or retraining in the preparation of many hospital personnel, the psychotherapeutic model served as a standard of reference until the mid-fifties. Thus directly or indirectly, psychoanalysis inspired a whole range of human relations technologies which, roughly speaking, might be called "institutional psychotherapy": group and milieu therapies, music therapy, dance therapy, game therapy, psychodrama, and so forth. The degree to which such techniques were used depended on how willing a particular institution was to experiment with new methods. Even when they were used extensively, it is hard to say whether or not conditions in the hospital were really altered very much.

Forward-looking members of the medical professions have lately shifted their hopes to a new set of methods, known collectively as "behavior modification" techniques. Based on the theories of conditioning (Pavlov) and behaviorism (Thorndike and Watson), these methods are aimed at extinguishing pathological behaviors and reinforcing desired behaviors. Gone is the ambition to treat the patient's personality as a whole; instead, the aim is to control his symptoms by the time-honored technique of administering rewards and punishments, in their modern guise according to a strict, scientifically conceived plan. Behavior modification is undoubtedly one of the most widespread and comprehensive forms of treatment in use in the United States today (see chapter

8); a closed institution such as a mental hospital is ideally suited to its application. Indeed, since the hospital staff can fully control the environment, behavior modification techniques provide a simple and, we are told, effective means of "normalizing" both the life of the institution and the behavior of its inmates.

To describe one of many similar scenes: in the day room of a chronic ward, ten or eleven patients are sitting at a table playing cards with two staff members. An old man with a vacant look lets the cards go by him. When the hand is over, a psychologist passes around a tray of cookies. But he does not serve those who did not play. The old man's gaze suddenly comes to life—does he feel pain, rebelliousness, or does he simply fail to understand? The next time, perhaps, he will play cards or sweep the floor, and then he will receive his reward.

The systematic application of such techniques is called a therapeutic program. Some wards keep a chart on each patient, ruled in three columns. The first lists the symptoms to be attacked; the second records the patient's likes (watching TV, smoking cigarettes, eating candy, walking on the grounds) and dislikes (cleanup duties, baths, etc.); the third indicates in step-by-step detail the program to be followed in reinforcing desired behavior and eliminating undesired behavior using the items in column two to attack the symptoms in column one: each time the patient manifests a symptom, the fact is noted and a suitable reward or punishment is meted out, in accordance with the subject's likes and dislikes. A more subtle version of the same technique uses tokens to mediate between the patient's behavior and the consequences of that behavior. The patient wins or loses tokens for each desired or undesired act recorded by the staff. For example, sweeping the day room or "discussing one's problems in a constructive way" wins the patient three tokens; he loses two if he sleeps late or complains about the staff's work. The patient can then use the capital he has accumulated in tokens to buy certain privileges. Such is his freedom.

According to the proponents of these techniques, whose faith in what they are doing is unbounded, behavior modification methods have the advantage of being individualized, simple, effective, and easy to use, even by relatively unskilled staff. With their widespread use we may see the realization of the old dream that underlay "moral treatment" in the nineteenth century: that is, the dream of manipulating even minute details of the subject's behavior in keeping with the manner in which the staff wishes the institution to be run. The assumption is that what is good for the staff and the hospital is also good for the patient, for if he has been a good patient he will leave the hospital as a well-adjusted member of society. This, then, constitutes the ideal of a truly therapeutic— as well as a truly "total"—institution. Unfortunately for today's technocrats, this pitch of perfection has not yet been reached, except in a few wards where the methods are particularly advanced. Practice in many mental hospitals is as eclectic as ever— drugs, electroconvulsive treatment, and psychotherapy are combined with socializing activities and authoritarian behavior modification. This eclecticism serves as a clumsy rationalization and incomplete camouflage for the same old functions: segregation, normalization, and control of the patient population. In some respects, however, mental institutions have been rationalized, modernized, and streamlined. To achieve these ends, they have had to adopt even more brutal methods—ruthlessly expelling some patients who had once found a pitiful refuge in the hospitals and adopting new techniques, techniques that shook up the old institutions but reduced the patients to playthings in the hands of progressive planners.

THE MANAGEMENT OF THE EXCLUDED

While the state mental hospitals are still the most important providers of inpatient care for certain segments of the patient population, they are merely one element in a system in which each type of treatment facility has a place, a specific function, a clientele, a method of intervention, and a history of its own. Figure 4.4, which covers patients institutionalized over a period of nearly thirty years, shows in a rough way how the relative importance of the main institutional elements in the mental health care system has changed over time.

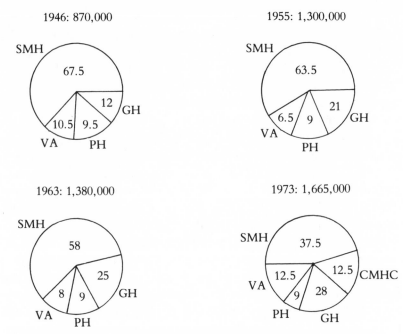

Figure 4.4: Hospital treatment incidents by type of institution. (Number of incidents equals number of patients present on January 1 plus number of admissions during the year.)

ABBREVIATIONS: SMH, State Mental Hospitals; VA, Veterans Administration Hospitals; PH, Private Hospitals; GH, General Hospitals; CMHC, Community Mental Health Centers.

SOURCE: Morton Kramer, "Historical Tables on Changes in Patterns of Use of Psychiatric Facilities 1946-1971," Biometry Branch, O.P.P.E., National Institute of Mental Health, October 1973; and National Institute of Mental Health Statistical Note no. 127, February 1976.

A recent comparative study has focused on the number of staff employed in each type of institution and, among the staff, the number of professionals. The results, reproduced in table 4.1, give a rough indication of the potential of each institution for providing treatment.

MENTAL HOSPITALS RUN BY THE VETERANS' ADMINISTRATION

In 1974 veterans could call upon 40,000 beds distributed among 113 different institutions, 27 of which were devoted exclusively to neuropsychiatric cases, while the other 86 were psychiatric wards within general hospitals. Along with St. Elizabeth's Hospital in Washington, D.C., these are the only mental hospital facilities financed entirely by federal funds. Because of the high proportion of chronic patients, the atmosphere in these places is close to that of the state mental hospitals, except for certain specific characteristics: the residents are all male, the facilities are located nearer large cities, and patients receive slightly more attention because the shortage of personnel before and especially during World War II was so scandalous, and the need for services had increased so much, that earlier and greater efforts were made (beginning in 1946) to expand the size of VA hospital staffs.[52] The demographic profile of the inpatient population in these facilities (see figure 4.4) reflects the changing situation, ranging from World War II and its aftereffects to Vietnam.

PUBLIC INSTITUTIONS FOR THE MENTALLY RETARDED

In 1976, 237 public institutions still sheltered 155,000 retarded adults of all ages, in facilities ranging in capacity from 10 to 3,000

Table 4.1 **Staff-patient ratio (in full-time equivalent) per 100 average resident patients in selected mental health inpatient facilities, January 1974.**

Type of Institution	Total Staff	Professionals
Psychiatric Units of Public General Hospitals	148.8	81.7
Private Not-for-Profit Mental Hospitals	139.8	78.8
Psychiatric Units of Nonpublic General Hospitals	114.9	64.8
Private For-Profit Mental Hospitals	110.2	54.4
Residential Treatment Centers for Emotionally Disturbed Children	77.2	49.7
Veterans Administration Psychiatric Services	67.1	33.4
State and County Mental Hospitals	57.1	18.1
Public Residential Services for the Mentally Retarded	67.0	12.0

SOURCE: Based on National Institute of Mental Health Statistical Note no. 129, May 1976, and R. C. Scheerenberger, "Public Residential Services for the Mental-Retarded" (Ph.D. diss., University of Wisconsin, Madison, 1976).

beds and providing the necessary minimum of qualified staff. A legacy of the time when the aim was to neutralize "oligophrenics" at the lowest possible cost, these facilities still serve mainly as custodial repositories for the most severely handicapped, notwithstanding the great improvements that have been made.

It is true that the 135 institutions in existence in 1965 have slightly reduced their average number of beds (from 1,185 to 1,037), and still more their average number of inpatients (to 732 in 1976), while 102 new facilities have opened their doors since 1965, with an average capacity of only 260 beds. More and more of these institutions are attempting to involve families and reintegrate their patients into society, mainly using behavior modification techniques, which have gradually been replacing the older work therapy.[53] Frequently, though, these places are like enormous warehouses, and living conditions are dehumanizing and depersonalizing. In 1973 suit was brought against one such institution, and the case (*Souder* v. *Brennan*) was to have a decisive impact on the future of patient labor in mental institutions. The scandal erupted over the case of a patient who worked sixty-six hours per week in the kitchen for wages of two dollars a month. A 1972 study was then produced showing that one-fifth of all patients in similar facilities worked under such conditions. The hospital was found guilty under the provisions of the Thirteenth Amendment, which prohibits slavery and peonage. In theory, this decision made it compulsory for all mental institutions to pay inmates for any useful labor they might perform, under the supervision of the Department of Labor.

Whether conditions in some facilities actually improved, however, is doubtful. In 1975, another suit was brought on behalf of 5,000 patients in the Willowbrook Development Center, the largest institution of its kind, located in New York state. The District Court found that because of "overcrowding and inadequate staffing at Willowbrook, conditions are . . . inhumane . . . [Testimony of parents] showed failure to protect the physical safety of their children and deterioration rather than improvement after they were placed in Willowbrook School."[54]

RESIDENTIAL TREATMENT CENTERS FOR EMOTIONALLY DISTURBED CHILDREN

In 1966 there were 149 centers serving fewer than ten thousand children. By 1974, 340 centers were "treating" approximately thirty thousand children (eighteen thousand already present and twelve thousand new admissions).[55] Given that these institutions are private and have only 10 percent of their beds vacant, that most youngsters are admitted directly upon request of their families with no preliminary psychiatric examination, and that the facilities are poorly staffed (see table 4.1, and compare the figures with those for state childrens' hospitals), it is clear that here we witness the emergence of yet another industry turning a profit on the general problems and contradictions associated with childhood and adolescence in American society.[56]

PRIVATE MENTAL HOSPITALS

Of the 180 private mental hospitals surveyed in 1975, nearly two-thirds were operated for profit. There were 35 for-profit hospitals opened between 1968 and 1975, while 6 nonprofit hospitals closed their doors. Thus we are looking at yet another growth industry, which saw the number of patients admitted increase by more than a third, and the number of residents rise by 10 percent in seven years. In 1975, 120,000 patients were treated in private hospitals, and 11,500 were resident inpatients.[57] Until 1965 most private hospitals were reserved for patients sufficiently well off to afford private insurance. Since the passage of the Medicare Act providing coverage for the elderly, however, the patient population has gradually been changing, expanding to include less fortunate strata of society. Still, many of these institutions depend for their survival and profit wholly on reimbursement through insurance, and few clients are financially able to bear the cost of a hospital stay longer than that covered by their policy, generally twenty-one days for Blue Cross, the most common type of insurance, and two months for Medicare.

As a result, treatments are chosen that provide rapid improvement in the patient's symptoms. At Gracie Square Hospital in New York, for example, a highly skilled team administers various kinds of shock treatments all day long, one after another: with or without anesthetics, with bilateral or unilateral treatment electrode placement, and even chemically induced (by inhalation of flurothyl). The staff justified this inundation of shock therapy by arguing that the terms of insurance policies made recourse to such methods inevitable. Psychotherapy is out of the question when insurance payments provide for only a few weeks' treatment. Only rarely will the insurance company doctor authorize an extension of the treatment period.

Some private hospitals have generally been able to avoid the constraints imposed by the insurance companies. These hospitals service clients wealthy enough to afford long stays, are financed by religious and charitable foundations, have advantageous arrangements with governmental authorities, or enjoy certain advantages thanks to the prestige of their founders, such as more "interesting" patients to choose from, the ability to impose a lengthy therapeutic regimen, and the services of highly skilled personnel who are eager to work in such prestigious institutions. This group includes such famous institutions as McLean's (Boston), Menninger (Topeka), Chestnut Lodge (Washington), and Hillside (New York). These hospitals and others like them have been in the forefront of experimentation and innovation, particularly in adapting psychoanalysis to institutional use. In recent years, however, they have tended to become more and more similar to run-of-the-mill private hospitals. For example, Hillside Hospital, originally financed by a Jewish foundation, entered into an agreement with the city of New York under which the city financed virtually unlimited stays for some residents. When this city coverage was subsequently reduced to cover only two or three months, however, the hospital was forced to change its procedures. As a result, it tended to draw more and more of its clientele from a limited area centered on the nearby community, and this tendency was reinforced by the fact that the hospital received federal funds for serving as a community mental health center. Hillside seems to have had surprisingly little difficulty adapting to its new role. Some of the same personnel who, ten years ago, were administering classic psychoanalytic treatment are today developing behavior modification programs. Business is business.

Thus even in the best hospitals, it is the question of financing that determines the therapeutic orientation. This is of course even more true of less prestigious institutions. The clients of private hospitals, who are not as poor as the clients of state hospitals, enjoy somewhat greater comfort, but the sort of treatment they receive is chosen in light of its dollar return.

PSYCHIATRIC WARDS OF GENERAL HOSPITALS

General hospital psychiatric wards all share certain characteristics, regardless of whether the hospitals are public or private (in this respect the U.S. and France are markedly different) or associated with a city or state government, a university, a charitable organization, or the like. Although they have relatively few beds (24,500 in 1974), they are serving more and more clients as a result of increasingly rapid turnover. Nearly a third of all institutionalized cases are treated in such wards, accounting for almost half a million patients each year. The financing is often better than for other hospital facilities, particularly where there are university ties. University-associated hospitals claim the bulk of the considerable amount of money allocated to research by such federal agencies as the National Institute of Mental Health, the Department of Defense, and others. The most prestigious general hospitals can only be described as "health empires" (see chapter 3), whose primary concern is to promote their own growth and to outstrip rival institutions. They are overstaffed with highly qualified personnel. Because capacity is low, and "interesting" patients are needed for teaching and research, these cases are skimmed off the top of applicants for admission. In addition, the general hospitals enjoy the prestige and benefits of being part of the university medical establishment. They were quick to welcome psychoanalysis and to set up interdisciplinary research teams, and since the turn of the century have been experimenting with new institutional structures including outpatient consultation and ambulatory care (see chapter 2). American general hospitals are therefore less rigidly wedded to psychosomatic and neurophysiological theories of mental disorders than are their European counterparts. In years past, while state mental hospitals vegetated outside the mainstream of medical progress, it was the general hospitals that saved American psychiatry from completely losing touch with what was happening elsewhere.

American institutions are more specialized than European institutions. Not only are there hospitals for the poor and hospitals for the rich, but also special facilities for the retarded, the young, the old, the dangerous, alcoholics, drug addicts, and delinquents (we shall have more to say about some of these later on). In recent years, moreover, there has been a noticeable tendency to return to the use of "medical" methods in running these institutions. The methods used are often aggressive, such as the administration of heavy doses of medication or the employment of behavior modification techniques. In all these developments, however, there is no sign that the isolation of mental patients is a thing of the past. With respect to the mental hospitals, in particular, in 1960 or so there was apparently a change similar to the one that paved the way for the advent of early nineteenth-century psychiatry. At the beginning of the last century, philanthropists rescued some inmates from their traditional confinement and put them into "special hospitals" where they could be treated separately. This philanthropic gesture was in fact a composite of three distinct operations: the parasites were eliminated, the categories of patients to be treated were redefined, and the old-fashioned general hospital was reorganized with the aid of new medical technologies. For the past twenty years, these same three strategies have been employed to transform American mental hospitals, and this effort is continuing even today. Undesirables are literally being thrown out of the hospitals. Increasingly, mental hospitals are specializing in the treatment and handling of certain groups (problem children and adolescents, violent and dangerous adults, etc.). Finally, experimental methods and new techniques are being tried, including psychodynamics, behavior modification, and others.

Thus cynical economic motives, managerial requirements, ambitions to "improve psychiatry," and suspicion of mentally ill and deviant individuals have all contributed to the modernization of the total institution. The new rationale is economic: mental hospitals were costly to run, even if they did no more than house the poorest of patients in the most miserable of conditions. The new rationale is also bureaucratic: these vast, overcrowded, ugly old buildings could not be effectively supervised. The new rationale is also medical: how is treatment possible under the conditions prevailing in the old hospitals? And finally, the new rationale is philanthropic: the idea of a right to treatment has lately won acceptance, despite ingrained habits and the opposition of self-interested parties, and thanks to humanitarian and progressive criticism of the status quo. Thus modernization has been guided by four distinct principles aimed at getting rid of dysfunctions and overcoming lags. With a rationalized development program and ample resources, the hospitals have recently embarked on a journey toward a new destiny. A priori, there would seem to be no reason to expect the era of the modern psychiatric hospital to end any more quickly than did the era of its now discredited nineteenth-century forerunner, the asylum.

CHAPTER 5

————•——

The Illusions of Community

The counterpart of the myth of deinstitutionalization was the myth of collective care. In 1961 the report of the Joint Commission on Mental Illness and Health stated, as though it were self-evident, that

> the objective of modern treatment of persons with major mental illness is to enable the patient to maintain himself in a normal manner. To do so, it is necessary (1) to save the patient from the debilitating effects of institutionalization as much as possible, (2) if the patient requires hospitalization, to return him to home and community life as soon as possible, and (3) thereafter to maintain him in the community as long as possible.[1]

These objectives once seemed attainable because they were a natural outgrowth of theoretical and experimental research carried out by the most progressive segments of the psychiatric profession.

During the Second World War, a fire destroyed the Coconut Grove nightclub in Boston, killing several hundred people. A Boston psychiatrist, Erich Lindeman, took it upon himself to provide intensive care to survivors of the blaze and families of the victims, to help them overcome and accept the trauma they had sustained. Whereas physical medicine treated only the body, and traditional psychiatry intervened only after abnormal behavior manifested itself, and then only as a palliative, the magnitude of the Coconut Grove tragedy as well as its unprecedented nature called for intervention of a new type. The problem was to deal with a pathogenic situation affecting the whole community rather than with an individual disorder. What was needed was on-the-spot treatment of reactions induced by the disaster, so as to prevent their hardening into permanent mental disorders.[2] Thus the concept of "crisis intervention" was born. A crisis is a time of stress in which an individual (or group, family, couple, etc.) comes to see a difficult problem as insoluble, leaving no escape but through irrational, uncontrollable, and usually catastrophic behavior. Such reactions can, however, be warded off if help is received from specialists having an intimate knowledge of the specific problem and its social context. Crisis intervention can produce rapid results by helping the subject reevaluate the problem, make rational choices, and accept what has happened. Once the crisis has been surmounted, it may even be seen as having played a positive role in the development of the individual or group concerned.

This new kind of intervention obviously called for new techniques with direct access to real-life situations, not cut off from society as traditional psychiatric techniques had been because they were tailored for use in institutional settings. Ultimately, what was needed was a rethinking of psychiatry from top to bottom, and this Gerald Caplan undertook to do in his work on preventive psychiatry.[3]

Caplan distinguishes three levels of prevention, in each instance emphasizing the relationship between the psychiatric problem and its implications in and for the community. "Primary prevention" is aimed at correcting pathological or pathogenic conditions in the community. It is based on knowledge of the demographic, sociological, and psychosociological characteristics of the population involved; on intimate familiarity with living conditions, economic problems, work situations, housing, schools, recreational activities, religion, and subcultures in the area; and on first-hand investigation of the various subgroups, institutions, neighborhoods, and other factors involved. To carry out a program of primary prevention, an effort must be made to determine what standard of living the population desires, what possible causes of trauma exist, and what groups run the greatest risk of mental disorders. The objective is to rank the community's needs in order of priority and to formulate a coherent program for the development of psychiatric services.

A primary prevention strategy may be carried out in a variety of ways. Consultations may be held, for example, with individuals and groups representative of the community, in order to help them analyze latent conflicts and cope with their pathogenic consequences. Such representatives may include teachers, clergymen, social welfare, employment, and housing agencies, neighborhood spokesmen, welfare workers, youth workers, recreation officials, physicians and other medical or paramedical personnel, policemen, judges and court officers, etc. In addition, classes may be held to instruct people not only about mental illness and mental health but also about general circumstances affecting the quality of their lives. Meetings, lectures, and debates can be organized, films shown, pamphlets, newspapers, and posters distributed, and the local press involved. Action can be taken to inform local politicians and bureaucrats about the needs of the community, and efforts made to influence and even to exert pressure on them to take certain decisions or establish certain priorities with the approval of the community. Finally, direct preventive measures can be taken with respect to groups deemed subject to especially severe stress, hostility, or problems of adaptation as a result of certain events or the general community environment. For example, black schoolchildren can be prepared for entry into integrated schools; discussion groups can be organized to help new college students by enabling them to speak with older students; and recent widows and widowers can be introduced to others who have learned to cope with their loneliness after suffering a similar loss. Clearly, primary prevention is an ambitious program. It aims at nothing less than a metamorphosis of psychiatry into a new form of social and political action.

Once this has been done, the next step is "secondary prevention," a program in which narrower, more specific objectives are targeted. Secondary prevention aims particularly at groups within the community that were spotted during the primary prevention phase as being particularly vulnerable to psychic disorders, manifested either in the form of abnormal behavior by individual members of the group or, more commonly, as abnormal group behavior. Thus, for example, psychological assistance can be offered to individuals suffering from chronic diseases likely to produce stress or disability, such as diabetes, hypertension and other cardiovascular ailments, obesity, etc. In addition, special education can be offered to problem children. Psychiatric personnel provide help in two ways. Indirectly, they work through the schools, offering support to teachers and counseling them on how to improve scheduling, curriculum, and teaching methods. They can also work directly with the disturbed children, thus offering a presumably warm and reassuring presence in the classroom and on the playground as an alternative to the sterner aspect of the educational authorities themselves.

"Tertiary prevention" is concerned with patients suffering from more traditional sorts of mental illness. Its purpose is to guard against the aftereffects of disabling pathological conditions, or at least to reduce their severity. Under this head we may include programs designed to help former inpatients readjust to their work situations, find housing, and register for welfare, as well as intervention of a more indirect sort, designed to help the family and associates of a mental patient tolerate his condition more easily. Other programs work directly with the patient, not to cure him but to help him accept his condition and overcome feelings of inferiority. Still other preventive measures are designed to improve relations between the patient and service providers such as mental hospitals, to make hospital conditions less pathogenic, and to prepare the way for eventual discharge of inpatients. Employers may be approached about accepting handicapped workers, for instance. Measures can also be taken to ease the patient's reintegration into society, both through community education and through consultations with patient and family members. Halfway houses can be set up and special rehabilitation or retraining programs established in order to help patients overcome the feelings of helplessness and maladjustment that all too often follow mental breakdown, whether acute or prolonged.

These preventive programs are obviously related to Lindeman's early work, though they have been pushed much further than Lindeman imagined. The crisis intervention begun after the Coconut Grove fire was nothing other than a primary prevention program designed to deal with a group of people who had been subjected to extreme stress. It also included a secondary prevention program for people affected particularly severely by the trauma of the fire. And finally, there was a tertiary prevention program designed to minimize the social and psychological consequences of the physical and moral shock sustained by the victims. To work effectively, all these programs required familiarity with the social, economic, and cultural background of each individual, group, and family involved.

Such a thoroughgoing reform of traditional psychiatric methods carried with it implications that were revolutionary—in appearance at any rate—in three respects: the personnel involved in the treatment, the client–therapist relationship, and the organization of the service-providing facilities.

1. Traditional psychiatric training did not provide a base of skills broad enough to enable psychiatrists to deal with all the new problems, whose solution required intimate familiarity with the populations involved. The therapy teams therefore took on new members, chosen for their ability to interpret the needs of the community: middle-class housewives, student volunteers and, above all, so-called paraprofessionals and indigenous nonprofessionals. Housewives and students are reminiscent of the volunteer workers in traditional charities, but the indigenous nonprofessionals were often drawn directly from the groups most likely to be demanding psychiatric services: they represented ethnic minorities, the poor, the unemployed, retired people without funds to fall back on, the physically and mentally handicapped, former drug addicts, and so on. By hiring such workers, the mental health care teams not only obtained additional staff at low cost and contributed to the fight against unemployment; they also hoped that the new personnel would serve to bridge the gap between professionals and their clients, and that the nonprofessionals would invent new roles and new functions for themselves, since they were intimately familiar with the problems of clients who lived day in and day out in the same community they did.

2. A second strategy for creating an organic tie between the mental health care team and the community was to involve representatives of the district served in the organization and administration of services.

Accordingly, community advisory boards were set up with several objectives in mind. First, the members of the boards could inform members of the community about the services offered by the mental health center. Conversely, the board could let the staff know what the community's real needs and priorities were, as seen by the users themselves. Through the board the community itself shared the responsibilities of planning and administering mental health services and exerted some control over the way the center operated. Furthermore, the board brought local support—political, psychological, and in some cases financial—to the centers.[4] Community involvement was codified informally at best, for in reality it was a phenomenon of broad scope, not limited solely to the area of mental health. Implicated was the whole ideology of community participation, which was bound up with the social movements of the early sixties and particularly with the civil rights movement (see chapter 3).

3. Clearly, the monolithic mental hospital based on the principle of custodial care in segregation from the community was not an appropriate institutional setting for the new psychiatric services. The community mental health center was envisioned as an alternative. Traditional inpatient care was now seen as just one of the five basic services that officially approved mental health centers ought to provide. Centers also had to offer ambulatory care facilities, emergency services, flexible residential units (day and night posttreatment facilities, halfway houses), and above all community advisory and educational services. To be truly comprehensive, a center was also supposed to provide five other kinds of services, which the sponsors of the legislation left optional (perhaps to their later regret): these were specialized diagnostic services, rehabilitation, preadmission, and posttreatment facilities for state mental hospital patients, research and evaluation of community needs, and staff training.[5]

In principle, then, the bold new approach to the problems of mental health involved setting up a variety of public facilities throughout the United States. These were to be accessible to all, administered and run in collaboration with the users themselves, and staffed by multidisciplinary teams including members drawn from the community. The new facilities were to be located in the community being served and not set apart in remote institutions. They were supposed to have an impact on the community as a whole, not just on individuals. And they were to emphasize prevention rather than treatment, indirect measures rather than direct intervention in cases where problems were manifest. As one article put it: "Actually no less than the entire world is a proper catchment area for present-day psychiatry, and psychiatry need not be appalled by the magnitude of this task."[6] Today, however, fifteen years after the passage of the Community Mental Health Center Act, disillusionment is widespread.

A statistic may help to give some indication of the failure of the project: of the 2,000 community mental health centers envisioned for 1980, only 400 existed in 1975; most of these were built between 1967 and 1972.[7] The most recent estimate predicted a total of 647 centers in operation by October 1978.[8] In 1973, the community centers treated only 12.5 percent of all inpatients and 28 percent of ambulatory patients. The hope that the centers would gradually replace the state mental hospitals has come to nought, as we have seen, since the hospitals were emptied out with little or no regard to whether community services existed or not.

This state of affairs is widely blamed on the policies of the Nixon administration. It is claimed that the Republicans cut funds for mental health and for welfare projects in general, and reoriented policy toward new goals:

> The Nixon Administration is exercising stringent control over the NIMH budget and its funding priorities, and, in something of a historical déjà vu, favors efforts once more aimed at those "special" populations (drug addicts, alcoholics, and criminals) which it perceives as the most threatening to American society.[9]

These allegations are not altogether wrong. The War on Poverty, of which the community mental health movement was a part, had fizzled, and Nixon's election was both the sign and the instrument of a shift in priorities back to "law and order" and defense of middle-class privileges. The truth in regard to mental health, the poor, fringe groups, and social deviants is not quite so simple, however. So sharp a distinction between the policies of the Republican and Democratic administrations would be valid only if the Democrats' generosity had been truly disinterested in its motives. As we have seen (chapter 3), this was far from true. The Kennedy Act itself was quite vague about the obligation of the new mental health centers to give free treatment to the poor, and the responsibility to care for former state mental hospital patients was left optional. Conversely, it was under Nixon's presidency that an amendment was passed in 1970 giving supplementary funding to poor districts, and it was under Ford's presidency in 1975 that further steps were taken that tended to give a new impetus to the community mental health center movement. The 1975 amendment reaffirmed that

> community mental health care is the most effective and humane form of care for a majority of mentally ill individuals. Federal funds should continue to be made available for the purposes of initiating new and continuing existing community mental health centers and initiating new services within existing centers.[10]

Even if there were changes at the federal level that worked against the community mental health movement, it would be incorrect to blame them entirely for the failure of a policy that required a number of different agencies and interest groups, often hostile to one another, to coordinate their activities. While the idea came from Washington, local communities were left to take the initiative and to bear much of the financial burden. Federal funds were appropriated only for a limited period of time, ostensibly to "prime the pump," while local authorities gradually assumed responsibility for operating expenses. The federal government undertook to provide only one- to two-thirds of construction costs and other necessary start-up expenses (under the 1963 act) and to contribute a steadily diminishing portion of operating costs and salaries for a period of eight years after the opening of each center; the federal share was to range from 75 percent of the operating budget initially to 30 percent at the end (under the 1965 amendment). The 1970 amendment increased the federal contribution to centers in poor districts from 75 percent to 90 percent initially and from 30 percent to 70 percent at the end of the eight-year contract period. The idea was that the federal government would supply "seed money," as it was called, long enough for each center to line up its own sources of financing. It is not hard to understand why some communities were reluctant to commit themselves to meeting such costs on a long- or medium-term basis, while others leapt at the chance to take federal handouts only to sabotage the spirit of the project later on by paying operating expenses out of fees charged to clients or through third-party payments, with the inevitable discrimination implicit in such arrangements.

Local authorities were allowed great latitude in organizing the new services: they were free to choose the location of the center, as well as the specific organization or agency responsible for its operation (city, county, public or private general hospital or mental hospital, district health center, association or consortium of various public and/or private health agencies, etc.). They were also free to arrange for election of a community advisory board, as well as to name the board of directors, sign contracts with existing service agencies and medical personnel, hire the necessary staff including "indigenous nonprofessionals," arrange for a division of expenses not covered by federal grants, client fees, and insurance payments between the state government and the administration of the center, and so on. Locally, the role of the regional offices of the National Institute of Mental Health and the state departments of mental health was limited to stimulation, coordination, and management supervision.

The possibilities for conflict in these arrangements are easy to imagine. To begin with, there was room for trouble between the states and the federal government. Some states took a dim view of Washington's interfering in their affairs or failed to see the benefits to be reaped from such an outlay of funds. Others saw federal intervention as a useful adjunct to their own efforts to keep the lid on explosive tensions (as in the South Bronx, for example, to which we shall return below), or as a way of economizing on state expenditures and thereby scoring political points (cf. the case of California, discussed earlier). Still other states, particularly in the South, continued to rely to a large extent on a system of welfare based on charity and personal relationships, and found it difficult to accept the notion of a centralized system of free mental health facilities. Finally, there were states that had themselves established community mental health care centers as part of their efforts to move toward deinstitutionalization. In California, for example, the Short–Doyle Act of 1954 provided state aid to pay 90 percent of the cost of setting up county mental health centers.[11] Minnesota picked up 50 percent of the cost of setting up similar facilities.[12] And Michigan, in 1963 but before passage of the Kennedy Act, gave its sanction to users' committees, which were to take charge of organizing community mental health centers.[13] Clearly, these states were better prepared to set up the new centers than were states that had had no previous experience with community facilities and had to create everything from the ground up (or else do nothing).

Still, the fate of the community centers was determined not by federal or state directives but at the local level, where the real operational choices were made; even where federal and state agencies coordinated their activities rather than bicker with one another, this was the case. The decisive influence was exerted by the pressure groups that participated in setting up a given center. Success depended on how the different groups involved interacted with one another, as well as on how they interpreted the official program in the light of their own interests. The "freedom" that prevails in American society inevitably produces this sort of situation, because bureaucratic constraints are not merely obstacles to overcome but frequently serve as levers to be used by one or more players in the pluralistic game of free enterprise. Two groups of actors played a central role in determining how the different pressure groups interacted and interpreted the program: members of the medical profession and members of the community. In each locality, the way the community mental health center was to be set up and run was determined by the nature of the compromise worked out by these two usually hostile groups. This explains the complexity of the resulting pattern of arrangements.

THE WEIGHT OF PROFESSIONALISM

Erich Lindeman, the father of community psychiatry, is the namesake of the monumental Lindeman Community Mental Health Center in Boston, an enormous, imposing edifice, the very architecture of which discourages its use by underprivileged residents of the surrounding neighborhoods, who are further discouraged by the traditional medical methods that predominate among the services offered. Boston backers of the community mental health center movement see this center as a symbol of the diversion of their ideas into traditional channels by the psychiatric establishment: "innovation without change," creation of "new and more efficient facilities for distributing the same old services"[14]—such is the disillusioned assessment made by those who had hoped to see radical changes. They felt that although calls for innovation were heard throughout the sixties, it was innovative talk that was encouraged while innovate *action* was resisted.[15] But who resisted, and why did they resist? When a model is coopted we must ask: "By whom?" And, "What kind of idea was it that lent itself to cooptation?"

The ideas of crisis intervention, general prevention, and above all direct community participation in setting goals for and running the new facilities all figured in the innovative talk of a handful of pioneers, who were encouraged by government backers of the War on Poverty as well as by the then potent ideology of Black Power and the civil rights movement. Most members of the psychiatric profession did not agree that these were wise ideas. Recall (see chapter 3) that the Joint Commission had worked out a rather traditional compromise between the professional self-interest of psychiatrists and the need to modernize the practice of psychiatry. The Democratic administration, which had new objectives of its own, gave this compromise an apparently progressive twist. But even the Kennedy Act mandated real change in only one area of the five compulsory categories, namely, consultation and education.

Thus the stage was already set for habit to win out over innovation when it came to concrete application of the new proposals. To base mental medicine entirely on community practice was a leap into the unknown so alarming that even the most committed were hesitant. People who had over many years and with great difficulty acquired some knowledge of individual behavior and dynamics, along with a few modest principles for changing certain limited aspects of the way individuals operate, were now being asked to turn their efforts toward understanding and changing whole segments of society. The prospect was frightening.[16]

From the first, most specialists refused to take on overnight the role of superexperts in economics, law, urban planning, education, sociology, and the like and would not work "in an undefined role, meeting undefined needs of undefined clients."[17] Accordingly, wherever no other pressure group mobilized in opposition, the psychiatrists, who in general were lukewarm to the idea of taking on a public service role, given the weight of professional traditions, were likely to provide no more service than was required to obtain federal grants, concentrating only on those areas that best served their own financial interests or enhanced their personal prestige.

In this connection, the history of the Metropolitan Community Mental Health Center in Minneapolis, Minnesota, is typical. In 1964, two neighboring but hitherto separate private general hospitals joined together in setting up a psychiatric unit. The state government refused to approve their application for a grant under the Hill–Burton Act (which provides federal funds for hospital improvement), because the proposed plans were not detailed enough to meet Minnesota requirements. The hospitals therefore took advantage of the new funding made available under the Kennedy Act and a few months later obtained directly from the federal government nearly a million dollars for the construction of a community mental health center.

According to MCMHC's administrator, "There was no real understanding then of a community mental health center. It was still thought of in terms of in-patient facilities. When we found out that Hill–Burton money couldn't be used for in-patient psychiatric service, we needed to rethink and to agree to provide more than just in-patient facilities."[18]

In actuality, however, the new center could scarcely be distinguished from an ordinary hospital. In 1968, luxurious buildings linking the two hospitals were completed, including a tennis court, a swimming pool, and costly furnishings, while across the street a multilevel parking garage and medical office building serviced the private patients of hospital psychiatrists and physicians, almost all of whom worked only part time in the hospital, as is the case in many public facilities. In 1969, however, the center received a federal grant to cover a portion of its operating expenses over a five-year period during which the federal contribution would gradually decrease. In 1970, still not satisfied, hospital officials submitted plans for a county mental health consortium, which would have resulted in a $750,000 state grant to the center. These plans were rejected on the grounds that the services proposed were too traditional and that neither primary nor secondary prevention programs were contemplated. Still, the buildings were built with federal money and their operation was financed for several years in part by federal tax dollars, though the center satisfied none of the federal regulations concerning users' control, decentralization of services, and variety of programs offered. However, the psychiatrists pocketed their fees and per diems paid by the patients or their insurance companies.

It is not unusual for community mental health centers to be run in this manner. The Mission Center in San Francisco, the Touro and de Paule Centers in New Orleans, the center in Amarillo, Texas, and many others were set up in the same way and underwent a similar evolution. According to a Chicago official of the National Institute of Mental Health responsible for checking abuses of this sort, these practices are the rule rather than the exception: "It's a rule of thumb that whenever you see a general hospital associated with a community mental health center, you immediately look to see if the inpatient facility has been co-opted by private psychiatrists."[19]

The bold new approach to mental health advocated by President Kennedy has clearly been unable to overcome the power of the hospitals, which offer treatment based on traditional ideas of mental medicine, doctor–patient relations, and private financing; it has been unable to reach out to meet the needs of the community. Community centers are often located within general hospitals or very nearby, and the hospitals often have few if any contacts with the community the center is supposed to serve. A high proportion of staff time is devoted to the treatment of inpatients (three-quarters of the total man-hours in the Minneapolis center as well as in San Francisco's Mission Center),[20] and inpatients account for a high percentage of the centers' clients (73 percent in Minneapolis, 66 percent in Amarillo[21])—two more signs that in essential respects the centers are no different from traditional hospitals. As the administrator of San Francisco's Mission Center put it, naively, the question was where the most people could be seen. According to him, the Center's main goal was to provide services, and outpatient programs were not as effective.[22]

Under the circumstances it is quite natural that treatment of both inpatients and outpatients should be be based on a medical model. When patients are chosen because their condition is acute and their prognosis good, and shock treatments are administered frequently (in Minneapolis, one patient in seven or eight receives electroconvulsive therapy), locked wards are a necessity (twelve of the fifty beds in the Minneapolis center were in locked wards),[23] and even isolation rooms are needed (Amarillo has nine, and means of restraint are available). Ambulatory care in many cases amounts to no more than prescription of drugs to the less interesting patients, who are rarely seen by the doctors, while other patients come in for regular appointments and receive standard psychotherapy.

Besides being based on the medical model, treatment is also influenced by the "private-care" model in several respects. Centers sometimes refer patients to private psychiatrists in the area on a contractual basis. At Burlingame (in California), for example, almost all direct outpatient care is provided by private psychiatrists, psychologists, social workers, and other aides affiliated with the center. Each client of the center has a private therapist, who is paid by the patient, his or her insurance company or, in the case of uninsured patients, directly by the center.[24] While such a regime has proved practicable in Burlingame, a residential suburb, it would be difficult to copy in poor areas where there are few if any private psychiatrists, and where the clients do not readily adapt to one-on-one relationships with professionals. It would hardly be profitable, moreover, to attempt such an arrangement in these areas where most clients are uninsured.

Although centers are not as a rule based on a private-practice model, such a model is commonly singled out as especially praiseworthy:

> The fact that a comprehensive community mental health center can be developed by private practitioners gives us hope that mental health programs and psychiatric patients can be included in first-class programs and as first-class patients in a national health plan.[25]

The director of the Metropolitan Community Mental Health Center in Minneapolis was even more explicit. He declared that the model for all treatment in the mental health center would be the model of the psychiatrist in private practice.[26] Yet the Minneapolis center serves a poor neighborhood. The private-practice model chosen by the professionals has therefore served to transfer middle-class values with regard to mental health, healing, treatment methods, and therapeutic relationships to elements of the population far removed from a middle-class way of life. Traditional psychiatry has thus not been reformed as a result of confronting the challenges of practicing in a nontraditional sociopolitical context; instead, the profession has attempted to impose its most traditional methods on situations of every kind.

Another consequence of reliance on the private-care model is that profitability becomes the criterion of patient selection. The original community mental health care legislation was quite vague as to the obligation to provide a reasonable level of service at nominal cost or free of charge to persons unable to pay.[27] In practice, this "reasonable level" has often been quite low:

> We have set up fiefdoms so that various people have their respective pieces of real estate to which they're supposed to provide service. What are the social regulatory mechanisms that are going to control this? What's going to keep them from operating, as some of the Hill–Burton hospitals do, entirely in the private sector? How are they going to stay

public? I see evidence that many of them are going to be private facilities.[28]

In New Orleans, the Touro Infirmary Mental Health Center operates like a medical cooperative. Most of the patients are private, and the indigent ones are sent to state or charity hospitals.[29] The Metropolitan Community Mental Health Center in Minneapolis accepts all patients who are able to pay, regardless of whether or not they come from the district it was designed to serve. Indigent patients can receive only ambulatory care, however, and then only if they reside in the district. Hence there are no indigent inpatients at this center. It is true, however, that the per diem cost of a hospital bed in 1972 ranged from $63 to $86, while ambulatory care was much less costly, ranging from $15 to $150 per *month*.[30]

Clearly, such centers are discriminatory in their selection of clients. Not only does the staff apply social and financial criteria in choosing patients, but clients tend to select themselves, except in cases where treatment is imperative. The center's location, rather far from certain neighborhoods it is supposed to serve, discourages its use by patients without private means of transportation. Above all, the fact that it is associated with a hospital projects an "establishment" image, which often drives prospective patients away, particularly when they come from the poorer classes. Finally, reliance on the private-care medical model eliminates most patients seeking long-term therapy rather than acute care, since therapy requires a great deal of time of both clients and staff, brings little prestige to the center, and demands a knowledge of local conditions lacking in most of the professionals of the center staff. Members of racial minorities in particular feel out of place at the center. One Minneapolis Indian claimed that the center was a nice place for the rich but one that he couldn't afford. There were no Indians on the staff, which couldn't understand the problems of Indians. He said that Indians were mistreated at places like the regular hospital, and were made to wait for hours for treatment. When the American Indian Movement asked the center to help improve conditions for Indian children in Minneapolis schools, "they didn't think it was an appropriate request."[31] No matter what their ethnic origins, poor people, when they are not kept out of the centers altogether because of lack of funds, generally react to them with similar feelings of distrust, claiming that the centers do not meet their needs, which are frequently more social than medical.

Problems that cannot be dealt with within the narrow bounds of medicine per se are also raised by young people in trouble with their families, schools, or society at large. It was no accident that free clinics flourished in the sixties: more official agencies found themselves unprepared to deal with the new clientele of alienated youths (see chapter 7). Alcoholics and drug addicts were also neglected. As the director of one center put it: "The reason we don't treat addicts or alcoholics is because they're not interesting to me. I'd rather provide services to patients who are of medical interest."[32]

Leaving aside questions of pecuniary motivation, we find that a particularly high value is placed on this notion of "medical interest" by personnel in community mental health centers associated with medical schools or prestigious hospitals, where strong emphasis is placed on teaching and research. In many instances these centers offer a broader range of services and employ innovative methods (see below for a discussion of the way Yeshiva University organized services in the Bronx). Regardless of whether a center is mainly interested in teaching or profit, treatment of the elderly, the handicapped, and chronic patients, including both former residents of state hospitals and those unfortunate enough not to have been admitted to state hospitals, requires a heavy investment in facilities offering little or no "scientific" return. These clients often come from the same underprivileged strata of society that have a hard time gaining access to the centers. There is an acronym that is commonly used to describe the typical client of private psychoanalysts: YARVIS, which stands for Young, Attractive, Rich, Verbal, Intelligent, and Sophisticated. This same acronym can be considered a caricature of the patients of community mental health centers as well. Though extreme, perhaps, this characterization is indicative of a certain tendency. The full significance of this tendency becomes clear when we compare these traits with those of the typical state hospital patient, bearing in mind that the centers were supposed to replace the state hospitals.

In itself professionalism is undoubtedly not an evil, but it encourages certain predilections: to defend the interests of the profession, for one, which is readily transformed in the minds of the more "acquisitive" members of the profession into a propensity to provide only those services that yield the greatest profits. For another, there is a predilection to adopt a paternalistic and self-important attitude to outsiders, bred by the belief that only members of the profession are competent to judge the needs of others. Everett Hughes has given an excellent description of what professionals believe: "They profess to know better than others the nature of certain matters, and to know better than their clients what ails them or their affairs."[33] Among the professions sharing such a view, the medical profession has probably carried the notion of what Elliott Friedson has called "professional autonomy" farther than any other, refining a set of techniques designed to widen the gap between professional practice and more popular or commonplace approaches to sickness and health.[34] Ultimately this propensity results in emphasis on the most highly technologized and specialized approaches in preference to other possible methods. Not all such approaches are worthless. We have chosen here to focus on extreme cases, cases verging on self-parody. When countervailing tendencies are present to offset the negative aspects of professionalism, professionals have developed methods to make improved care available to more patients than ever before, for which they deserve full credit. The problem, however, is that there is no way to force the profession to share responsibilities with the community, which is presumably the goal of community psychiatry.

THE CONTRADICTORY DEMANDS OF THE COMMUNITY

The meaning of the word *community* is overdetermined in common American parlance. "Community participation" was the great myth of the sixties, but it has deep roots in American history and society: traditionally, America has given greater weight to grass-roots organizations than to governmental agencies; the various Protestant sects have long played an activist role ranging far beyond religious activities per se; ethnic groups have been of fundamental importance; and there has been a tradition of mutual aid and of seeking local solutions to social problems. It may have been attempting the impossible to take a notion so charged with ambiguous meaning and use it as justification for an institution that was the result not only of deliberate planning but of action by the authorities farthest removed from the community, namely, the federal government. The truth is that much of what is ambiguous about community psychiatry results from the multiple meanings of the word *community,* which readily lends itself to ideological distortions of one sort or another. Community participation was meant to establish contact with specific groups at the grass roots of American life. What usually resulted was an artifact of bureaucratic logic.

In the first place, the community was defined geographically by designation of a so-called catchment area to be served by a particular center. These areas were chosen to contain between 75,000 and 200,000 inhabitants. The backers of the Community Mental Health Center Act admit that these figures were chosen empirically, that is, in large part arbitrarily. "There was no real reason behind the limits . . . 50,000 seemed too small and 300,000 too big. We felt that 75,000 to 200,000 was about right."[35] In laying out the boundaries of the catchment areas, the authorities often tried to take account of social, demographic, and cultural factors, as well as formal and informal patterns of communication, exchange, and socialization. Easier said than done. Previously existing medical and social services, if any, also played a decisive role in the planning, even though they may not have been located in such a way as to best serve the needs of the population.

Furthermore, it is a myth that community residents are really concerned about what goes on inside a community mental health center. Basically, two groups of people were involved in the planning. One included professionals and other mental health workers such as health service personnel, educators, welfare workers, and "gatekeepers" who served as go-betweens between the service agencies and their clients (e.g., police officials, clergymen, representatives of charitable organizations, pharmacists, etc.). The other group consisted of the direct consumers of mental health services, who as a rule had to put up with whatever system was available. In theory this second group should have included all potential clients of the mental health system, i.e., ultimately everyone. In fact, however, it is clear that the two groups were not equal. The mental health workers and their peers all shared a similar cultural and educational background, performed similar functions, and took a similar view of social problems. The patients, on the other hand, whether current or prospective, were drawn largely from the most vulnerable and underprivileged groups in the society, whose way of life and cultural background could not have been more different from that of center officials.

Accordingly, when the time came to decide who to consult about any given problem, the most natural thing was for one professional to turn to another. This tendency was only reinforced by the fact that many clients shared the prejudice of the professionals: why should they tell the doctors what to do? In many cases, they often did not know themselves what they wanted or needed. Clients were also apt to believe that their being asked to participate was only a sham, which was most likely true. In any case they could hardly help being suspicious of a new agency that was connected with institutions with whose paternalistic attitudes' they had long been familiar.

If community participation was not entirely precluded by the objective differences between the two principal groups involved, these differences tended to shift attention away from the three original goals of the community mental health movement: these were to inform district residents of what services were available in the centers, to inform psychiatrists and their coworkers of the desires, needs, and priorities of people in the community, and to involve clients in organizing and running the facility.

Schematically, then, we should expect at first sight that, because of these kinds of problems, the idea of community participation would have had little chance of success, beyond its use as a slogan by demagogic politicians or a pious hope by daydreaming bureaucrats. In reality, though, the interactions that actually took place were often quite complex. The nature of the interaction depended on a variety of factors: the homogeneity of the community; the difference—ethnologically speaking—between community residents and the center staff; the history of psychiatric services in the area, if any; the attitudes of the professionals; the social and political consciousness of the clients; the personalities of neighborhood leaders; the balance of power among the various pressure groups; and so on. These factors combined in various ways to produce different types of centers, the most common of which we shall attempt to characterize. Specifically, three formal mechanisms of participation gave rise to informal communication between the staff of the mental health center and the residents of the community, communication whose content was complex, ambiguous, and often contradictory. One of these formal mechanisms revolved around the department of the center responsible for community consultation and education; another around the community advisory board; and a third around the hiring of volunteers, paraprofessionals, and indigenous nonprofessionals to work with the center staff.

1. "A unique characteristic of the Community Mental Health Centers Program is its fifth mandated service, Consultation and Education (C & E) which serves as the foundation of the centers' preventive care program and weaves mental health services into the fabric of other human resources in the community."

This general definition appears at the beginning of a statistical report issued in September 1974 by the National Institute of Mental Health.[36] The figures presented in the report, however, combined with the description of what "consultation and education" services are actually offered, belie the promise that mental health services would be woven into the community, showing that in fact these activities were quite limited in scope. In February 1973, all services grouped under these two headings accounted on the average for only 5.5 percent of the total man-hours worked in the 325 community mental health centers that had been in operation for more than a year and a half. Less time was devoted to prevention in the year the report was compiled than in the previous year. Nearly half the activities counted in the C & E category involved staff consultations concerning individual cases, while less than a third were devoted to discussions of long-range plans, and less than a quarter to development work and to on-the-job training of consulting teams. Approaches to school officials accounted for a third of the time, while only 3 percent was devoted to the elderly. The rest of the time was divided up more or less equally (10 percent or so for each category) among consultations with welfare departments, agencies responsible for dealing with alcoholics and drug addicts, court officials, other mental health agencies and medical facilities. Only 15 percent of this already limited time (or less than 1 percent of the team's total man-hours) was allocated to such activities as consultation with representatives of grass-roots organizations (e.g., neighborhood groups, community leaders, citizens' committees, clients' associations, etc.).

This is a far cry from the bold new approach to the problems of mental health through prevention. Under the actual system, community demands for technical assistance and cooperative planning are handled by high-level contacts between specialists. The centers respond accordingly, bypassing the clients. The response to community demands focuses primarily on pathological individuals rather than on what is pathogenic in the community. Children are a primary service target, owing to the commonly held conviction that "early intervention" is more effective than programs to eliminate environmental "risks" (see chapter 7).

2. Community advisory boards were instituted in order to facilitate interchange between clients and staff. The boards were supposed to make the staff aware of the population's needs and, if necessary, see that they were attended to. Conversely, the boards were to inform the community of the services available at the centers. In other words, the boards were supposed to embody the notion of "community control" over the organization, administration, and operation of mental health services. Like

other organizations and agencies created during the sixties for the purpose of promoting community participation, the community advisory boards were important because of the federal government's stated intention to give a voice in government and decision-making power to the most deprived groups in the society.

As we have seen, however, the administration's motives were in fact more complex than its stated intentions indicate: the War on Poverty, of which the community mental health center program was a part, had two other important objectives, namely, to win minority votes and to neutralize the more dangerous radicals in the community by integrating them into the system. Some radical leaders were not deceived. One black neighborhood in Harlem refused to allow a mental health center to be opened for reasons that were explicitly political: the center was seen as a new way of controlling the black population and forcing it to accept middle-class values, even though it was to be run by blacks—this was seen as perhaps the most insidious aspect of the project. The job of the radicals in defending their opposition to the center was made easier by the fact that, initially at least, disadvantaged social groups generally tend to demand the most traditional sorts of medical service and to accept the most stereotypical image of the doctor—an image that even minority group physicians are quite willing to embody.

In areas where mental health centers are organized and operated by the community (i.e., in the Harlem case, by the blacks predominant in the area), services tend to be no more revolutionary in conception or execution than in centers elsewhere, though they do tend to be more comprehensive. San Francisco's Westside Center, for example, is a consortium of nineteen previously existing agencies. The board of directors, consisting of one representative of each agency and an equal number of members of the community advisory board, manages and coordinates all the center's services, most of which were already available before the center was set up in 1966. This center services an officially designated poverty zone, and almost all of its officials are members of minority groups (blacks and Asians). Among the services provided are emergency care for adults (including crisis intervention, suicide prevention, home visits, and temporary residential treatment in emergency cases), hospitalization for acute cases, day-treatment centers, overnight facilities, a ward for medium-length inpatient care, liaison with the Napa Valley State Mental Hospital, consultation centers, and ambulatory care; for children, both inpatient and outpatient care are available, along with day-treatment centers and more specialized services (such as advice for single parents); there are also services for drug addicts, including emergency treatment, orientation, counseling, total or partial hospitalization, methadone maintenance (see below), and job counseling. All these services are available at twenty-five different locations throughout the area, conveniently available to all residents of the district. No community mental health center offers a more comprehensive and wide-ranging spectrum of services, and yet nothing at Westside goes beyond the bounds of standard forms of medical therapy.[37]

Westside is often described as a successful community mental health center. In certain respects this description is accurate: the center offers a variety of services, an important role in running the facility is played by people who seem to be representative of the community, and the center is accessible to all and free of discrimination. In other words, this center is painted as one of the few in which both professionals and community advisors play a role in running a center which, if it has not completely revolutionized the existing system of mental health care, has at least made what seems to be a range of decent services available to social groups previously denied access to that system.

Elsewhere, however, the mere fact that the community advisory boards play more than just a formal role does not necessarily mean that they give voice to the desires of the populace. What often happens is that an alliance is forged between medical professionals on the one hand and important social service officials and responsible community representatives on the other, the upshot of which is a center that is run in an authoritarian and discriminatory manner.

Consider, for example, the Mountain Mental Health Center,

which is located in the town of Prestonburg in Appalachia. The inhabitants of the area earn their livelihood mainly from coal mining. In the wake of mechanization in the thirties and competition from oil in the fifties, the number of people employed in the mines has declined steadily, and the profits made in coal are often invested in more booming areas. The population is poor, aging, handicapped by illness and work accidents, and subject to what is known as "East Kentucky syndrome" (the equivalent of "North Africa syndrome" in France), which local doctors dismiss contemptuously as a set of symptoms feigned in order to obtain welfare benefits. The few doctors there are concentrated in the cities, and they generally devote little time to Medicaid patients, force them to buy drugs from their own pharmacies, and in some cases hospitalize patients in for-profit clinics that require the poor to pay their bills in advance. Doctors are part of the region's small ruling class, along with teachers, lawyers, bureaucrats, and public service employees. The poor majority looks upon these community leaders as being in league with the mine owners, which in many cases is true, if not economically then at least ideologically: some doctors and lawyers have worked for the mining company, elected officials have had the support of the company in their campaigns, and so on. The Regional Committee on Mental Health, which was set up and organized by the center, is made up exclusively of such people. Explicitly, the reason for this is to give the center a respectable image in order to assure its acceptance by the middle classes. But the services offered by the center are looked upon as a program for the poor and are not used by those who can afford to go elsewhere. Nevertheless, the poor are not satisfied. They complain that the services they need are inaccessible or dispensed in an authoritarian manner, and that no attention is paid to their demands and grievances.

The fact is that most of the center's activity in this "poverty zone" is given over to individual psychotherapy. Although 75 percent of the center's patients are below the poverty line (set by government experts at $5,500 annual income for a family of four), and although many of the problems with which the center must deal are social in origin, nothing has been done to attack these problems at their roots. The dozen or so paraprofessionals hired by the center, most of whom work in small, mobile groups that travel around this very spread-out region, have not been given the support they need to provide satisfactory service. By contrast, a satellite of the center has been opened in the residential suburb in the area.[38]

This type of community involvement (or, rather, noninvolvement) is not unusual. Initially, area leaders take charge of organizing a community mental health center, thereby imparting an image of respectability and establishing operational standards. Thereafter the running of the facility is entrusted to the medical staff.

Another area of potential conflict is between the personnel of the community mental health centers and the representatives of the community. Broadly speaking, the antagonism may take one of two forms: either the community or the pressure groups that speak in its name may refuse to agree to the installation of facilities that are seen as not particularly wonderful or even as threatening in some way, or highly motivated users' groups may organize around the fight for services in order to overcome the resistance of recalcitrant professionals.

An illustration of the first type of conflict may be found in the misfortunes of the Mission Center in San Francisco. This center serves a particularly cosmopolitan area, a traditional haven for immigrants in which the various nationalities have refused to mix, instead maintaining their native cultures. The heart of the area, the Mission district itself, is a poor ghetto, while the outlying neighborhoods to the east and west, once rather well-to-do, have increasingly mixed populations.

Created in 1968 by psychiatrists of the San Francisco General Hospital (an association that deterred many residents of the area from using the center), the Mission Center attempted to decentralize in 1971 by setting up two satellite centers, one to the east, the other to the west. This project precipitated a battle in which the opposing forces were out to capture far more than just formal control of the center. The backers of the decentralization plan seem to have been in the majority: these included the center staff itself, as well as the board of directors, the clients, other welfare agency employees, white middle-class liberals, and minority group representatives, in particular the Mission Coalition Organization, an umbrella group representing most of the neighborhood organizations working to improve ghetto living conditions. The opponents of the project, on the other hand, seem to have been few in number, being mainly small, scattered groups of property owners, merchants, and real estate agents. Their strategy was coordinated to perfection, however, by powerful business groups, one of whose leaders was a man who was a landlord and creditor of many of the opponents of the project and exerted pressure on them that was anything but moral persuasion: he threatened rent increases, evictions, calling in debts, and business boycotts if they did not support his position. They themselves had strong reasons for opposing the project, reasons apt to draw widespread support: although the official party line mentioned fear of the deleterious influence of drug addicts on the children of the area, this was not the real reason—no drug treatment program was contemplated for the satellites—so much as the fear that property values would suffer if the neighborhood were invaded by undesirables.

This pressure group succeeded in mobilizing opposition to the decentralization plans and in getting around local agencies favorable to the project. By pressuring city officials and using smear tactics (such as reporting a priest who had openly supported the project to his bishop), the opponents of decentralization succeeded in scotching the plans. The composition of the center's board of directors was changed to include a larger number of representatives of the more well-off neighborhoods to the east and west at the expense of ghetto representation.

These tactics, some of them reminiscent of strong-arm gangster methods, could not have succeeded without the support of a large segment of the population. The same pressure group also prevented a group of black doctors from opening an office and blocked creation of a methadone maintenance center for heroin addicts, as well as a dispensary for young drug addicts.[39] Community participation does not always result in an idyll of democracy. Problems of this sort have caused so much concern that the leading names in community psychiatry recently held a conference to discuss "community intolerance of the mentally ill."[40]

Sometimes, though, the opposite occurred: representatives of the community instituted new services as part of an effort to combat the elitism of the medical establishment. Doubtless the best example, owing to the prestige of the institution, is Boston's Massachusetts Mental Health Center. In 1912 it became the first state hospital to open its doors to outpatients and to offer outside consultation (see chapter 2). As both a state hospital and a teaching hospital associated with a prestigious university (Harvard), its status was unique in the United States. Although all comers were welcomed, only cases deemed to be of interest for teaching purposes were actually admitted, the remainder being sent to another mental hospital some fifty miles away. The institution was dedicated to the training of students in medicine and psychiatry, instruction being carried out by extremely well-trained, multidisciplinary teams. In 1972 teaching and research still accounted for 90 percent of the total budget. Many officials of the center had been strong backers of the new ideas that emerged in the late fifties; they had participated in the work of the Joint Commission on Mental Illness and Health and had been among the first to put the new community-based policies into practice. But they had gone into community mental health with the same elitist and "scientific" spirit that had always governed their practice: that is, services and patients were chosen on the basis of strictly medical criteria, intervention of the most highly technical kind was preferred, there was general indifference to social problems and groups not likely to stimulate scientific advances, and so on.

The center was located, however, in an area much affected by the hippie movement of the late sixties, and several highly motivated and politicized neighborhood organizations were at work nearby. These groups took control of the community advisory board and insisted that wards be opened for the elderly and retarded even though these groups were without scientific interest; they also called for a new type of relationship between specialists and clients. Accordingly, they challenged one outpatient clinic chief whose professional style was deemed too "technocratic" and "bourgeois" for patients drawn from marginal groups; he was replaced. In 1972 the governor appointed a new state commissioner of mental health, who went all-out to support efforts to democratize the center. This led to open conflicts with the professional staff. The commissioner changed budgetary priorities, cut into allocations for research in order to finance services demanded by the users of the center, pushed for improvements in the training of nonprofessional staff, and so on. At the time we visited the center in 1974, the conflict was raging in the open. It is worthy of note that some of the promoters of the "psychiatric revolution" of 1963 were among the bitterest opponents of the new policy orientation and threatened to resign if their judgment of what was fundamentally best for the center continued to be challenged.

This crisis in one of America's most prestigious medical institutions was fairly unusual, however. It could happen only because of an unprecedented alliance between determined consumer groups and a state commissioner who insisted on enforcing the letter of the new democratic health policy even at the risk of antagonizing the very people who were supposed to implement it. Other cases demonstrate that even a genuine mobilization of the populace is not enough to challenge the traditional powers of hospital administrators and doctors. In Philadelphia, for example, the clients of the Mental Health Consortium, which was dominated by the University of Pennsylvania, waged a long battle to change the priorities of the consortium in keeping with the needs of the most disadvantaged groups in the society, but these efforts ended in failure.[41]

Our inventory of examples may have left the reader feeling that he is faced with a puzzle, the pieces of which have yet to be put together. The point is that it is impossible to evaluate the effects of community participation on mental health policy in a few words without oversimplification. The pattern of services in each area depends on the local balance of power. The general picture is therefore a mosaic of individual cases, which we have tried to investigate by looking at a few of the most typical ones. Broadly speaking, what we find as a rule is pseudoparticipation rather than genuine community involvement in setting the crucial priorities in mental health policy and in running mental health care services on a day-to-day basis. Even in the best of cases, the rhetoric of community participation was used as window dressing for a reorganization of mental health care that left the power in the same hands as before. As we shall see next, more or less the same conclusion applies to the results of another measure designed to bring mental health services closer to the people, namely, the employment of paraprofessionals.

3. As part of the War on Poverty, the primary official reason for hiring nonprofessionals was

> to give work to millions of the unemployed; to create social service jobs that cannot be replaced by machines; to rehabilitate the poor by giving them worthwhile work to do; to give more services to the poor, and services that are readily available to them; to reach those who could not be reached before; to limit job reductions in health, education, and welfare; to free professionals for more creative roles in supervision, planning, and training.[42]

Compared with these stated aims, the results obtained seem ridiculously meager: as of January 1, 1974, only 10,800 mental health workers were employed in the 400 community mental health centers then in operation. Some centers refused to hire nonprofessional workers. Overall, nonprofessionals accounted for less than one-third of the medical staff in the new facilities.[43] Even if we include nonprofessionals employed by other social service agencies (some 40 percent of the total number of nonprofessionals),[44] the result achieved is far from the millions of new jobs hoped for at the outset.

It is true, however, that the efforts to give preference in hiring to minority group members were more successful: in a sample of 380 nonprofessional workers, 46.4 percent were found to be black, 21.7 percent Mexican-American and Puerto Rican, 3.7 percent Indian, 2.8 percent Asians, and 2.6 percent of other origins. Forty percent were men, although traditionally few men have been employed in health jobs at this level. If, however, we look at the same sample and ask what the cultural background of the workers involved was, we find that 90 percent had finished high school and half held college degrees. Looking at their professional backgrounds, we find that fewer than one-tenth had never worked before and that only one-quarter had been on the welfare rolls.[45] The obvious conclusion is that paraprofessionals were not recruited from the poorest strata of ethnic minorities. The point is that, although the definition of paraprofessionals stipulated that no prior training be required, center officials wanted employees "carefully selected" from among "specially talented members of deprived groups."[46] Quite often those hired were the least representative of the community, the closest to conforming to middle-class standards: "The principle that emerges is that if you must coopt members of the opposition, at least coopt those who are going to cause you the least amount of trouble."[47] Finally, paraprofessional employees had been promised training that would enable them to rise through the ranks and eventually acquire professional status. In fact, the money and above all the interest were lacking to make such training programs broadly available and effective. It may well have been naive to expect a group of professionals to help undermine their own privileged status. In any case, except for on-the-job training, theory and practice were rarely taught, and where instruction was offered, it was limited to a select group among the nonprofessionals. The main emphasis was on inculcating middle-class, professional values and models. Only to a limited extent did such programs open the way to career advancement, and paraprofessionals almost never rose to high-level professional positions.

As for the services performed by the paraprofessionals, although it had been expected that community residents would serve to establish a link between the center staff and the community, and even that they would improvise new roles and new treatment techniques better suited to the needs of the populace, in fact they were usually used to relieve professionals of the most disagreeable chores, of jobs that required the least skills, such as tying children's shoelaces, for example, helping people fill out forms, taking patients from one place to another, and so on.[48] The bridge that the paraprofessionals were supposed to provide between the staff and the community turned out to be a one-way affair: deprived groups were exposed to the dominant social values via the paraprofessionals, who served as models of respectable behavior, as emissaries to the socially deviant.

> The family agent is also expected to serve, in a subtle fashion, as a role model for the family. She (most of the agents are women) is supposed to be an agent of acculturation—in other words, an agent of change—and a means of helping the family become assimilated into the larger society.[49]

Sometimes assigned to do unpleasant drudgery and deprived of all power and initiative, and sometimes regarded with suspicion along with the rest of the center staff by members of the community, nonprofessionals were all too likely to be treated with condescension by professionals and clients alike: one client described a paraprofessional as "a meddler, an 'Uncle Tom,' an opportunist, a tyrant."[50] "Worker and consumer, force for change and member of the system, critic of professionalism and aspirant professional,"[51] paraprofessionals are so entangled in contradictions that they risk total paralysis.

Some nonprofessionals have tried to overcome these handicaps, however, by taking a political view of their situation. A report presented to the National Council for New Careers in 1968 set forth an ambitious strategy for an attack on the private sector, the division of labor, and bureaucracy, an attack based on a radical critique of professionalism, which charged that the professions as they were then practiced were elitist and authoritarian in their very conception, and therefore antidemocratic and conservative in their effects.[52]

Those who attacked professionalism tended to espouse the views of minority movements and groups working for popular control. The *New Careers Newsletter* summed up the position of the new careers movement for which it spoke in 1969 as follows: "It is more concerned with new services, a new voice inside the system, new forms of participation, and a new responsive professional practice. . . . It does not want to patch up a system which is alien to the community, the poor, the consumer, the citizen."[53] In 1970 the name of the journal was changed to *New Professional:*

> For years workers have been stigmatized by being called a variety of names from paraprofessionals to nonprofessionals and so on. New Professionals feel that their work is no less critical than that of professionals, and in fact are primarily concerned with the delivery of quality services in their respective fields.[54]

It is difficult to measure how widely these aspirations were shared by the paraprofessionals as a group. Still, some of the radical critiques of the paraprofessional role and calls for revolutionary changes went beyond mere rhetoric. The crisis that hit New York's Lincoln Hospital in 1969 is an extreme example of the way the new mental health workers worked to change conditions in mental health facilities. If the contradictions at Lincoln were so glaringly apparent, perhaps the reason was the obvious gulf between the way the people served by the center lived and the way the facility was designed to function.

The neighborhood involved, the South Bronx, is in fact one of the poorest not only in New York but in the whole United States. The population is 70 percent Puerto Rican, 20 percent black, and 10 percent white. Each group inhabiting this desolate urban landscape is more miserable than the next. Rival gangs roam the streets, which are rife with violence and even death. Two members of one psychiatric staff of thirty were killed within a year. The police ignore unobtrusive delinquency and intervene only when the gang violence flares up into open warfare. The unending turmoil took on political overtones during the sixties, when groups of political militants moved in alongside the traditional gangs. Further aggravating the situation is the rivalry between blacks and Puerto Ricans. All things considered, then, this was an ideal place to wage the War on Poverty, given the ulterior political motives involved. Federal, state, and local governments were prepared to be munificent to health and social workers willing to move in to such an area.

In 1963, a group of psychiatrists from the Albert Einstein College of Medicine, affiliated with the prestigious Yeshiva Univer-

sity—one of the leading centers of psychoanalysis in the country—
founded the Lincoln Hospital Mental Health Services in the southern part of the South Bronx, the poorest area in the ghetto. Led
by highly trained, progressive psychiatrists and financed by a variety of public and private agencies affiliated with the War on
Poverty, this facility was a model of the new social psychiatry
even before the idea had gained currency in official circles. Though
lacking any real hospital facilities (there were never more than a
few beds), the center included facilities for part-time inpatient
care, therapy groups, professional training, drug addicts, emergency cases, and crisis intervention. One of the most innovative
services was the walk-in clinic, which offered immediate treatment
to all comers without appointments or other formalities, with a
team of specialists constantly on call.[55] Contacts and consultations
were undertaken with neighborhood associations and other social
service agencies in order to try to integrate the new center into
the community and to assist residents of the ghetto in obtaining
welfare, housing, and jobs. In 1964 the center began hiring local
nonprofessionals (70 were employed in 1969, out of a total staff
of 166). Carefully selected, they received not only on-the-job
training but also intensive theoretical and practical instruction to
enable them to qualify for higher level posts.[56]

Yet it was in this very center, in many respects a paragon, that
a serious crisis erupted in March 1969. Paragon though it was in
regard to technical organization and probably also in quality of
care, the center was nevertheless operated in a paternalistic manner, if we are to believe the assessment of general public opinion
reported by the paraprofessionals. All the power was in the hands
of a well-intentioned elite determined to do what was good for
the neighborhood. A flyer handed out on June 9, 1968, "told it
like it was":

> We're gonna see what you do with what you think is your center. You
> honkies complain that we don't respect authority and we don't want
> any compromise. Damn right. Your authority is no good and we've
> been compromising too damn long. So now you listen to what working
> people are saying loud and clear. And you better listen: Cause now
> we're not working *for* the center any more. We and the community *are*
> the center.[57]

This threat was made good on March 4, 1969, when the Lincoln Hospital was occupied by paraprofessionals, who chose new department heads from their own ranks, threw out anyone who did not support their cause, and demanded that the administration take certain concrete steps: rehire workers who had been dismissed, provide for the election of a community committee with real decision-making power, apply union rules to insure that employees would henceforth be promoted on the basis of seniority and competence, establish a training program leading to professional careers and not requiring students to work in the center while attending courses, reevaluate and reorganize all departments of the Lincoln Hospital Mental Health Services, and provide the community with substantial information about the facility and the way it operated. After fiteen days of occupation and some rather confused negotiations, the demands were almost completely met. The Lincoln Community Mental Health Center changed its name and became independent of the hospital and its psychiatric department. A new director was named with the consent of the remaining staff and the community.

However temporary this victory of the paraprofessionals over the doctors with all their professional prestige may have been, it was more than just symbolic. In a concrete way the possibility of a radical change in the way things were done was demonstrated by one team organized at the time of the crisis by a nonprofessional administrator and an immigrant psychiatrist. New members were selected by the entire team after observation of their work and evaluation of what they might contribute to the team as a whole, not so much in the way of technical competence as of sociopolitical analysis and commitment. Clients were treated by whatever workers were available, regardless of formal training. New methods were tried out in family and group therapy, methods based not on psychological reductionism but on comprehensive analysis of the situation. Collaboration with practitioners of "alternative" forms of medicine popular among minority groups was contemplated: for example, mediums popular in the Puerto Rican community were contacted, and patients were referred back and forth on the basis of criteria established in an atmosphere of mutual respect and confidence. The staff supported militant groups in their struggles for minority rights. It may well be that a truly novel form of community participation cannot be imagined until the staff has been faced with community protest, demonstrating the place of mental illness within the overall sociopolitical context. It may also be that it was necessary to work within a milieu in which pathology was obviously related to the existence of unsatisfied basic needs, so that the subjective nature of the problem could be put in perspective rather than denied. This also had the effect of putting the skills of the specialists into perspective as well, since those skills were exclusively in the realm of psychology and did not touch the larger problems of the community.

In other poor ghettos in the United States, however, nonprofessionals have also been employed by community mental health centers and yet innovation has not been forthcoming. Even the Lincoln experiment did not prove viable in the long run. With the exception of the group for drug addicts, which continued until recently to operate on the same radical basis (see below, chapter 6), services at Lincoln have since 1975 gradually been returning to a more traditional mold. Many obstacles stand in the way of the radical changes desired by the leaders of the New Careers Movement:

> It will require facing such issues as professional resistance, institutional vested interests, racist social policies and practices, community demands that exceed community cohesion, paraprofessional satisfaction with a larger slice of the status quo, and the limitations of knowledge in the mental health field.[58]

Most commonly, poorly paid nonprofessionals assigned to lowly jobs and ineligible for promotion have done no more than help bring low-grade psychiatry to the poor. At first a token of community participation, nonprofessionals later became hostages within the community centers, which continued to operate under the aegis of professionalism.

FROM KENNEDY TO CARTER

What social and political prerequisites had to be met in order for the new psychiatry to succeed? To answer this question we shall examine a paradoxical and probably unique example in which community psychiatry was indeed successful. What we will learn by studying this special case is how hard it was to meet these requirements in other cases. It will also become clear, further, that recent developments in community psychiatry indicate not so much that the original goals have been abandoned as that there is a tendency now to take a more realistic approach in a changed political context.

The case we propose to study is the psychiatric department of the health services of the celebrated Massachusetts Institute of Technology (MIT). Its staff provided individual therapy and crisis intervention to the personnel of the Institute (students, teachers, researchers, administrators, and other staff) and also served in an advisory capacity in areas within the university that had little apparent connection with problems of health. Under these circumstances the psychiatric staff developed a novel type of practice. This grew out of vigorous criticism of standard forms of therapy, including psychoanalysis. The MIT psychiatrists looked upon both traditional nosology and Freudian concepts as abstractions: like philosophical universals, they gave no direct hold on specific, concrete situations. While a specialist can treat only one patient at a time, still he must understand the client's situation thoroughly in order to interpret what he hears, and he must refrain from forcing the client's testimony into the Procrustean bed of preestablished theory. This sort of criticism of traditional medical attitudes need not imply that treatment should be administered by nonprofessionals, quite the contrary. In fact, a very high level of training, experience, and technological knowhow is required if the therapist is to grasp the full complexity of his patient's experience. Dealing with human relations in the here and now demands a multidimensional approach that is at once psychological, social, and political. This is far more difficult than interpreting a symptom in the light of a doctrine, psychoanalytic or otherwise.[59]

This kind of therapeutic method demands not only that therapists be well versed in the use of sophisticated techniques but also that they be immersed in the same milieu as their clients. If therapists and clients truly form an endogamous community, then the boundaries between personal problems and social problems vanish; the personal and the social become merely polar points on a spectrum, and therapy can deal with the whole spectrum by working to transform the individual and his surroundings at the same time. The psychiatrist treats individual cases, but he is also an expert in human relations in the community. He helps to keep both individual and institutional relationships in balance for the good of the community as a whole as well as of its individual members. Such methods are a concrete realization of Caplan's vision, combining crisis intervention with preventive action in the community.

The psychiatrist's role in this situation is ambiguous, however. Suppose, for example, that students in crisis receive individual treatment. In the course of administering this treatment, the therapist may learn that a certain course or teacher is having deleterious effects on the health of the students. Is it then up to the psychiatrist and his associates to suggest reforms? How far should they go? Should they report the troublesome professor to the appropriate dean? If they choose to do so, are they then to become involved in choosing a replacement, redesigning the teaching program, and so on? Where does technical intervention end and political action begin? In such a context, the distinction between the two is clearly untenable. In order to administer effective treatment, the psychiatrist must either have the power to impose reforms on the institution for the sake of its members' mental health, or he must be able to inspire those in power to undertake such reforms. In other words, he must be either the prince or an advisor to the prince—there is no other choice.

Anyone in such a position may well be faced with difficult problems of conscience, and such an ambitious mental health program is likely to be costly in other ways as well. It can be effectively implemented only in exceptional circumstances, of which the MIT case is a prime example: the mental health group there had access to all the power centers of the institution and was dealing with a community that was largely homogeneous. A psychiatrist working in a black ghetto, by contrast, is faced with a far more difficult problem: alienated from the community in so many ways, how can he possibly hope to understand its problems? How can he possibly hope to monitor the effects of his actions? Ghetto communities, as we have seen, put forth a large number of ill-defined demands, to which professionals tended to respond either in narrowly medical ways, as a means of self-protection, or else, in a few cases, in a political way, a possibility that was enhanced because the mission of mental health care was so vague and its methods so uncertain.

The only way to avoid such widely divergent responses and achieve the goals of social psychiatry is to make a wide range of resources available to mental health workers. Americans have been reluctant, however, to make the necessary sacrifices to establish public facilities on a continuing basis, not only in medicine but in other social services as well, in part because such facilities are costly, in part also because centrally controlled, federally run public services are viewed with suspicion. In times of crisis, like the sixties, temporary special measures have been taken. It was undoubtedly not very realistic, however, to think that a project as sweeping in its objectives, as costly to run, and as centralized in its organization as the Kennedy Act could have been carried out as planned. Once the situation had been stabilized, the temptation was to go back to the old internal modes of regulation, to private initiative, and to local control. The recent tax revolt by the middle classes[60] is a spectacular illustration of the broad consensus that exists for a reduction of state intervention and of allocation of manpower and resources to public services. It may well be that scattered resources can be mobilized and coordinated in an interdependent system of heterogeneous facilities that will be just as effective as, and cost less than, a comprehensive system built from the ground up by the federal government and run by it from Washington. Accordingly, the new leaders of the social psychiatry movement, like leaders in other areas of American society, have since the seventies been impressed by the argument that there is a need to subdivide and individualize the demands of the community and to meet those demands with more highly technical and less costly responses better tailored to local requirements.

In 1972, nineteen states, including Georgia, of which Jimmy

Carter was then governor, hit upon the idea of unifying the various "human services" they offered their citizens. In each district, one building was to be designated to house health and mental health services, welfare offices, public housing agencies, employment services, and sometimes even representatives of the courts.[61] Not only would this mean a savings in time for both clients and service workers, but now there would be a centralized source of information. Efficiency would be enhanced, and at the same time control would be tightened over each individual user. Under the new arrangement the superspecialist who processed each client and put him or her in touch with the right service providers for his or her particular case would no longer be a psychiatric specialist well versed in the problems of the community but rather a human resources generalist, an expert in dealing with social problems on an individual basis in the purest case-work tradition. Thus psychiatrists and their aides were induced once again to focus on their medical and technical speciality rather than try to reform society. No longer was psychiatry in danger of slipping into political involvement; rather, the goal of attacking community problems across a broad front was achieved in part through the use of more limited means, by coordinating and rationalizing human services across the board.

Legislation passed in 1975 under Gerald Ford exhibits a similar tendency to offer a broad range of specifically targeted services. Expanded mental health services were authorized, but each new service was aimed at a specific group within the population: there were special facilities for children, for the elderly, for alcoholics, and for drug addicts, as well as expert advice fot the courts, prehospitalization examination of mental patients, posthospitalization services, half-way facilities designed to bring down the number of patients in institutions, etc. Clearly, the failures of previous measures were taken into account in drafting this new legislation. Health services were diversified and expanded through contractual arrangements with existing public and private facilities, marking a new stage in the evolution of the mental health care system.

The new direction is best illustrated by the report of the President's Commission on Mental Health named in February 1977

and chaired by Rosalyn Carter.)[62] The focus on coordinating
services already in existence indicates a step backward from the
ambitious plans of the sixties to construct a new system from the
ground up. The goals remained the same, however, even if the
route now proposed for reaching them was based on a more
realistic assessment of the obstacles. As for the populations to
which services were directed, the monolithic notion of a "community"—scarcely allowing for differences between ghettos and
white neighborhoods or between urban and rural areas—was now
supplanted by a new recommendation: look at the needs of each
subgroup individually, and provide resources tailored specifically
to blacks, Hispanics, Indians, Asians, minorities of European origin, women, children, the elderly, the handicapped, alcoholics,
rural populations, divorced people, people living alone, battered
women, victims of rape and rapists, etc. Another explicit recommendation was to focus on meeting—not to say creating—a
new set of demands centering on complaints of depression, de-
moralization, and other problems of daily life, rather than limiting
treatment to well-defined pathologies. "Passages" has become a
new vogue term, replacing "crises," and it has now become ac-
ceptable to prescribe psychiatric care for people faced with life's
familiar trials and tribulations, even where no traditional pathological etiology or breakdown was in evidence.

Another point was that psychiatric care should no longer be
dispensed only in places specifically associated with mental health
in a traditional sense. Psychiatry could also be practiced in the
family, the school, neighborhood organizations, bureaucracies,
welfare offices, police stations, and courtrooms; employees could
become aides to the psychiatrist. Psychiatrists were urged to mobilize all existing resources—public, private, charitable, and even
"alternative"—"on the basis of genuine cooperation, not co-op-
tation and control."[63] Among the resources to be called upon
were self-help groups; free clinics; hot lines for runaways, drug
addicts, and would-be suicides; religious cults; *curanderos* (healers);
spiritualists; and so on. It is not hard to see that the government
stood to save a great deal of money if the help of such resources
could be enlisted in running the mental health care system, for

most of them were independently financed and privately managed. With all these auxiliaries helping out, moreover, psychiatrists themselves would be free to concentrate on developing their own specialty, whose autonomy had been threatened by the community-participation ideology. For the community movement had undermined the psychiatric profession in two ways. On the one hand, the importance of technical expertise had been downgraded in comparison with the emphasis on sociopolitical commitment. On the other hand, this had provoked a defensive reaction on the part of some members of the profession, who were led to advocate a rigid reliance on strictly medical forms of treatment.

It would have been impossible to redefine mental health policy in this way without a number of new initiatives between the Kennedy Act of 1963 and the recommendations of the Carter Commission in 1978. During this same period, moreover, a number of new institutions were set up, and experiments were conducted with new techniques. Most of these prerequisites to the redefinition of federal policy were worked out independently of earlier policy and in some cases even in opposition to it (see chapter 7). Since that time, these innovations have been integrated into the revised federal policy on mental health care, which says a great deal about both the capacity of American society to digest "countercultural" experiments and about the special relationship between the public and private sector in the United States. We shall have more to say about this later on (in the conclusion to this book). At this point, however, we are in a position to perceive the underlying reasons for this special relationship and to appreciate what benefits it has to offer at the present juncture.

One such benefit is economic: privately run services cost federal and state governments virtually nothing. Another benefit is political. As was mentioned earlier, one of the purposes behind the community psychiatry program—its strategic function, if you will, within the War on Poverty—was to use medical services of a new type as a way of establishing a governmental presence within certain communities and as a way of exerting governmental control over certain fringe groups. In its more ambitious (and costly) versions, this program was designed to set up new facilities in certain target areas and to grant them extensive powers to attack social problems with medical means. Social psychiatry rests on equivocation about the meaning of the word *social*. It is concerned about the role of social factors in causing mental illness, which implies that society is conceived as a pathogenic environment requiring "treatment" by medical specialists trained to recognize the pathology. This induces a shift in the definition of *social*: rather than refer to objective political realities, the word comes to refer to that which "social psychiatry" is capable of treating. Society becomes the space within which a medical norm can be imposed. In trying to understand the political consequences of this shift, we need not impute any sort of Machiavellian scheme to the practitioners of social psychiatry. Their view is merely one-sided, denying the validity of the social and political conditions responsible for society's sufferings, imbalances, and disorders, so that the methods of "social medicine" can be applied.

The same social and political factors can also be invalidated in another way: the government may choose a strategy of offering a bewildering variety of services, each focused on one tiny problem or minute aspect of a problem. The individual is then "serialized" [to use Sartre's term—TRANS.] or broken down in accordance with the dictates of a series of specialized agencies responsible for dealing with, say, one particular age group, type of handicap, ethnic minority, etc. Clients are sent from department to department and cut off from their personal support networks; specific problems are forced into a mold shaped by the agency's own priorities. The bureaucratic classifications do not correspond to real groups within the society but merely to an arbitrary administrative breakdown of necessary sdrvices and to exigencies of management and institutional definition. This strategy harks back to time-honored American traditions of charitable assistance. From the beginning, charity has been doled out from a multitude of sources, public and private, local and regional, broken down according to the vagaries of geographical, jurisdictional, and bureaucratic boundaries (see chapters 1 and 2). This case-by-case, sector-by-sector policy helps to keep relief recipients in a dependent status, impeding the development of collective consciousness and forestalling mass action. This tradition can be traced back to the days of "moral evaluation" and social case work: each individual is evaluated personally to determine whether or not he or she meets the criteria set by the institution. Accordingly, the social and political reasons for which the person might have been driven to seek assistance are never analyzed.[64] At first sight it may seem paradoxical that the most far-reaching federal effort to unify the mental health care system, which culminated in the passage of the Kennedy Act, was ultimately undone by the introduction of a broad range of new, "psychology-oriented" services. This change in policy, however, does not necessarily mean that all of the federal government's goals of the early sixties were abandoned, if it is true that the basic objective, then as later, was to help defuse an increasingly explosive political situation and to help certain victims of the disintegration of American society to accept their status in life.

It is therefore an exaggeration to say that the community psychiatry movement ended in failure, as many of the professionals and administrators involved in its inception now tend to do. The community mental health center movement changed the mental health scene in the United States in ways no doubt less fundamental than its sponsors might have wished, but nonetheless in ways that were essential.

1. Community psychiatry can be understood as being part of a general effort to bring psychiatric practice as close as possible to the life of society. In the private realm, the first step in this direction was taken by the mental hygiene movement (chapter 2). Later, federal backing was obtained, and elements of the public mental health care system were enlisted in the movement. Although the program was never carried to completion (i.e., to the point of replacing the asylum altogether) and although there now seems to be a growing reluctance to create a broad range of new services from the ground up, much public outpatient care of mental illness is now practiced in a community setting (on the order of one-quarter of the cases receiving medical attention). For better or for worse, a new type of mental health care facility has been created to fill the gap between the old-style asylum and private psychiatric practice.

2. Much of the treatment dispensed by community-based facilities is

directed to population groups different from those treated by the old mental hospitals. The pathologies treated are generally less serious, and the patients often come from less underprivileged backgrounds than do patients for whom the mental hospitals are the last resort. The recent recommendations of the Carter Commission confirm that one of the purposes of federal policy is to draw into the orbit of the mental health care system—for better or for worse—new groups of clients, who are offered assistance that certainly would not be available if these facilities did not exist.

3. The movement provoked a serious crisis within the psychiatric profession. Attention has already been called to the persistence of defensive reflexes on the part of the profession. These defenses were put to a severe test, giving rise to an atmosphere of crisis and factionalism; some psychiatrists compromised themselves by becoming engaged politically, for which they would long bear a stigma. The profession lost the unity it had had when it was sure of its therapeutic mission (or when disputes were at worst limited to issues of technique or theory). Furthermore, while many community mental health centers merely offered the same services as traditional mental hospitals, community practice did in some instances produce an unusual combination of circumstances that enabled the more innovative centers to develop new techniques of mental medicine.

4. The crisis that now besets the movement will not necessarily lead to an abandonment of its main objectives. As we have seen, there have been two responses to the difficulties that community psychiatry has encountered. On the one hand, there has been renewed emphasis on professionalism and a return to modes of practice based on the medical model, which the movement had once sought to replace. On the other hand, community psychiatry has been integrated into a new "human services" system. Psychiatry has thereby lost some of its autonomy; this phenomenon is not limited to the United States, and the reasons for it have to do with a decline in the once-exalted status of psychiatry, as well as with the fact that mental health care is now one of many services included within the "human services system." Similar developments have occurred in Canada.[65] In France, the latest developments in the *politique de secteur* also suggest that the ambition of the sixties to establish a modern, accessible mental health care system has been toned down to fit into a more complex program involving the medical establishment, government, and the private sector. These policy changes do not reflect a retreat from a strategy of treatment coupled with social control but

rather the opposite: public services are coming to rely increasingly on psychology. Thus, public mental health care is not the only way to extend the range of a welfare system that performs functions of control, surveillance, and normalization, and it seems likely that it is no longer the preferred way. Our next problem will be to discover what new strategies are being used to extend the influence of the system.

PART THREE

Psychamerica

With the advent of mental medicine, the lunatic came to be seen as a patient suffering from a malady. For the first time, a distinction was made between the mentally ill individual and others belonging to such miscellaneous categories as social deviants, delinquents, vagabonds, vagrants, debauchees, wastrels, idiots, criminals, and others guilty of violating social and sexual norms. Before people could conceive of mental alienation (and hence of psychiatry as a discipline), they had to learn to identify stable clusters of symptoms associated with specific disease entities (nosographies). At first these symptoms were related to intellectual shortcomings, but later they were broadened to include emotional and behavioral disorders. Presumably, nosologies have something to do with "scientifically" established etiologies (which may be either somatic or psychic), and the associated pathologies, we are told, are amenable to treatment by qualified specialists (namely, psychiatrists) affiliated with specialized institutions (at first asylums and later mental hospitals).

The nosographic classifications of mental illness have always been dubious, however. They are based on the assumption that there is a clear dividing line between people who are "ill" and therefore within the purview of psychiatry, on the one hand, and people who are "normal"—though they may come under the jurisdiction of some other repressive agency, such as the courts—on the other hand. Ever since the nineteenth century, when this sort of dichotomy was found to offer a workable way of limiting the number of patients accepted for treatment, the boundary between the normal and the pathological has become less and less clear, with the consequence that the scope of mental medicine has steadily broadened. In the United States the area in which psychiatry is thought to be applicable has expanded in four ways.

First, the mental hygiene movement and, later, community psychiatry moved toward social forms of practice and thereby extended the influence of psychiatry into areas from which it remained excluded so long as its practice was confined along with its patients to impregnable institutions. This required a reworking of the nosographic categories and institutions of mental medicine itself. Fighting mental illness continued to be the objective, even after the emphasis shifted to prevention as a way of obviating later treatment. The expansion of psychiatry's influence was based on the conviction (ostensibly substantiated by epidemiological studies shaped by prevailing medical ideology, purporting to show that there are always more people in need of treatment than are actually being treated) that there were patients awaiting treatment and diseases waiting to be prevented, coupled with the idea that the germs of these diseases must be traced to their sources in social life.

Second, psychiatry also extended its influence by taking responsibility for categories of individuals who came under the jurisdiction of the courts or other social agencies. This, too, occurred quite early. Thinking about criminals, mental defectives, sexual perverts, psychopaths, runaways, and other such groups has traditionally wavered between two extremes, one legal, the other medical. Today, things are different in two respects. First, treatment programs have been extended to new categories, such as alcoholics, drug addicts, children with learning disorders, etc. Second, even criminals who are caught and sent to prison are likely to be placed in treatment programs, which have increasingly been supplanting old-fashioned incarceration as it becomes necessary to justify punishment and lend plausibility to hopes of eventual rehabilitation (chapter 6).

The third way in which psychiatry extended its influence is somewhat more baffling at first sight: it took advantage of the resistance of certain groups within the population to the official mental health care institutions. Countercultural movements of one sort or another posed new problems. Among them were problems related to drug use by middle-class youths, feminist and homosexual demands, and so on. Traditional psychiatrists were accustomed to working with nosologies that proved inappropriate for diagnosing the difficulties that people in these new contexts were experiencing. These people refused, moreover, to seek help from official mental health care facilities, which for them symbolized the authoritarian and bureaucratic institutions they were fighting against. Accordingly, a number of alternative institutions, such as free clinics and self-help groups, were set up to enable the counterculture to take care of its own, as it were. The problem was to establish a setting in which the patient's humanity and personality could be respected even though the malady from which he was suffering placed him in a situation of dependence. The paradoxical nature of the problem accounts for the ambiguous fate of the alternative institutions: although they did in some respects represent a move away from some of the more rigid features of traditional medical facilities, at the same time they added a new link to the chain of available mental health care facilities (see chapter 7).

Finally, the influence of psychiatry was broadened in a fourth way: while some submitted to and others resisted the encroachments of mental medicine, still others chose freely to accept it—or thought they did. Typical of the free-choice situation is the doctor–patient relationship in the private-practice setting: in principle, the patient freely chooses a doctor and pays for his treatment, establishing a relationship of reciprocity between them. In private practice the medical model is not forcibly imposed on a dependent patient population; instead, a service is offered to consumers. In the United States, however, demand for services of this kind has long since exceeded the available supply of private psychiatrists and psychoanalysts. The extraordinary proliferation over the last ten or fifteen years of new kinds of therapy (family therapy, sex therapy, behavior modification, bioenergetics, Gestalt therapy, primal scream, transactional analysis, and various encounter group techniques ostensibly unconcerned with therapy as such) is one sign that medicopsychological models of treatment have made deep inroads. These developments bring us into the postpsychoanalytic era. The people who seek these new services exhibit symptoms that are signs not so much of a specific pathology as of a malaise in daily life: exaggerating somewhat, one might say that what must be cured is normality. Now that we have reached the point of "therapy for the normal," virtually all of social space has been opened up to the new techniques of psychological manipulation (see chapter 8).

CHAPTER 6

The Psychiatrization of Difference

DELINQUENCY: CURE AND PUNISHMENT

The delinquent, in the course of his life, comes into contact with the three principal components of the penal justice system: the police, the courts, and the prison. We shall look at each of these institutions in turn in order to analyze how the way they operate in the United States has been profoundly altered by medicalization.

The Police

During the sixties, a time of constant conflict between the police and minority groups that culminated in the great ghetto riots, a new approach to maintaining law and order was worked out, an approach involving "mental hygiene." Police collaborated with mental health specialists in three main ways: psychologists, psychiatrists, and sociologists were called upon to help train officers to deal with community relations problems; the police themselves learned to employ psychological and psychosociological techniques; and police officers and social workers worked together in the community.

At the time of the Watts riots in 1965 a number of police publications indicated the need for "sensitivity training" to help police officers modify their behavior. The Presidential Commission on the Causes and Prevention of Civil Disorder, which studied the riots of the sixties, called in 1969 for "the establishment of sensitivity training in each police department for each level of officer"[1] Courses for patrolmen devoted a good deal of time to this kind of training. The National Institute of Mental Health lent its support to efforts to "make better policemen," as the title of one of its publications put it, by financing several training programs. The main objective was to teach policemen how they might improve their understanding of ghetto life and how they might tactfully try to head off a riot or cool down a disturbance in its early stages. The political significance of this training is made crystal clear by the statement that "a police officer can, in the regular course of his duties, obviously help to change the attitudes of ghetto residents not only toward the symbols of authority but toward the white community as a whole, for better or for worse."

The training offered relied heavily on role playing. To give one example, two police officers were asked to act out a situation in which the members of a gang are stopped for questioning (the gang members were played by other officers). The youths hurl insults at the officers. One of them knocks one of the youths against a wall. This is followed by discussion, role reversal, etc. A secondary, but by no means inconsiderable, benefit of this kind of training is that young white recruits are taught to speak the language of the ghetto—the method is reminiscent of the immersion techniques used by some language schools.[2] Another program arranged for officers to visit ghettos and meet people of various social and ethnic backgrounds: "Plans are being made for each of the officers to spend time in the home of a minority group family as part of his training and perhaps eat a meal with that family."[3]

On one occasion in Seattle, a training class attended by forty-eight police officers was interrupted by a telephone call announcing that a riot had just broken out in the ghetto. Several policemen were injured (as were many more ghetto residents), but the officers who had taken part in the group training session were congratulated for having taken a "humane" approach during the confrontation.[4] Despite opposition from many old-line officers, higher-ups encouraged their subordinates to act as advisers and arbitrators in order to involve the police in the community and fight against the "pig" image—the commonly held belief that racism and brutality are rampant among policemen—that helped exacerbate tensions. It should not be forgotten, however, that even while the police were taking this new line, they were also physically doing away with the most radical militants, such as the Black Panthers.

Thanks to these training programs, the police started to use techniques reminiscent of those used by mental health workers. Consider, for example, the officer trained in family crisis intervention. In many cities officers receive training modeled on the crisis intervention techniques pioneered by preventive psychiatry (see the preceding chapter), which are designed to enable them to deal with family disputes (and bear in mind that situations of this sort were responsible for 22 percent of police deaths in the line of duty in 1974). In California the department responsible for dealing with juvenile delinquency financed programs in which police officers did counseling, gave courses, and offered assistance not only to youths but also to their parents and others in the neighborhood. The 1978 report of the Presidential Commission on Mental Health reaffirmed the need for police officers to learn and apply modern mental hygiene concepts and techniques.

We also find cases where police officers have worked closely with medical and psychiatric personnel. In many police departments social workers are on call around the clock. There are "roving medical teams" which include a psychologist and an intern who work with the police. This gives mental health personnel access through the police to people who would never have thought of seeking psychiatric help on their own, particularly in the ghettos and other poor areas. In addition, the mental health worker can proceed, after the crisis has been quelled, to administer treatment, which seems to be particularly effective in these conditions:

> This early treatment is beneficial, too, because people in serious trouble are frequently quite receptive to treatment and help with personality reorganization immediately after crisis. They are often not as receptive a long time afterwards because they have had a chance to erect defenses, rationalize (neutralize) their behavior, or make patch-work, bandaid repairs which usually do not last long.[5]

Thus the ideas of Lindeman and Caplan (see the preceding chapter) have found novel application. Psychiatrists come upon some of their choicest cases through collaboration with the police, while the police borrow some of the psychiatrists' choicest methods for use in their own work: a first-rate illustration of the workings of what Nicholas Kittie has called the "therapeutic state."[6] But what happens in the heat of crisis when psychiatrist and police officer both rush to the scene is merely illustrative of a more far-reaching interaction of medical and repressive functions that is typical of the entire American penal system.

The Courts

Psychiatric concepts were aided in making their way into the legal system by two models that were first elaborated in the nineteenth century and further developed by the mental hygiene and social psychiatry movements: the model of individualized treatment and the model of prevention.

Individualized treatment was developed primarily in connection with the treatment of disturbed children (see chapter 3). To deal with wayward urban youths made rootless by rapid immigration, charitable institutions resorted to some rather heavy-handed techniques; in addition, the juvenile court system was created. Even before the end of the nineteenth century, efforts were made to establish clear lines of demarcation between the juvenile courts and their adult counterparts. The stated intention was to avoid traumatizing young offenders by sending them to jail, relying instead on less drastic and more humane measures: private consultations, informal discussions with the child about the motives for his reprehensible actions, evaluation of the likelihood of rehabilitation, and so on. As a result, the young delinquent's whole life was laid open to scrutiny. This was the first step away from punitive and toward preventive penology. Emphasis shifted from punishing specific violations of the law to examination of the subject's regular behavior, reputation, and motives, even in cases where no crime had actually been committed. A whole range of activities was accordingly opened to scrutiny and subjected to vaguely defined sanctions: these included sexual promiscuity, drunkenness, frequentation of pool halls, loitering, and so on. Judges wore the spectacles of doctors and educators, and even in the nineteenth century their language was embellished with medical and psychological metaphors, like "We do not know a child until we have examined him fully," and "We must plumb the depths of the child's very soul." Judges apparently saw their task as one of establishing the whole truth about the child, in much the same way as the doctor seeks to uncover all the symptoms of the patient's condition.[7]

Reformatories were also based on the idea that their residents could be completely resocialized. Some reformatories were organized like obstacle courses: the young prisoner had to overcome one obstacle before being allowed to proceed on to the next. As he advanced his behavior was monitored and appropriate rewards and punishments were meted out. This system was a late nineteenth-century forerunner of present-day behavior modification techniques (see below). Sentences to such institutions were of indeterminate length, so that administrators held all the cards and could manipulate every aspect of the inmates' lives by linking release time to good behavior while in prison.

These innovations, inspired by psychology and first perfected in the juvenile courts and reformatories, have since been extended to the entire criminal justice system, transforming it from top to bottom.

The confusion or failure to differentiate between penology and psychiatry can be seen most clearly in the treatment of mentally defective delinquents and sexual psychopaths. Massachusetts state law defines a sexual psychopath as a person "whose misconduct in sexual matters indicates a general lack of power to control his sexual impulses, as evidenced by repetitive or compulsive behavior and either violence or aggression of an adult against a victim under the age of sixteen years."[8] According to Maryland law, a defective delinquent is an

> individual who, by the demonstration of persistent, aggravated antisocial or criminal behavior, evidences a propensity toward criminal activity, and who is found to have either such intellectual deficiency or emotional unbalance, or both, as to clearly demonstrate an actual

danger to society so as to require such confinement and treatment, when appropriate, as may make it reasonably safe for society to terminate the confinement and treatment.[9]

These attempts at clear definition conceal the fact that the behavioral categories to which they refer are poorly defined, at variance with the usual criteria of both psychiatric nosography and the criminal code. Hence it is unlikely that persons classified as psychopathic or defective will receive any treatment specifically tailored to their conditions. Those falling into these special categories of "criminally insane" can nevertheless be incarcerated for unlimited terms in special institutions whose medical label is no more than a convenient cover. The statutes cited, moreover, were drafted in the heat of public outcry after certain notorious sexual crimes were committed in the late thirties. Since that time, they have been used as a pretext for coming down hard on largely minor offenses committed by docile individuals, guilty of exhibitionism or of acts between mutually consenting adults.[10] Finally, the characterization of the offenses in psychiatric or pseudopsychiatric terms has served as a way of getting around the guarantees written into criminal proceedings. Preventive detention on the basis of a psychiatric illness for which no defined treatment exists, and the use of competency examinations for punishment or to exclude the possibility of bail are two examples. When an individual is thus shunted from the legal system into the mental health system, he risks having to serve a longer sentence and will most likely be incarcerated in an institution that is medical in name only.

Similar remarks apply to offenders found "not guilty by reason of insanity" or judged "incompetent to stand trial," whose day in court is postponed until they have been released from the hospital (see chapter 4).

Besides the confusion of pathology and criminality that has beset these borderline cases, the regular legal system has also seen a recent increase in the role played by psychiatry and psychology. In the first place there was the development of so-called indeterminate sentencing. California, which has the most crowded state prison system in the United States (21,000 prisoners),[11] began experimenting with indeterminate sentences, under which an individual can be sent to jail for an unspecified period ranging from, say, one to fifteen years for breaking and entering. At the end of the minimum sentence (in this case one year), the prisoner appears before a special commission. Prison officials then decide whether or not to release him, and increasingly they are helped out by psychologists, who base their evaluation on the prisoner's personality. The prisoners, however, do not have anything to gain from this "individuation" of penalties: the average prison term is longer in California than in any other state, and the rate of imprisonment is the highest, 1.45 per 1000 inhabitants. Recently, however, the state changed its mind about the wisdom of this system and went back to the old "flat sentence" system.[12]

Then, too, the increasingly widespread practice known as "pretrial diversion" has contributed to the growing influence of psychology in the courts. Diversion allows the accused to go free while awaiting trial, sometimes without restrictions, sometimes on condition that he submit to supervision by the court. The supervision required may take the form of compulsory visits to a mental health center, a drug-addiction treatment program, or the like. After trial some defendants are placed on probation and are required to participate in programs that offer the advantage of not forcing them to go to prison—this at the price of submitting them to constant supervision and continuing reeducation. In some of these prison-substitute programs, several categories of offenders are treated simultaneously, which shows that it is not so much the objective nature of the offense that is being attacked as it is the personality of the offender. Operation De Novo in Minnesota, for example, treats thieves, drug addicts, alcoholics, prostitutes, and others, all at the same time. Each individual in the program sets certain goals for himself in cooperation with his counselor. If he achieves these goals, the charges are dropped. If not, he must appear in court.[13]

These innovations are so many signs of a comprehensive new penal policy—a policy made necessary by the rising crime rate, which has swamped the prisons. In Florida, for example, 6,969 persons were imprisoned in 1965, compared with 8,840 set free on probation or parole. By 1975 the number of prisoners had climbed to 11,335, while the number of offenders not sent to prison rose to 52,412, an increase of more than 500 percent![14]

To be sure, not all lawbreakers diverted from the traditional prison system are "treated" in any psychiatric sense—far from it. Most programs amount to little more than a few visits each month to a counselor. Other, more elaborate programs also make use of group techniques coupled with social activities. The preliminary evaluations of the results of these programs give cause for skepticism: the recidivism rate is as high as for individuals sent to prison, and the results are not significantly different for offenders whose cases are followed up more closely.[15] Just as in the case of the psychiatric policy inspired by the Kennedy Act of 1963 (see chapter 4), it seems that the main purpose of programs offering a "community alternative" to prison has been to extend official surveillance and control to a larger number of people. Despite the ingenious efforts of judges and administrators, the rate of imprisonment has remained more or less constant at around one prisoner per thousand Americans: 166,000 in 1950, 212,000 in 1960, 203,000 in 1971.[16] What has changed in recent years, however, is that now imprisonment is only one of the implements used to check juvenile crime, and in quantitative terms it is of secondary importance. The number of young Americans in trouble with the police each year has been estimated at four million, with two million cases actually resulting in arrest. But only half of these go to the courts, and only half of the cases referred to the courts actually come to trial. Finally, 100,000 youths are sent to prisons and reformatories, while 400,000 under indictment remain out of prison but under court supervision.[17]

American courts confront a basic contradiction. Unable to mete out the prison sentences provided for by law, they discharge their responsibilities by sending lawbreakers to community treatment programs, most of which the judges know to be shams. What makes this deceit credible is that the concept of "treatment" is invoked—in other words, the contention is that techniques based on medicine will be used to help rehabilitate delinquents. Were it not for this safety valve, perhaps the fiction that justice is being done by the courts would have been exploded long ago, and people might then have been willing to look more closely at the foundations of a legal system (and a society) so conceived that nearly a third of the nation's young people violate its laws.[18] Rather than raise basic questions about the system, people have cast about for dubious alternatives to what are ostensibly the most brutal forms of punishment. What is paradoxical about all but a few[19] of these "alternatives" is that they have done nothing to empty the prisons while augmenting the number of people mixed up with the courts.

It may well be that alternatives to prison have made the system of justice even more unjust. In this connection, the results of a recent study are worthy of serious attention. Conventional wisdom has it that members of minority groups, blacks in particular, are the most dangerous or, at any rate, the most asocial members of society. Proof of this contention is said to lie in the fact that the proportion of blacks in prison is far higher than the proportion of whites, which is true. But a study has shown that

> States with a high incidence of persons living below the poverty line tend to have a *lower* crime rate but a *higher incarceration* rate. . . . There is no significant correlation between a state's racial composition and its crime rate but there is a very great positive relationship between its *racial composition* and its *incarceration* rate.[20]

Thus there is good reason to think that more flexible punishments have been applied in a very selective fashion, leaving the most deprived members of society to populate the prisons. One consequence of allowing for psychological factors in judging criminal offenders is thus to stigmatize more systematically than before those people whose life patterns and values are farthest removed from those of the middle classes.

The Prisons

The broadening of community programs for prisoners is based on the assumption that prisons will continue to exist, at least for criminals deemed to be "high risk" cases. Recent thinking among penologists, however, shows that they are uneasy about incarceration of high risk prisoners, a practice which nearly all of them suspect perpetuates and even increases the dangers it is supposed to combat. Here again, the individual treatment model provides an out. Even within the prison itself, the patent failure of punishment by example has led to increasingly systematic reliance on the treatment model, under which lawbreakers are treated as though they were patients.

According to a former director of the California Department of Correction, "Crime is certainly in part a mental trouble. We hope also that prisons are becoming more like hospitals."[21] Once again California is out in front, employing a broader range of psychological and psychiatric techniques in its prisons than any other state. Psychiatric services are today fully integrated into the California penal system. Consider the fact that *before coming to trial*, any person indicted for a serious crime must submit to a series of tests administered by one of two state diagnostic centers. The results of this pretrial investigation are conveyed to the judge within ninety days. The judge makes use of them in deciding whether to hold the defendant in prison or to release him provisionally on condition that he participate in one of a number of available programs. *After sentencing*, convicted criminals are evaluated over a sixty- to ninety-day period prior to being sent to one of the thirteen penal institutions in the state, which to some extent specialize in accepting certain types of prisoners and offering certain types of services.[22]

In prison 20 percent of the inmates are supposed to receive psychiatric treatment. California prisons instituted group and environmental therapy in 1955. Today, even transcendental meditation is being used at Folsom Federal Prison, where seventy-five prisoners are involved in a meditation program.[23] Above all, however, it is the Vacaville Correctional Medical Center that has made the California prison system famous. It is from Vacaville that the leaders of the Symbionese Liberation Army, which became notorious after the Patricia Hearst kidnapping, emerged. Conditions at Vacaville had turned out a group of fanatical revolutionaries. Vacaville is a prison hospital with 400 beds for acute cases and facilities for 550 patients to receive intensive psychotherapy (for chronic cases, there are 600 beds at the California Men's Colony). Vacaville has been in the forefront of experimentation. In the Jenner Homosexual Unit, for example, several kinds of drugs were used in behavior modification experiments: antitestone, which causes the testicles to atrophy and thereby suppresses the sexual impulse, and anectone, which paralyzes the muscles and can even cause respiratory difficulties (it produces an effect that inmates compare to the feeling that one is drowning). Apart from attempts to "cure" homosexuality, other drugs were in wide-spread use, including prolixin, which alters the personality (and which in 1971 was administered to 1,093 Vacaville prisoners).[24]

Psychosurgery was also practiced in California but on too mod-est a scale to satisfy the Corrections Commissioner, who in 1971 asked for appropriations to fund a more systematic program: all violent inmates were to be examined at Vacaville; if brain abnor-malities were deemed to be the cause of their violent behavior, psychosurgery would be performed. The project was abandoned after the Prisoners' Action Committee publicized it.[25]

Not only is psychiatric "treatment" administered during the inmate's term in prison, but psychiatric evaluation is used to de-termine when the inmate should be released. All inmates diag-nosed as suffering from mental disorders are required to submit a psychiatric report when applying for parole. In 1968, 8,000 such reports were submitted in California. Parole is often granted in such cases on condition that the ex-convict submit to regular psychiatric observation. In case of a "relapse," the parolee can be returned to prison.[26]

Elsewhere in the United States, we find the same spectrum of techniques, but rarely are they applied as systematically as in Cal-ifornia. According to a 1972 study, four out of five prisons make use of group techniques, whose purpose is, they claim, to give prisoners counseling and guidance and to inculcate a socially ac-ceptable image of themselves and of their community. These tech-niques include group therapy, guided group interaction, discus-sion and counseling groups.[27] At the time, one-quarter of the institutions using these methods had nearly all their inmates enrolled in at least one program of this type, and over the years the number of such programs has increased.

Psychiatric techniques are often introduced into a prison after it has experienced a riot or other violent episode. At the Kansas State Penitentiary, for example, an awareness training program was financed by the National Alliance of Businessmen. Prisoners also enjoyed access to transactional analysis, yoga classes, and transcendental meditation. They could play music, paint, do theater and gardening.[28] The new policy was inaugurated after a series of riots beginning in 1969. Over a six-month period, three hundred prisoners deliberately mutilated themselves for life by cutting their Achilles' tendon, as a way of protesting the way the prison was run.[29] The new programs, inspired by psychotherapy, were introduced to change the atmosphere of rebellion.

It may be objected that the use of such methods is harmless: they help prisoners to pass the time, and inmates quickly learn to take advantage of the programs for their own purposes and to adjust to the idiosyncracies of the various specialists. But psychological programs are also ways of policing the institution. In group therapy sessions, everything that has gone on during the day or week comes up in the course of ostensibly therapeutic discussion. The effects of transactional analysis, the technique most widely used in the prisons, have been described by one inmate as follows:

> But what happens is that outside of the "Game" the men seem to get distant and paranoid of one another, in the mess hall or on the yard the men are afraid to be honest with one another for fear of having something thrown up in their face when they get back into a "game" situation. Maybe that doesn't seem very important, but I've seen times when a close brother was afraid to talk to me about something because another close brother who was in his "game" was sitting at my table with us. TA has also got the men into policing themselves.[30]

Some inmates recognize that transactional analysis is a way of brainwashing them, of turning them into "middle American dudes." Not all are willing to play this game, as is shown by the following dialogue between two prisoners who are discussing the death of a thief killed by the police. Who is to blame? The first inmate, a black serving time for robbery himself, says that society is responsible. The second inmate replies, "You took transactional analysis. You know you can choose to be a winner or a loser. Mr. B. chose to be a loser." To this, the first prisoner responds, "He chose to be a loser in the same way I chose to be black. If you stay legal, you stay poor. The legalest man in the world is the poorest."[31]

These methods may have ulterior motives, but at least they have the advantage of being comparatively liberal. Behavior modification, on the other hand, represents a step toward coercion. In the vocabulary of this new disciplinary technique, punishments become "negative reinforcements" and solitary confinement becomes "time-out therapy." Just as in mental hospitals using these techniques, the routine of daily life is programmed by a system of rewards and punishments. The tokens awarded for good behavior buy such "privileges" as the right to possess a comb, to take a shower, or to have a transistor radio in one's cell. Aversion therapy has also been widely used on "hard-core" inmates and sexual offenders, particularly homosexuals. At Somers State Prison in Connecticut, electrodes were attached to the skin of child molesters and a shock was administered each time a photo of a naked child was projected on a screen in front of the prisoner. At Atascadero State Hospital, aversion therapy techniques included the injection of succinylcholine and the use of electric shock treatments to punish homosexuals who "misbehaved" within the institution.[32]

At the Iowa Security Medical Facility—"an institution for persons displaying evidence of mental illness or psychological disorders who require diagnostic services and treatment in a security setting"—apopmorphine was used in aversion therapy of "behavioral problems," that is, in cases of infractions of institutional rules, such as refusing to get up in the morning, insulting guards, or concealing weapons, drugs, etc. In a cell equipped with a basin, a male nurse injected the drug, and the inmate receiving the injection would vomit for anywhere from fifteen minutes to an hour, often experiencing cardiovascular difficulties at the same time. In 1973 inmates filed suit to halt this program. They won because the judge found that there was no way to determine whether or not the use of apomorphine was a recognized medical treatment.[33]

In other words, the legal criterion for accepting or rejecting experimentation of this sort turned on the degree to which the technique in question was genuinely "medical." This may explain why what is probably the most systematic application of behavior modification principles, the program in Maryland's Patuxent Institution, has never been challenged. Opened in 1955, this institution is neither a prison nor a hospital but a combination of the two. The director is a psychiatrist and the staff includes forty psychologists and other professionals for four hundred inmates. According to the institution's charter, its purpose is "to protect society from this segment of the criminal population who will again commit crimes if released on the expiration of a fixed sentence. . . . If they cannot be cured, such indeterminate sentence accomplishes their incarceration for life." Thus inmates are committed for an unspecified term and on the average remain incarcerated for a longer period than if they had received the legally mandated sentence for their crime. The system according to which the institution is run is based on a hierarchy of "ranks," and inmates climb from one echelon to the next in reward for good behavior. Each patient also participates in a therapy group. According to the *Patient's Handbook*, "participation is voluntary. . . . You hold the key to your own future by participation in the institutional program."[34] In fact, both inmates and staff are perfectly aware that the only way to get out of Patuxent is to take part in group therapy and perform satisfactorily during the sessions.

If these systematic disciplinary techniques fail to achieve the desired results, there remains the ultimate weapon in the arsenal of "hard" technologies: psychosurgery, which has already been discussed in the case of California. Of late, there have been increasing numbers of court challenges to the use of psychosurgery. In 1973, for example, the Medical Committee for Human Rights brought suit against the Lafayette Clinic in Detroit, which was accused of performing psychosurgery on prisoners. The court ruled that such operations are legal only if the patient freely chooses to undergo them. When institutional constraints play a part in the decision, the choice is not free.[35] The limitations of the legal remedy are apparent: it is not the principle of psychosurgery that is being rejected but rather the conditions under which it is performed.

As in the case of mental hospitals, then, it is not quite accurate to say that deinstitutionalization describes the new techniques for dealing with criminality and deviance. From 1972 to 1978 the number of prisoners in federal and state institutions actually increased by 50 percent.[36] The main target in institutions has been the repeat offender, of whom the National Commission on Criminal Justice Standards and Court Goals had this to say:

> He is found in virtually every type of institution. He represents a constant danger for the other prisoners and prison personnel as well as for the public, on account of his repeated attempts to escape. Although he is not psychotic, he resists every attempt to control or change him. He reacts with pronounced hostility to the least admonition to behave reasonably. He frequently urges other inmates to rebel and uses physical intimidation to achieve his ends.[37]

The irreducible hard-core prison population very likely does consist largely of this sort of inmate, a hybrid in whom the signs of delinquency, pathology, social maladjustment, and political rebelliousness become more and more blurred as time goes by. Such individuals are obviously an embarrassment to optimistic ideas of rehabilitation. In spite of this contradiction—the symbol of all the other contradictions of the prison system—research aimed at perfecting new methods of treatment goes on, research whose ultimate aim is to hide from public scrutiny behavior in the prisons that is nothing less than an act of self-defense against society and a rejection of its alien values. When a citizens' group raised doubts that it was really possible for prisoners to submit voluntarily to psychosurgery, the head of California's Department of Justice responded by evoking the plight of criminals sentenced to life terms and asking, "What else can they do?"[38] Perhaps. In that case, however, it is pointless to disguise the cynical purpose of the surgery beneath the rhetoric of humane medicine.

The flaws in the criminal justice system have become so apparent that they are now recognized even by official experts. The commission named by President Carter, for example, observed that

> historically, changes in justice system procedures which have replaced what appear to be severe, inflexible, and formal sanctioning processes with more humanitarian and informal substitutes often trigger unintended consequences, either in the direction of (1) increasing the number of guards surrounding their imposition ("widening the net"); or (2) removing incentives and facilities for official responses to persons with real service needs ("avoidance response").[39]

THE DRUG ADDICT

The use of drugs, particularly heroin, has been a major social problem in the United States in recent years. According to a National Institute of Mental Health study, there were 45,000 heroin addicts in the United States in 1959 and 250,000 ten years later. In 1976 the number of daily users of heroin was estimated at 400,000, half of them in New York City alone.[40] Between two and four million Americans were said to have tried heroin at least once.[41] In 1971 President Nixon branded the drug "public enemy number one." In 1973 New York Governor Nelson Rockefeller, known for his liberal leanings, instituted extraordinarily repressive measures providing life sentences for pushers of hard drugs.

According to some estimates, however, the number of addicts was most likely higher in the early twenties than it is today, perhaps nearly as high as one million.[42] But addiction was not yet recognized as a social scourge. What has happened lately is not so much a drug "epidemic"—a term suggestive of the medicalization of the problem—as a stepping up of coordinated efforts to control certain social groups. Efforts to stamp out opium use in the late nineteenth century are an earlier example of the same strategy. The West Coast experienced a heavy influx of Chinese immigrants beginning in 1850, and opium use was associated in the popular mind with the "yellow peril." Chinese workers played an important role in building the railroads and competed for jobs with other laborers. The fact that they smoked opium apparently did not prevent them from working, but it was used as a pretext for branding them as "different." In 1887 the anti-Chinese lobby secured passage of a law prohibiting importation of opium by Chinese but not by Americans. Even after all opium imports were banned twenty years later, morphine and heroin continued to be sold freely for several years: they were not yet recognized as drugs.[43] In retrospect, the nineteenth and early twentieth centuries have been called a "drug addicts' paradise": morphine and heroin were widely used both for medical purposes (in the treatment of alcoholism, as sedatives, and for "women's troubles") and simply for pleasure.[44] The definition of a substance as a drug is a social act and goes hand in hand with efforts to restrict its use.

Ideas about drug policy in the United States have constantly wavered between two extremes, one medical, the other criminological. Actual policy has been the result of a compromise between the two approaches. The Harrison Act of 1914 prohibited unlicensed sale of opium, morphine, and heroin. Some forty-odd dispensaries were opened where addicts could obtain the drugs legally. Prohibition, however, soon gave rise to a black market that outstripped the legal traffic, and more strenuous repressive measures were instituted. In 1923 the last dispensary was closed, and thereafter narcotics were treated for the most part as illicit contraband. Even the two "narcotic farms" opened by the federal government at Lexington, Kentucky, in 1935 and at Fort Worth, Texas, in 1938 were not so much treatment centers as prisons, to which inmates were referred by the courts and which produced very low cure rates. The American Medical Association steadfastly opposed ambulatory treatment for drug addicts until the late fifties.

Beginning in the early sixties, drug policy once again veered toward the opposite extreme, accentuating the medical aspect—although now the generally approved form of treatment was closely connected with legal incarceration or compulsion of some sort. In 1961 a California state law was passed setting up rehabilitation centers for drug addicts and even for people "in danger of becoming addicts." Members of the public could apply for admission even if they had committed no crime. In 1966 the Narcotic Addict Rehabilitation Act extended this type of policy to the federal level. Funds were provided to state and local governments to develop treatment and rehabilitation programs. More and more addicts were "sentenced to treatment" by being obliged to participate in these programs for indeterminate periods ranging up to ten years. The choice sometimes offered addicts between such programs and prison terms is illusory. To cite one example, the California Rehabilitation Center, the largest treatment facility in California, is surrounded by a double wall topped by two watchtowers. Inside, it is against the rules to move from one closed cellblock to another, and some of the staff are armed. Just as in the case of the criminal justice system analyzed earlier, addict treatment programs have been used not so much to provide more humane ways of dealing with drug addiction as to broaden the range of cases subject to official control. At the Abraxas Foundation in Pennsylvania, for example, only 15 percent of the inmates are heroin-dependent. The rest are users of alcohol, hallucinogens, marijuana, or glue and other inhalants. According to one member of the staff, most of the youths sent to this program would have preferred to go to prison.[45] But many of them had not committed offenses that warranted prison terms.

Treatment of drug addiction has been based mainly on two models. One of these was developed by nonprofessionals, usually reformed drug addicts. The purpose of this type of treatment was to change the addict's personality and transform him psychologically and morally by structuring his life in the context of a "therapeutic community." The other treatment model, which was developed more recently and which has lately seen increasingly widespread use, is conceived along more traditional medical lines. It is based on the controlled use of a substitute drug, methadone.

The prototype of the therapeutic community for addicts is Synanon, founded in 1958 by a former addict, Charles Dederich. From the outset, treatment at Synanon was antimedical in conception: self-help was the rule, and this was to be fostered by group activities and isolation from "straight" society. The community was supposed to be a large family living in economic independence from the rest of the world. Today it owns real estate valued at several million dollars, and branches have been established in a number of cities across the United States.[46] As of 1971, ten to twelve thousand addicts were said to have passed through Synanon's facilities. The Synanon idea has served directly or indirectly as inspiration for many other communities, such as Daytop Village, Phoenix House, and Odyssey House in the East, each with several branches, and Delancey Street in San Francisco, where two hundred fifty residents manage seven businesses—restaurants, garages, moving companies, and so on—from which they earn their livelihood.

Synanon's techniques are also widely imitated, especially the "Synanon game." In this game the drug user is induced by group pressure to change his life and drop his street image. The goal, often reached only after violent confrontations, is to break down the addict's ego defenses and then reconstitute a "normal" and disciplined personality. The underlying philosophy is this: "Synanon views its members as emotional infants and through a combination of concern and firmness guides them to emotional maturity."[47]

Most therapeutic communities use "behavioral learning" techniques based on obedience and discipline, the point of which is to make each person monitor his own behavior by forcing him to monitor the behavior of all the others. Community residents generally advance through a hierarchy of echelons. Upon entering the community, each person is assigned to the lowest echelon, which means that the most menial jobs fall to him. Advancement through the ranks is supposed to correspond to progress toward a cure; progress in both respects is gauged by how closely the individual fits the norms of the community and how well he handles a series of tests in which other members of the community witness and comment upon his behavior, criticizing any signs of nonconformity, if need be. This is referred to as showing a "responsible concern" for others. Survival of the community and respect for its norms are regarded as absolute values. To cite one example, two individuals sent under court order to the Phoenix

House on Hart Island (New York) filed habeas corpus writs asking that they be released. It was pointed out to them that taking such a step injured the morale of the other residents and had a deleterious effect on their capacity to benefit from the program. This sign of a negative attitude was said by one member of the staff to be "a malignant cancer that had to be cut or squeezed out of the house."[48]

If a resident violates one of the rules of the community, he may be expelled (which in many cases means being turned over to the police or the courts) or demoted to a lower echelon. Sometimes he may be forced to bear some mark of his crime (such as a shaved head, a degrading article of clothing, or a sign recording his misdeeds). Conversely, conformity is rewarded handsomely, the ultimate success being appointment to the supervisory staff of the institution. In some therapeutic communities, such as the Phoenix House, the majority of the staff is made up of former addicts.

Is *psychiatrization* really an apt word to describe such therapeutic communities? Because of the lack of any real psychiatric or psychoanalytic treatment for drug addiction, it has been necessary to use nonprofessionals, often recruited among addicts themselves. As we shall see in the next chapter, the free clinics that were founded in the sixties faced the same sort of situation: when official institutions are incapable of coping with a problem, there is a certain freedom for marginal outsiders to try new approaches. But this freedom is subject to strict limitations. Addicts are perfectly aware, even when they choose voluntarily to enter a therapeutic community, that they are at the end of their rope, being wanted by the police and the courts on the outside. When an addict is allowed by a judge to choose between entering one of these communities and going to prison, the judge knows that such apparent laxity involves no great risk, since the communities, though not run by government officials like the prisons, are nevertheless "total institutions." They subject the deviant individual to a carefully devised system of constraints, designed to drive home the stringent rules that are supposed to govern normal existence.

Thus, despite the frequently antimedical ideologies of these communities, they have in their own way reinvented the old principles of moral treatment on which traditional psychiatry was based. In a crude but effective way they have fashioned their own teaching style involving rewards and punishments: behavior modification therapy is merely a more "scientific" version of the same thing. It is hardly surprising, then, that the predominantly coercive methods worked out in these self-styled "antiprofessional" institutions have been taken over by the psychiatric establishment. The Synanon game and similar techniques have been used in traditional institutions and therapeutic communities such as Crossroads near Chicago.[49] Antidrug programs such as the Illinois drug abuse program have used Synanon-type techniques in conjunction with the most traditional psychiatric methods in multidimensional approaches to drug-related problems. Similar techniques are now being used to deal with an ever wider range of cases. Originally designed for use with hard drug addicts, for whom a therapeutic community was a last resort, the same methods are now applied to juveniles accused of abusing alcohol, amphetamines, or hallucinogens.

This model for treating drug addiction is of secondary importance, however. It has been estimated that no more than 5 percent of all addicts enter therapeutic communities.[50] The number of cases treated successfully is more difficult to evaluate. Most of these institutions claim a high cure rate, on the order of 80 percent, but individuals who drop out of the program prior to completion are not counted in the figures. Furthermore, the communities cannot exist without individual and local initiative. They are hard to incorporate into a comprehensive policy, and it is open to question whether the techniques are effective when used outside the context of an isolated, self-supporting community and without the presence of a charismatic leader. For these reasons, the other strategy for dealing with drug addiction has become increasingly popular: the strategy based on the medical model.

In 1963 two doctors at New York's Rockefeller Institute began research into the effects of methadone, a synthetic narcotic discovered by the Germans during World War II as a substitute for morphine. Taken orally once a day, methadone quells the addict's need for heroin and eliminates the symptoms of craving for the drug. The researchers concluded that around 80 percent of hard drug addicts could be rehabilitated by use of methadone.[51]

The discovery of methadone came to light at a critical moment, when large numbers of blacks and Puerto Ricans were migrating to large cities, particularly New York, and the federal government was launching its War on Poverty, in part because of the need to establish control over social fringe groups and cope with the fear they aroused in the rest of the populace (see chapter 3). Accordingly, middle-class New Yorkers were first sold on methadone as a drug capable of controlling deviant behavior and consequently of enhancing the security of the city:

> If a way could be found to transform street addicts into productive citizens, society would not only be spared the cost and indignity of massive jails, but would also gain support for families now being carried by public funds, and, with improvement of neighborhoods, would diminish the rate of new addictions. . . . With a narcotic blockade [like methadone] patients can be made indifferent to heroin and capable of functioning as normal individuals in free society.[52]

What was at first a big-city problem involving relations between the middle classes and ethnic minorities later became a national problem when drugs moved beyond the ghetto and, eventually, with the Vietnam War, infiltrated all the pores of American society. In 1971, the year Nixon declared his war on drugs, it was estimated that one out of five Vietnam veterans was a drug addict.[53] In the same year the Pentagon directed that the urine of all servicemen be analyzed for signs of drug use. One official document listed the following virtues of methadone:

1. Elimination of Illegal Drug Use
2. Adoption of a Productive and Self-fulfilling Life Style
3. Elimination of Criminal Behavior
4. Stabilization of Clients on Methadone Maintenance.[54]

In fact methadone itself is far from harmless. *The New York Times* estimated in 1973 that more people in New York City died of methadone than of heroin. Compared with heroin, however, methadone has two decisive advantages in connection with drug control policy: there is no withdrawal, so users are less likely to be driven to violent crime in search of drugs or money to satisfy their craving, and users become dependent on methadone and are thereby forced to submit to daily scrutiny by the medical personnel who dispense the drug. Official documents recognize the fact that methadone users are in a dependent state and hold that this is one key to its effectiveness. One stated that many addicts have difficulty forming close relationships, and if they were not dependent on methadone, they would find it difficult if not impossible to go to the dispensary every day and establish a long-term relationship with the staff. Thus the dependence created by methadone is crucial to establishing a potentially therapeutic and rehabilitative relationship with the addict.[55]

Again, this a situation that people must be forced to accept. It is estimated that only one-quarter of the people enrolled in methadone programs volunteered for the treatment. Most federal programs classed as "treatment alternatives to street crime" were quite coercive, despite the lip service paid to treatment. After arrest, suspected drug abusers are tested and, if found to be addicts, placed in a treatment program, either while being held in jail or under a provisional release program, in many cases before their cases have even come to trial. More than thirty thousand addicts had been treated under this program by 1977.[56]

Methadone research has also led to the development of narcotics antagonists, drugs such as naltrexone, cyclazocine, naloxine, and others, which block the effects of specific narcotics. In 1973 the director of the Special Action Office for Drug Abuse, a government agency, suggested using these substances in a preventive program designed to "immunize high-risk populations". He thought that doctors and community officials might use these techniques on high-risk populations in the same way that x-rays have been used to test groups that run a high risk of contracting tuberculosis. In this way they could uncover heroin users before they became addicts. Once identified, these potential addicts could be temporarily immunized by means of a daily treatment.[57] Another scheme was to place antagonist drugs in the water supply in certain high-risk neighborhoods such as Harlem.[58]

Not surprisingly, these programs met with a hostile reception from knowledgeable leaders of minority groups, who charged that methadone was "therapy directed against the black community" and even "a kind of genocide," an "instrument of colonialism." In 1971 a national congress of black doctors and health workers declared that methadone was "an attempt to control large segments of the nonwhite population by reducing them to a state of dependence."[59] Some minority organizations, such as the Detox Center in the Bronx (see next chapter), attempted to deal with their own drug problems by making a political analysis of their situation. Radical groups such as Health Policy Advisory Center (Health P.A.C.) in New York also criticized the political implications of methadone and similar programs.

This kind of resistance to treatment had considerable influence on Governor Rockefeller's decision to toughen antidrug policy in 1973. Once again, this move illustrates how the approach to the problem tends to swing back and forth between medical and legal remedies; in reality, it is clear that the two alternatives are merely different forms of the same policy. The law mandating mandatory life sentences for drug pushers was unconstitutional, yet it impelled many addicts to submit to treatment against their will.[60]

More than 80,000 addicts are now being maintained on methadone in 450 clinics. (Doctors cannot prescribe methadone for private patients.) Treatment of addiction relies more and more on medical methods. Originally the urine of addicts receiving methadone was checked to make sure they actually swallowed the drug. Lately, more and more tests are being administered to addicts receiving methadone, including tests for hepatitis, venereal disease, general physical condition, and so forth. As one researcher ironically put it, "this is more in keeping with the medical model."[61] At the same time, this involves a tightening of control over "high-risk populations"—known in Europe as the "dangerous classes"—and the feeding of more and more information about them into computer data banks.

THE ALCOHOLIC

The history of the treatment of alcoholism in the United States parallels that of drug addiction and exhibits the same shifting back and forth between medical and criminal approaches. As early as 1780 Benjamin Rush considered immoderate use of distilled beverages a pathological symptom and estimated the number of deaths due to alcohol at 4,000 each year, out of a population of 6 million.[62] Today the number of "problem drinkers" is said to be on the order of 9 million.[63] In 1965, 40 percent of all arrests were for public drunkenness or driving under the influence.[64] Estimates of the percentage of alcoholics among hospital patients and particularly mental hospital inmates range from 10 to 50 percent.[65] These are very rough figures and depend largely on whether alcoholism is taken to be a primary diagnosis or a symptom associated with another "disease."

The prohibition movement, always strong in the United States, is evidence of the moral animus against alcoholism. In 1833 there were more than 6,000 local temperance societies with more than a million members. The Prohibition Party was organized after the Civil War, and laws passed in several states made antialcohol propaganda mandatory in the schools. In 1919 the Eighteenth Amendment to the Constitution inaugurated prohibition, which remained the law of the land until 1933. Alcohol could be prescribed by a doctor as a "therapeutic agent," however, and in 1928 the whiskey laws were worth 40 million dollars a year in income to American physicians.[66] Prohibition remained in force in Mississippi until 1966 thanks to the support of religious groups, and there are still many "dry" counties in the South.

Not until 1947 was a federal law passed mandating treatment and rehabilitation for alcoholics, who were still defined in moral terms. According to the law, an alcoholic is a "person who chronically or habitually uses alcoholic beverages . . . [until he has] lost the power of self-control [and/or] endangers public morals, health, safety, or welfare."[67] According to this law, judges can remand alcoholics to special treatment programs. In 1956 the American

Medical Association declared that "alcoholism is a disease that deserves medical attention" and recommended placing alcoholics in hospitals rather than prisons. The Vocational Rehabilitation Act of 1965 allocated special funds for the diagnosis, treatment, and eventual return to society of alcoholics. The Uniform Alcoholism and Intoxication Treatment Act of 1971 aimed to make new funds available for the decriminalization of alcoholism and for setting up detoxication centers in various parts of the country.

Court decisions reflect the hesitation to decide whether alcoholics are criminals or victims of disease. Initially, the Supreme Court decided that alcoholics could not be punished for exhibiting behavior judged to be a pathological symptom. As a result, 3,400 habitual drinkers in Washington alone were issued a card stating that they were chronic alcoholics and could not be arrested for drunkenness.[68] But in 1968 the Supreme Court issued a conflicting decision that made it legal to arrest chronic alcoholics for being intoxicated in public.

The question remains clouded because medicine has not demonstrated a capacity to deal with the problem—far from it. The most effective treatments, apparently, are those administered not by professionals but rather by private groups such as Alcoholics Anonymous, which was founded in 1935 and which now has some thirty thousand affiliates throughout the United States.[69] In institutions where medical approaches are preferred, group therapy techniques have been tried. Hypnosis and behavior modification have been coupled with the usual sermons about the pernicious effects of alcohol. Antiabuse treatments have not proved particularly effective.

Once again, medicine and psychiatry have been used as camouflage for attempts to identify and control groups that pose threats of one sort or another to law and order, even though the problems are hard to define and no effective treatment techniques exist. "Problem drinker" is certainly as ambiguous a category as "addict" or "abnormal personality," and there is just as little psychiatric knowledge to justify any particular definition. Nevertheless, a new type of repression, referred to euphemistically as "treatment," has been developed to deal with alcoholic cases that the court system can no longer handle. In this connection we should mention one of the most recent measures taken in the battle against alcoholism in the United States. The Alcohol Safety Action Program has since 1971 been administered by the Department of Transportation. A driver arrested while under the influence must undergo a series of tests designed to find out if he is a "problem drinker," a "social drinker," and so on. Depending on the results, the judge can sentence the person to detoxification, psychotherapy, or court supervision. That these measures result in a "cure" is open to question. Recent evaluations, in fact, show that their effectiveness is almost nil.[70] But their purpose is to intimidate and control the daily behavior of drinkers.

In view of the foregoing, two general methodological remarks may be made that hold good whether we are studying delinquents, drug addicts, alcoholics, or, more broadly, deviants of any sort. First, the different institutions availabe for dealing with these problems—including police, mental health centers, prisons, parole officers, therapeutic communities, detoxification centers, etc.— must not be analyzed independently. The "soft" institutions cannot function without the "hard" ones, and vice versa. The whole spectrum of services constitutes an instrument of social control, and frequently a particular subject is shifted about from one point on the spectrum to another. For example, the addict who misbehaves in a therapeutic community can easily find himself back in prison, while a prisoner may find himself released for good conduct on condition that he submit to medical supervision. No matter what type of facility we look at, we find transactional therapy groups and awareness training groups. We find behavior-modification drugs that addicts have the dubious privilege of testing. Among the staff we are likely to find former police officers who have taken courses in prison education and who now do primal scream therapy with the inmates. Just as the various institutions support one another, so, too, do the roles of different specialists overlap. Similar techniques are used in many different institutions. When one solution fails, another can be tried; a hard approach can be taken after a soft one has failed to produce results, or vice versa. Trial and error continues until a slot in the system has been found for each deviant.

Our second methodological remark is this: the labels used by recent reformers to camouflage the old repressive machinery should not be taken literally. Undoubtedly, the use of medical and psychological terminology in connection with surveillance and control techniques designed to deal with deviance, delinquency, and alienation is more than mere window-dressing: the terminology has important practical implications. But the new vocabulary has not eliminated the brutality that is endemic in American prisons, and massacres such as the one at Attica have taken place at the same time the "humanization process" is going on. The new techniques have made it possible to tighten surveillance and control and extend their range. If prisons are beginning to look like hospitals, this means that their claim to provide therapy is not incompatible with their repressive function.

CHILDHOOD, THE PRIMARY CONCERN

As everybody knows, an ounce of prevention is worth a pound of cure—and what better time to practice prevention than early childhood? Childhood has attracted the attention of all the professions that specialize in suspicion: examiners, testers, and detectors of all sorts of anomalies. And children have found themselves enmeshed in a web of surveillance and techniques of behavior control.

Early childhood intervention was first the province of specialized institutions (where it is still practiced). As we have seen (chapter 4), the children's wards of mental hospitals and residential treatment centers for emotionally disturbed children are among the few institutions whose populations are still growing. For children even more often than adults, psychiatric labels are often thin disguises for difficulties in adjusting to specific social, family, or scholastic situations rather than descriptions of clear-cut pathologies. It is relatively easy to commit children because many states allow the parents to do as they please, as long as the child is under eighteen and a medical certificate has been obtained. Recent court decisions have begun to alter this picture by establishing that children above the age of thirteen or fourteen have certain rights to be heard by the courts before they are placed. The American Psychiatric Association has opposed these developments, however, on the grounds that court hearings may upset the child and because in its view there is a fundamental social interest in preserving the integrity and autonomy of the family unit.[71]

Along with families, social service agencies are largely responsible for the institutionalization of "problem children." A typical example: a black woman in Louisiana applied for welfare because her husband had just left her. The welfare department decided that four of her eight children must be placed in homes. Accordingly, a two-and-a-half year-old boy was sent to live in three different foster homes, one after another, and was then found to be emotionally disturbed and placed in an institution in the state of New York, more than a thousand miles from his home. Three years later he was moved to another institution in Texas. "Every time I asked my case worker when Joey could come home, I was told that he was too sick to come home, he was too emotionally disturbed."[72]

The child returned home after his mother filed a class action suit. Thanks to the trial of this case, 700 Louisiana youngsters were "found" in Texas institutions. It has been estimated that 20,000 children have been similarly placed in institutions outside their home state.[73]

A child might well be "emotionally disturbed" by the conditions commonly found in some of these institutions: unventilated concrete buildings, isolation of stubborn children for periods lasting up to several weeks, use of knockout drugs, etc. Two attendants testified in 1974 before a Senate committee that they had been dismissed from a Florida home for refusing to administer injections of carbon dioxide and urine as punishments.[74]

Optimistic readers will no doubt take the view that such horrors are remnants of another age that is rapidly dying out. In our view, it is more accurate to say that, on the contrary, institutional so-

lutions to the problem are still being proposed, with some modifications, especially for the poorest classes of society. The new
methods that are the heart of the modern approach overlap the
old methods without replacing them. The present goal is not
merely to segregate abnormal individuals but also to detect potentially troublesome cases early on. One element of the new
strategy is to examine everyone belonging to certain specific social
groups or age categories.

In 1969 President Nixon asked his Secretary of Health, Education, and Welfare for an opinion on a report prepared by his
personal physician suggesting that "the government should conduct mass testing of all children between the ages of six and eight
in order to identify those exhibiting violent or homicidal tendencies." Those found to have "delinquent tendencies" would
undergo "corrective treatment"—psychological counseling, treatment in a mental health center, and for high-risk young criminals,
a stint in a special camp.[75] The director of the National Institute
of Mental Health answered on behalf of the secretary that the
identification technology was not yet sufficiently advanced to
make the results of such testing reliable. Still, there are already
systematic examinations of smaller groups thought to involve
special risks.

To give one example, all children receiving Medicaid benefits
(i.e., children of welfare families) undergo what is known as an
"early periodic screening and diagnostic test," which includes
medical, dental, and other examinations, as well as, in certain
states, psychological and behavioral testing beginning in early
childhood. In Baltimore, for instance, several thousand schoolchildren, mostly from the ghetto, were tested in 1973 for "mal-
adaptive tendencies" and "potential delinquency." In California's
Orange County schoolchildren identified as potential delinquents
by their teachers were assigned a counselor responsible both for
assisting and for supervising them. On the pretext of prevention,
the concept of "predelinquent" and similar notions were used to
justify surveillance of large numbers of youths, many of whom
had never been in trouble with the law. The idea of "diverting"
individuals away from prison, already discussed in connection

with adult offenders, reaches the height of absurdity when coupled with the ideology of early childhood intervention: it has been used to justify the intrusion, without the usual legal guarantees, of specialists into the lives of youngsters who have committed no crime. Under one delinquency prevention program in Oakland, California, for example, counselors were sent to speak to the brothers and sisters of youngsters who got into trouble with the police.

Today, however, it is the school system, backed up by the family, that has become the center of an impressive and growing system for detecting behavioral anomalies and treating them medically. It is common knowledge that the American educational system is particularly inefficient in some areas. Perhaps this is why cause and effect are often reversed, and pupils are made responsible for the poor performance of the school system—a conspicuous example of blaming the victim. More than in other countries, there is in the United States a tendency to diagnose failure and maladjustment as effects of individual problems or maladies; psychological therapy and/or drugs are then prescribed as appropriate treatments.

In 1970 the Undersecretary of Health, Education, and Welfare for Education proposed a plan under which in each school there would be a diagnostic center to which all children would be brought by their parent or tutor at the age of two-and-a-half. The objective of the center would be to gather all possible information about the child and his environment, in order to establish an individualized educational program. Examinations would include an educational diagnostic, a medical diagnostic, and home visits by a competent professional who could become the counselor of the child and the family. Once this information was gathered, the center would know all that it needed to know about the child— his living conditions and family situation, his cultural and linguistic inadequacies, his dietary and medical needs, and his overall individual potential. After processing by computer, this information would be transmitted to a team of specialists that would work out a set of detailed prescriptions for the child and, if necessary, for the family.[76] This information was supposed to be updated every six weeks between the ages of two-and-a-half and six, and every six months thereafter. It was to be made available to municipal health services or the family doctor, as well as to other medical, educational, or welfare service providers that might be of help.[77] Similar programs are now being tested in France.

The American program was not adopted in its original form, however; the utopia of exerting complete technocratic control over childhood has not yet been achieved. "Technocratic control" is nevertheless an apt description of the aims of the childhood intervention policy now being put in place. Dozens of research programs, hundreds of experimental projects, thousands of special courses of instruction for teachers, and millions of tests, diagnostics, and evaluations of children are gradually bringing us nearer the day when childhood will be totally regimented by medicine and psychology. In New York, for example, a typical student file contains no fewer than a dozen cards, including information ranging from the results of dental checkups to personality, behavioral, and aptitude evaluations, as well as a record of all rule violations. Schools are increasingly being used to separate the wheat from the chaff, the normal from the pathological, and growing numbers of specialists are being trained to assist, counsel, and treat what might be called "abnormal pupils." The Carter Commission in 1978 reiterated the need for complete, periodic evaluations of every child's development. It also called for "the development of a community-based health and mental health delivery system in which public schools are the locus of responsibility in providing, obtaining, or assuring preventive and rehabilitative care for children and their families."[78]

Medical metaphors—prevention, rehabilitation, prescription, diagnostic, treatment—have found their way into teaching manuals. A official government publication in 1969 predicted that by 1980 or so "it would be more correct to refer to teachers as learning clinicians."[79] In one Pennsylvania school that accepts only "normal" children, all pupils must take a battery of tests, on the basis of which they are divided into three groups: the "oedipally conflicted," the "developmentally arrested," and the "ego disturbed." For each of these groups there is a specific recommended teaching strategy. Already, then, both the patterning of the pupil's day and the methods of instruction are being shaped by psychoanalytically inspired clinical categories, the appropriateness of which we shall have occasion to judge in what follows.[80]

Whether psychoanalytic ideology will in the future be able to justify medicalization of this sort is open to question, however. It now seems that psychoanalysis is being edged out by two other treatment technologies: drugs and behavior modification.

Five hundred thousand to one million schoolchildren are being "maintained" on drugs. Most are classed as hyperactive or as suffering from so-called minimal brain dysfunction. Both diagnostic categories have been subject to severe abuse. The most commonly used drug is an amphetamine derivative known as Ritalin (methylphenidate hydrochloride), which is marketed by Ciba Laboratories. Originally, the use of Ritalin and similar products was limited to the treatment of chronic fatigue and slight depression in adults. Research on children was financed by large appropriations from the National Institute of Mental Health and by grants from pharmaceutical laboratories. After Ciba-Geigy launched a major advertising campaign in 1970, sales increased at a dizzying rate, and indications for use of the drug were broadened to include emotional disturbances in children. "Is your child hyperactive?" asked an advertisement in one New York newspaper. A youngster who shows signs of excess energy and is very agitated, aggressive, and impulsive is often seen by his parents as "just a typical boy" or a "little devil," the ad continued. It warned parents that such behavior may have a hidden cause, which would have serious consequences on the social development of their child when he or she grew older. Parents were advised to consult their doctor if they thought their child might be hyperactive. The sooner the problem was identified, the sooner parents could get help to aid their child in his problems of social adjustment. The ad stated that there are drugs that can be of great help in treating the hyperactive child, and asked the parent or doctor to give the drug company a call.[81]

Drug company lecturers showed films to audiences of parents and teachers. Before Ritalin treatment: an impossible monster.

After: a little angel. If your child is wearing you out, see your doctor and buy tranquillity in pill form. As one doctor observed in testimony before a Senate committee: "That a disorder usually believed to be relatively uncommon should suddenly become a major affliction of childhood is a mystifying matter. . . . We seem to have a plague of hyperkinetic [hyperactive] children on our hands."[82]

What exactly is this disease that is so susceptible to treatment with the aid of drugs? The notion of "minimal brain dysfunction" emerged in the twenties, when a connection was established between behavioral problems in school and a neurological etiology in connection with work on aphasia.[83] Little more was heard about it until 1965. The notion is a bastard one whose inconsistency is no doubt its great virtue: a presumptive link is established between a "minimal" brain lesion and a functional disorder. That this is the correct etiology remains to be proven. The main research effort was actually focused on linking together the symptoms that supposedly constitute the "MBD (minimal brain dysfunction) spectrum phenomenon."[84] Most of the clinical symptoms are behavioral irregularities that are in no way suggestive of an organic lesion. One writer, summarizing ten years of the medical literature on the subject, draws two conclusions: she notes, first, that

> Hyperactivity is a nonspecific symptom in children. It may appear in a child with a mild adjustment reaction or in one with severe brain damage or schizophrenia, or it may accompany any disturbance of intermediate severity. . . . [And second] hyperactivity is certainly not synononymous with a diagnosis of organic brain syndrome.[85]

The "positive" effects of the drugs seem to have been verified in an equally careless manner. Leaving aside secondary effects (dependence, weight loss, and arrested growth when used for prolonged periods), it has often been noticed that the "symptoms" of the disease disappear during school vacations even when the child stops taking the drug.[86] Whatever the drug's effects, it does not cure the disease or pseudodisease but in most cases merely covers up the symptoms.[87] Two alternatives are available: either the medication must be continued indefinitely or else discontinued, whereupon the child lands back in the original situation—provided no permanent damage has been done in the meantime by the so-called treatment.

Because of the controversial nature of the disease and the problems connected with identifying its symptoms, in particular the inconsistency in the definition of the minimal brain dysfunction syndrome, the Food and Drug Administration in 1975 decided that there were insufficient medical grounds for recognizing the syndrome as a disease for which treatment with a specific drug is indicated. The major symptoms of the disease—short attention span, hyperactivity, impulsive behavior—are still being treated, however, and there is no longer any need to refer to a pseudo-organic lesion as justification. Thus it seems clear that the real target of the treatment is the child's disruptive behavior per se. The therapeutic excuse for the use of these drugs has been abandoned, and they are now openly accepted as instruments of control. As one pediatrician has put it, the object of medication is to improve the functioning of the brain so that the child becomes more normal in his thinking and responses.[88]

The changeover from therapy to pure control has been accentuated by the introduction of behavior modification techniques into the school and family. Because these techniques are focused exclusively on symptoms and not at all on underlying causes, and because it is easy for laymen like parents and teachers to participate in the behavior modification program and even to run such programs themselves, these techniques have found wide application in the educational field. Completely rationalized individual educational programs based on behaviorist precepts have thus been created. Not only has this approach been used to restore discipline in the classroom and to rationalize the learning process (see chapter 8); it has also served as a way of involving parents in the correction of their child's undesirable behavior in accordance with criteria, requirements, and prohibitions laid down by the schools.

Education of parents is a flourishing business in the United States. Parent Effectiveness Training, for example, employs 8,000 teachers (generally retrained social workers), who, for a fee ranging from $50 to $90 per course, have already trained 250,000 parents in parent-child "conflict resolution." An even larger number of parents have read the organization's publications. Another school for parents, the Parent Training Program, is more narrowly focused on the use of behavior modification techniques. Parents are taught to standardize their child's behavior, with a series of objectives marked out at regular calendar intervals on a large chart—ample proof of the scientific seriousness of this experimental method. Every move the child makes, whether sitting at the dinner table or walking in the woods, at work or at play, is interpreted as positive or negative in relation to the goals that have been set. Desirable behavior is rewarded, undesirable behavior punished. Many other teaching manuals are also available to parents, some of them based on B. F. Skinner's behaviorist learning theories.

Thus, apart from those children who are placed in special institutions, whether because they are suffering from more severe disorders or because they come from underprivileged backgrounds, childhood in general has become the prime target of an indiscriminate hunt for anomalous behavior. At school and in the family, teachers and parents have taken on the role of unpaid aides to doctors, psychologists, and other trained professionals, helping to correct ever more minute behavioral irregularities. It will be objected that the school and the family have always been places where standards are set and enforced. The difference now, though, is that more and more refined techniques are being used to track down "abnormal" behavior. The result is that today, millions of children are no longer considered to be part of the general run of mankind—children who are more tranquil or more active than normal, children who are too agitated or too slow—but are instead thought of as being qualitatively different from the normal population and as forming a separate group because they suffer from minimal brain dysfunction, hyperactivity, or functional behavioral disorders.[89]

William Ryan has used the phrase *blaming the victim* to describe the ideologies and practices that have been used in the United States against deprived groups and individuals suspected of menacing law and order. This is how it works:

> First, identify a social problem. Second, study those affected by the problem and discover in what ways they are different from the rest of us as a consequence of deprivation and injustice. Third, define the differences as the cause of the problem itself. Finally, of course, assign a government bureaucrat to invent a humanitarian action program to correct the difference.[90]

Ryan may be overly optimistic on one point: describing the programs thus invented as "humanitarian." This is the adjective he applies, in particular, to the War on Poverty of the sixties, a period during which generosity was frequently mixed up with ulterior political motives. Since that time, some of the ambiguity surrounding federal policy has been dispelled. The purpose of that policy is now clearly to reduce social conflict and shore up weak spots in the social order, and increasing emphasis has been placed on providing efficient, value-neutral treatment bathed in the prestigious aura of science. There are lessons to be drawn from these developments.

First of all, there is now a range of "technical fixes" available for dealing with social problems. Take delinquency, for example. In 1973 the federal government sponsored a program in Springfield, Missouri, that was designed to serve as a model for prison reorganization: the so-called START, or Special Treatment and Rehabilitation Training program. Prisoners were first deprived of all amusements, such as reading matter, radio, and television. They were then constantly watched to monitor their progress toward "correct" behavior. As they advanced toward the goal through eight different stages, their harsh living conditions were gradually improved. Total planning of prison life in keeping with the precepts of behavioral "science" was supposed to solve the problem of running the prisons while at the same time preparing prisoners for reentry into society.[91] Meanwhile, at the annual congress of the American Correctional Association held in the same year, a small device was shown which could be attached to the wrist of a parolee so that the police would always know his whereabouts. Behavioral manipulation almost mathematical in its precision for use in the prisons, technical gadgets for controlling deviance on the outside—the technologies now exist and await their users.

There is also constant pressure to apply these technologies to new groups within the population that remain outside the sphere of influence of the courts and standard medical practice, whose traditional concerns have been exclusively with overt criminal behavior and cases of clear pathology. The psychiatric model elaborated by Caplan (see chapter 5) has been pressed into service elsewhere: to prevent emotional disorders, to identify potentially dangerous situations as quickly as possible, and to deal with disturbances before they become too severe. The strategy of combatting "social scourges" requires the means to intervene, if merely to pinpoint the problem, *prior* to its manifestation as pathological or criminal behavior. Accordingly, investigation has been overstepping the bounds of privacy, naturally in the name of the general interest: signs of potential trouble must be detected even if doing so requires penetrating to the sphere of subjective feelings. Investigative inquiry has also blurred the traditional dividing lines between individual pathology and social conditioning, between criminal behavior and political activity. If trouble is to be avoided, particular vigilance must be exercised with regard to certain high-risk groups. As though by accident, these just happen to be social groups with objective reasons for dissatisfaction with the existing social order. This, however, is a political consideration that value-neutral technocrats need not take into consideration. After the 1967 race riots in Detroit, for example, three well-known doctors proposed in a letter to the *Journal of the American Medical Association* that the arrested rioters be examined to see if any of them were suffering from brain lesions that would be likely to lower their "violence threshold," and if so that they be given special treatment.[92] The USSR is not the only country in which the boundary line between social and political dissidence and pathological or criminal behavior is blurred.

To date, organized resistance to the use of these new techniques has been directed against their spread. For instance, the START program was postponed after prisoners staged a sixty-five day hunger strike, which was backed up by a press campaign. This protest paved the way for challenges to the introduction of behavior modification techniques into other prisons.[93] Other proposals, such as the project to systematically identify all potentially dangerous children, were never instituted for fear of provoking hostile reactions. Nevertheless, these projects have not been permanently laid to rest, and periodically they reemerge in one new guise after another. There is no lack of objective scientists who are ready and willing to head out into the field, as it were, to help perfect the latest behavior control technologies, which were first worked out in laboratory experiments on rats and chimpanzees. And there are always government officials ready to embrace such technologies as the solution to all their problems. All this is done in the name of progress, knowledge, efficient management, and of course the public interest. Hence it is likely to become more and more difficult to mount an effective opposition. As long as authoritarian repression of nonconformist behavior was carried on in the name of an openly repressive ideology, what was at stake politically was clear. But when repression is carried out in the guise of treatment offered to the victims of society, there is a temptation to believe in the good intentions of those offering to provide services. If we are right in thinking that we are now witnessing a transition to a new and more effective level of technological manipulation of marginal social groups, then criticism of social control policies must also shift its ground to focus on the manipulative uses of the "scientific" approach.

CHAPTER 7

Alternatives to Psychiatry and Psychiatrization of the Alternatives

Thus far we have tried to examine the consequences of policies inspired mainly by official agencies—federal, state, and city bureaucracies, established psychiatric organizations, and the courts—and aimed at changing the way the mental health care system is organized. But changes in the system have also been influenced by initiatives of a quite different kind, which grew out of protest movements that originated outside the system. What we have in mind is the counterculture movement that flourished during the sixties.

During this period American society went through a crisis. At the risk of being overly schematic, we should like to identify two tendencies in the movements that emerged in response to this crisis. One tendency was more explicitly political and attacked the very foundations of American society (this included such minority group organizations as the Black Muslims and Black Panthers, radical white student groups such as the Students for a Democratic Society and some antiwar groups, and more traditional Marxist groups such as the Socialist Workers Party). The other tendency had a more countercultural orientation, identifying its enemy not as capitalism per se but rather as bureaucracy, technology, authoritarianism, and hierarchy. Led by middle-class youths, this "revolution" gave prominence to the struggle against an authoritarian social order that impeded the formation of authentic interpersonal relationships. The objective was to abolish alienation by seizing control of the basic social institutions responsible for the production, consumption, and transmission of culture and services. Concretely, one approach to this goal was community organizing, based on methods worked out earlier in the civil rights movement. The procedure was to analyze the needs of the community, take control of power locally in its most routine guises, and organize around specific objectives. The primary strategy was to set up alternative institutions, such as communal farms, self-managed cooperatives, alternative schools, and various consumer co-ops run by the consumers themselves. Taking control of everyday social functions would call forth a new type of sociability, which was supposed to do away with exploitation and foster individual growth.

In contrast to the transparent, "liberated" social relations characteristic of this utopian ideal, mental institutions served as a kind of countermodel, exhibiting rigid hierarchy, authoritarian control, formalistic relationships between clients and staff, and an ideology of professionalism. It is therefore appropriate that mental institutions have been a prime target of the countercultural offensive. Unlike movements in other countries, and particularly France, where similar ideologies have since 1968 been motivating criticism that has rarely moved beyond mere rhetoric, the American movement deserves credit for having spawned practical initiatives impressive for their number and variety. Free clinics, feminist and gay therapies, "radical" therapies, self-help groups, and organizations of present and former mental patients have provided outlets to many people who had been looking confusedly for new kinds of treatment but who had been unwilling to be branded as "mentally ill."

Now that similar attempts are being made in Europe, we feel that these American efforts deserve to be treated at length. Though minority movements, they nevertheless represent genuinely new approaches, and their impact on the official mental health care system has been far from negligible. Another reason for taking a long look at these alternative programs is that after ten years of operation we can begin to ask, in the light of certain recent events, what the future holds for them: Do they represent alternatives to psychiatry or a psychiatrization of the alternatives? It is probably no accident that, in the late seventies, *State and Mind*, an American journal that reports on these alternative movements, devoted a great deal of space to European "alternatives to psychiatry," whose inspiration is more political.[1] It seems that the American alternatives, which got off to an earlier start and have gone farther in practice, have now arrived at the critical stage where they are beginning to ask how their actual accomplishments compare with their initial aims.

THE FREE CLINICS: THE SUMMER OF LOVE

It was sometimes called the "summer of love." Thousands of adolescents, most of them of middle-class origins, turned their backs on the comforts of the suburbs and headed for San Francisco in the summer of 1967, in search of themselves, free love, hallucinogenic drugs, "good vibes," a new culture, and a revolution that would bring down the walls of the old world.

It was in 1967 in San Francisco that the first free clinic was founded, the famous Haight–Ashbury Medical Clinic located in the heart of the hippie district. The clinic was needed because "tripping" brought with it a spate of medical and social problems and an increased incidence of infectious and venereal diseases, due to unstable life styles, to an absence of hygiene, and above all to the use of drugs, which were often taken by people ignorant of their effects. Two of the founders of another free clinic that opened the following year in Boston, when the hippie wave broke on the East Coast, put it this way:

> There were many casualties among the kids that summer and following summers. Not only from the harassment of police, but from the terrifyingly free lifestyle they led. Sexual freedom can be oppressive, particularly when one is unclear about one's needs and desires and is responding to the social pressure to be liberated. Acid makes you crazy. It may be the craziness of immense creativity and joy, or it may be the craziness of unimaginable terror and disorientation. Unlike the peyote-eating Indians of the Southwest, the kids had no tradition of myth and

ritual to make sense of their mind-changing experience. They were like explorers of a foreign planet without maps or compasses.[2]

The new demands confronted traditional medical institutions with challenges they could not meet. Nor did they wish to meet them, because the prospective new clients were peculiar: young men with long hair and girls in Indian dresses, kids who were not sick in any standard sense, who were seeking food and a place to sleep more than professional attention, and who in any case were unable to pay for the services they were after. Then, too, the traditional institutions were quite often unprepared to deal with the new syndromes associated with drug use, the "bad trip" and the "freak-out," to which their initial response was to administer heavy doses of drugs that left the youngsters in psychological disarray when they did not cause serious physical damage. Conversely, the new clients, rightly or wrongly, were suspicious that health officials were cooperating with the police, and they were unwilling to abide by the bureaucratic regulations laid down by the institutions.

The free clinic alternative to psychiatry was born out of the movement itself. Thomas Szasz's criticisms of the concept of mental illness, Erving Goffman's attack on bureaucratic mental institutions, and David Cooper and Ronald Laing's attempt to describe schizophrenia as a valid existential experience and to link politics to personal experience all provided theoretical underpinnings to the self-help philosophy. The prevailing values of the counterculture are epitomized in the word *free*. The "free" in "free clinic" refers not only to the fact that services are provided free of charge but also to a philosophy that emphasizes freedom and authenticity in interpersonal relationships. These values were supposed to be reflected in the organization of the clinics:

> In the origins of the free clinic movement, a major issue was freedom from "bureaucratic tangles" and freedom to treat people as human beings rather than criminals, a particularly important issue in regard to the drug abuse population. . . . The free clinic philosophy implies a minimum of red tape and other barriers between doctors and patients, and also freedom from applying conventional labels and value systems to individuals regarded as "deviant" by the dominant culture.[3]

This general attitude was reflected in certain more specific characteristics of the movement, such as its goals of challenging the medical hierarchy and of calling into question the differences in status between patients and staff and between professionals and untrained volunteers. Another aim was to demystify technological fixes and medical knowledge:

> Experience of your own life, of others' lives, and the experience of other truly radical "therapists" is what counts. (And we mean mainly non-professional "therapists.") Those are not things you learn in psychiatry training, psychology training, or any other institution; those are things that we share with one another in terms of sensitivity to suffering, a world view of the society and its victims, and awareness of what we can do to help. We trust our gut feelings a lot. We have helped many people get through emotional crises through that trust—trust flows between people when it is real.[4]

What was being attacked was the very notion of "expertise," the idea of technical competence associated with professional status, in a generally anti-intellectual climate that emphasized the primacy of feeling, experience, spontaneity, and immediacy of shared feelings.

The movement also opposed the way traditional relief services were dispensed, the requirement that applicants for welfare submit to humiliating investigations. In the free clinics services were dispensed as a gift. The privacy of clients was respected, and often patients were listed in the files by code number rather than name. The atmosphere was friendly and informal. Traditional notions of normality were called into question, and the various forms of "deviant" behavior—mental illness, homosexuality, drug-induced states, sexual promiscuity, and refusal to work—were accepted without judgment. The free clinics at first seemed to tolerate anything and everything, and alienated young people rushed from every quarter to seek refuge in these no man's lands in the battlefield of the sixties.

Since the clinic staff and founders were themselves part of the "movement," the atmosphere of the clinics was naturally convivial. Most staff workers were young college dropouts who had begun work in the field of mental health and who viewed their commitment to the free clinics as a way of straddling the fence: they could maintain contact with the counterculture but at the same time compensate for their disillusionment with direct political action, an avenue many of them had explored. As many as two-thirds of the professionals who got involved with the new clinics were former civil rights activists who felt out of place in establishment institutions and who were curious to explore this presumably more rewarding alternative. They donated several hours of their time free of charge each week to the clinics (though some of them, as we shall see shortly, looked upon the free clinics as a potential source of new clients).

The magnitude of the movement is difficult to measure quantitatively. In 1970 tens of thousands of young people were served by around three hundred free clinics. Most were located in two areas that were magnets to young dropouts, the San Francisco Bay area and the environs of Boston. Free clinics caught on rapidly because they provided certain specific services to a very special public, services that were difficult if not impossible to find elsewhere. One such service was the hot line, where around-the-clock advice could be had about where to find a place to sleep or what to do to come down from a bad trip. The hot lines spawned a new service, drug counseling, or advice about the effects of specific drugs. As the need arose, the range of problems dealt with was broadened to include sexual counseling, legal advice, and so on. A distraught caller was sure to find a sympathetic listener on the other end of the line, someone who would refrain from making any sort of moral judgment.

Another service offered by the clinics was information about where to find a place to sleep off the streets—a "crash pad," in the argot of the times—and out of reach of the police, who combed the cities looking for runaways. In the crash pads no questions were asked and there were no rules: the slogan was "do your own thing," and the atmosphere was relaxed, the antithesis of the strict homes the young people were fleeing.

A third type of service offered was counseling, which revolved mainly around group activities. There were two reasons for this.

Groups were necessary to cope with the heavy demand, and they fit in with the reigning counterculture ideology, according to which group activities were an important element in the process of cultural change. "We solve problems in groups instead of in individual therapy because we feel that teaching people to act collectively is a vital part of our work as community organizers."[5] Therapy groups were often hard to tell apart from work or living groups. Group leaders generally had little technical training, and most groups (rap groups) were open to all comers, with the membership changing from session to session as moods and affinities varied and individuals came and went.

Free clinics usually offered all three services, along with certain others, primarily emergency treatment. Often a team was on call, ready to respond to outside emergencies. The emergency staff handled medical examinations and lab tests and prescribed and handed out medication. Special attention was paid to drug education, and detailed information about the nature, effects, and counterindications of various drugs was widely distributed. Visitors to the clinics were not lectured about drug use, but they were made aware of the dangers and taught how to prepare for a "trip." Warnings were issued when bad drugs were known to be on the market. All this is in sharp contrast to the measures taken by establishment institutions, which tried to talk the youth out of using drugs by spreading false and alarmist information, such as "marijuana kills," "LSD can cause blindness," and so forth. Free clinics also offered feminist and homosexual counseling before these became available elsewhere, as well as pregnancy and abortion counseling at a time when abortion was still not legal in the United States. All these services were designed to make medical information in plain language widely available. Practical advice was offered on how to help people out of difficult situations, prevent suicides, deal with crises, "accompany" people on bad trips, and so forth, all of which flew in the face of the ideology of professional competence. Information of this kind was often passed on by the so-called underground newspapers and movement publications. One of the most fully equipped free clinics, Boston's Project Place, employed as many as 80 persons full time along with 150 volunteers to administer 7 programs, ranging from an around-the-clock reception room to preventive counseling of one sort or another.

The free clinics apparently created a new type of community. Nostalgia for this communal spirit was later expressed by a former staff member of one of these clinics: "There were days when I would never leave the place because all my needs were met there. Friendship, care, clothed, housed, fed, sex. I didn't have to go anywhere to find it. It was all right there."[6]

Located near campuses in church basements, run-down buildings, and sometimes even in ghettos, the clinics bore the marks of the self-imposed poverty dear to the counterculture: a few beat-up armchairs covered with Indian bedspreads, a second-hand couch, perhaps a water bed. But the colors were bright and there was always coffee on the stove. The clinics gave the impression that the post-revolutionary paradise had already arrived, that the old discipline had been done away with and the new society was in the process of being ushered in. People were willing to believe that a new philosophy of human relations could by itself abolish inequality and hierarchy and open the way to new forms of sociability, from which conflict was banished. Many free clinics reflected this utopian idealism in their names: Changes, Genesis House, Pequod, and Project Eden, to name a few. Changes was a therapeutic community and self-help center. In the words of one of its members: "Changes people are into each other—we're a community for ourselves, feeling that except for the phone service the best way to be useful is to let people into our own good thing (which means that both for them and for us we want a good thing for us)."[7]

THE FREE CLINICS: THE AUTUMN OF THE UTOPIAN DREAM

The missionary zeal of the clinic staffs was nevertheless vitiated by certain contradictions. First of all there were money problems. It took some time for the need to be felt, because at first gifts flowed in abundantly: from local liberals (whose children were often among the runaways), from the universities, from churches that donated space, from private foundations. Musicians gave concerts, retiring physicians donated equipment to fit out emergency rooms, and so on. Initially, moreover, the members of the staff were not looking out for themselves and were willing to live on almost nothing, enjoying the emotional closeness of the group. As we shall see, however, it was not long before the need for funding led to acceptance of increasingly strict outside controls.

But money problems were only one aspect of the tenuous relations between the clinic insiders and the outside authorities: doctors, police, judges, and politicians. Some clinics set up boards of directors to give themselves credibility in the outside community. But then community leaders who served on the boards had to be persuaded to protect the clinics from harassment and keep the police at bay. In many cases the clinics themselves enforced an unwritten law, forcing dangerous clients, such as hard drug addicts, to leave the premises. Other clinics asked incoming guests to leave any drugs they may have brought with them in a box at the door, which was emptied every day by the police: in this way, peaceful coexistence was maintained—this may seem surprising, but it shows that all parties stood to gain by the arrangement.

On the other hand, in some clinics, such as Boston's Project Place, growing awareness of outside constraints on their activities led to radicalization of the staff, one of whose members claimed that they were still dealing with a broad range of human problems, every day seeing an endless tide of unhappiness, poverty, loneliness, anger, and fear. The injuries suffered by their clients often dated from long ago, and they were aware of the limited possibility of changing deep-seated attitudes through short-term treatments. Often they saw their best intentions thwarted by circumstances beyond their control: racial and class discrimination in schools, jobs, and housing.[8]

Once the staff became aware of these problems, it tried to take a greater interest in the problems of the black ghetto in which it was located. As a result, however, the clinic lost most of its financing. Liberalism has its limits.

There were also political differences within the movement. Most of the free clinics shared in the somewhat facile ideology of the counterculture, according to which authority and hierarchy were the ultimate evils and personal growth and loving group relationships the ultimate goods. A political outlook of a more traditionally anticapitalist sort did, however, take shape around one journal, *The Radical Therapist*. The staff at the Berkeley Radical Psychiatry Center felt that therapy must be a political act, that "adjustment" was reactionary, and that to cure was to bring about change in and through social struggle. In practice, however, "radical therapists" were likely to adopt the rather standard techniques of transactional analysis and group psychotherapy, with the claim that "all persons competent in soul healing should be known as psychiatrists."[9] It was not long before a split occurred between one faction, which continued to make use of therapy and to work toward humanizing existing psychiatric institutions, and another, which felt that the first was too middle class in its outlook and which doubted that any kind of therapy could be radical. This latter faction, which tried to link up all the various institutional struggles with other anticapitalist political movements, started a journal of its own, *Rough Times*, which was published in a Boston suburb.[10] Meanwhile, the Berkeley group put out a new journal, *Issues in Radical Therapy*.

An even more serious split developed between white and black, or, more generally, "third world" clinics. Minority activists had actually opened a different kind of free clinic. Located in poor neighborhoods, these were designed to provide poor people of all ages with the basic medical services they had never received. Black, Chicano, and Indian leaders were generally not critical of the traditional institutions per se. Rather, they complained about the absence of traditional services in the ghettos and demanded treatment equal to that given the white population, but under the control of the community. These clinics faced more serious administrative problems than their countercultural equivalents, both because of the lack of qualified nonwhite personnel and because of the greater difficulty of finding volunteers willing to work in the ghetto. Ghetto workers found a realpolitik approach attractive, and they therefore made demands of a different kind from those put forward by their white counterparts. They were critical, moreover, of the ultraradical ideology of certain white clinics.

> These free clinics which are located in poverty areas serve a critical need because for some of these people, the free service will have been the first medical, dental, or well-baby clinic care they have ever received in their lives. The critical need that is often evident in the poverty areas is one wherein Third World people feel that they will accept federal funding for their people no matter what the source.[11]

At issue were two different conceptions of politics and two ways of relating to the powers that be:

> A free clinic staff . . . would not be true to their cause if they failed to raise pertinent political issues. The goal of free clinic workers should be to remove the necessity for their existence (as far off in the future as that may be). Such a situation will never come about until the consciousnesses of oppressed minority communities are raised to the point where they demand the provision of quality and in depth health services without regard for income status.[12]

Even in the "white" clinics, however, the apparent consensus concerning the values of the counterculture actually hid a number of contradictions. There was, first of all, a contradiction between the egalitarian ideology and the hidden hierarchy. Counterinstitutions generally claimed to be self-managed and to apportion tasks in a democratic manner. In theory this was not impossible, at least where the methods used did not require long periods of training. Most clinics, however, were founded by charismatic figures. Almost invariably there was an inner circle around this leader, which made most of the decisions and had access to the really crucial information. Although open meetings were held, these generally played the same role as in therapeutic communities, namely, to perpetuate the ideology of democratic participation, while the key decisions were made elsewhere. The proof is to be found by examining moments of crisis, such as periods during which there was a shortage of funds. The leader and his inner circle then assumed sole responsibility for saving the clinic, in some cases shutting down on their own authority.

Second, there was a contradiction between the declared political ideology of the clinics and their actual organizational dynamic. In principle the free clinics shared the values of the women's liberation and minority civil rights movements. What is more, there were many women on their staffs, since women often preferred work in "alternative" institutions to the sexist atmosphere of official institutions. But they frequently found the same sexist relations in the counterinstitutions. We find, for instance, evidence of discussions of the propensity of males to dominate at meetings, of unequal division of labor between the sexes, and of the double standard in sexual liberation that left women free chiefly to be dominated by men. Antiracist rhetoric was as tough as antisexist rhetoric, but the fact is that even clinics situated in areas dominated by minority groups found it impossible to work effectively with and for the community. New white ghettos grew up within the ghettos of other races and ethnic groups as microsocieties of alienated youths settled in the midst of blacks or Puerto Ricans themselves living on the fringes of society.

Third, there was a contradiction between the permissiveness that reigned within the clinics and the constraints imposed from outside. Thus a clinic might have to choose between keeping hard drugs out and closing its doors. Even leaving such extreme cases aside, counterinstitutions were for the most part too weak and threatened to establish concrete rules and procedures for settling internal conflicts. Hence the internal history of most permissive institutions is shot through with scenes of violent conflict, factional disputes, attacks on the motives of rival groups, and sectarian splits. The group that founded the Berkeley Radical Psychiatry Center, for example, tried on several occasions to expel rival factions by arguing in favor of sectarian tactics that would have combined political terrorism with the categories of psychopathology. The contradiction was overcome in the end when the leader of the center, who also owned the house in which it was located, simply locked its doors.[13]

Finally, there was a contradiction between the antiprofessional ideology and the actual dependence on professionals. In spite of efforts to demystify medicine and combat hierarchy, the help of professionals was gratefully accepted. Certain services could not have been provided without them, and in addition they provided the cover necessary to protect the clinics from hostile elements in the community. This cover was all the more necessary after the medical establishment in several states (including California and Massachusetts, the two main centers of the free clinic movement) counterattacked by lobbying for the passage of laws imposing severe limitations on the practice of medicine by nonprofessionals. At this point many free clinic workers were faced with the choice of either giving up the work they were doing or else becoming professionals. Many chose the second option. But for a few exceptions, the clinics that survived did so at the price of more or less completely disavowing their more innovatory aspects. It was not long before the American Psychiatric Association was calling for doctors to take part in the work of the free clinics in order to improve the quality of care. Because of this new status, however, it became possible for medical inspectors in Chicago, for example, to gain access to medical records in the clinics.[14]

In view of the foregoing, it would be possible to give a fairly pessimistic assessment of the impact of the free clinics on the structure of the mental health system, particularly if the results actually achieved are compared with the initial expectations. Initially, the people who set up the free clinics hoped to bring about profound changes in the mental health care system, but in fact what actually happened was the reverse.

A turning point in the history of the counterculture came in 1972. McGovern, whose candidacy drew part of its support from the idealistic young, was decisively beaten by Nixon. A guilty conscience over the war in Vietnam lingered on in the national mind. Among its other effects, the war had loosed a new group of drug addicts on American cities. Harder drugs came into vogue (mainly barbiturates, alcohol, amphetamines, and heroin) and the streets turned tough. Middle-class junkies and "polyaddicts" took the place of the tripping flower children of the sixties. At the same time, such insignia of the counterculture as music, clothes, and drug paraphernalia, ostensibly symbols of rejection of bourgeois values, became consumer items on the capitalist marketplace.

In these changed circumstances many countercultural institutions simply scuttled themselves on the grounds that the changed climate was incompatible with their ideals and prevented them from carrying on with their work.

> Our philosophy was people were supposed to come in and work on personal issues. In fact, people were just coming in and hanging out and getting into the same jivey rap one night after another. Counselors didn't understand what their role was. When they loosened up, things got violent. There were a lot of rip-offs and fist fights.[15]

There was little to stand in the way of the inclination to close the clinics down, because most clinics were organized in a largely undemocratic fashion. Leaders became depressed or "burned out" after coping with difficulties year after year and simply walked out. Yet no one else in the organization had enough training and initiative to keep it going.

A good many free clinics closed when forced to comply with standards set by the medical establishment and the bureaucracy. When the movement was in full force it was possible to deal with these requirements and overcome crises by mobilizing the resources that were then available. Once enthusiasm waned, however, the old rules and regulations were dusted off and in some instances beefed up. In some places the health department decided to enforce health and safety regulations and had no difficulty finding violations aplenty: lack of cleanliness, cats in the kitchen, missing fire escape, etc. More commonly, the "quality of care" argument was trotted out for use against clinics lacking a medical cover. One scholar wrote: "No clinic dependent on outside financing can violate current medical regulations. Nonhospital services can only defend themselves if they function like community hospital or if they are affiliated with the federal government."[16]

The third possibility was to take the bull by the horns and reshape the organization of the clinic, the staff, and the services offered to fit the new requirements. The cost of making such changes was that political problems were redefined as technical problems. Most of the free clinics that survived were forced to comply with professional standards. There were two ways of complying. On the one hand, establishment-certified medical personnel took control of counterinstitutional services. On the other hand, one-time nonprofessionals became "preprofessionals" by enrolling in courses designed to enable them to catch up on what they had missed while doing movement work. The movement bowed to ouside pressure because there was often no other way to obtain government funding, particularly after the Nixon administration cut the budget. The changed attitude also reflects the fatigue of the clinic staffs, whose members had grown tired of activism and become concerned about their material well-being in a time of economic crisis. Their frustration led to the idea of viewing the years spent in activism as a sort of pretraining period, during which, it was argued, former activists had become acutely sensitive to new therapeutic possibilities embodied in the values of the counterculture: "Just as psychoanalysts spend four years in a training analysis, young nonprofessionals or preprofessionals require some time and space for questioning and self-exploration."[17]

The medical establishment was ready to listen to this sort of argument—or at least its liberal wing was ready. As one liberal psychiatrist put it:

> Free clinics also serve as social institutions where alienated youth can find a place to participate in meaningful work experience. Many young people have acquired skills as medical paraprofessionals, drug counselors, administrators of medical programs, apprentices to lab technicians, and in a variety of other jobs that have helped them re-enter the dominant society in a constructive way after leaving the free clinic.[18]

These changes in the clinics of course meant changing the kinds of services that were offered. Rather than organizations for social change, the free clinics now had to become purveyors of certain kinds of therapy: sex therapy, family therapy, individual counseling, group therapy for smokers, for the overweight, and so forth. If the clinic successfully made the changeover, its clientele also changed; the new clients were wealthier, more middle class. The few clinics that kept faith with their original purposes were forced to deal with much tougher cases, with clients nobody else wanted to touch: chronic mental patients evicted from the hospitals, tough youths, and drifting rebels without a cause. These new clients were not easy to handle. They often carried knives along with their hypodermics and brought the violence of the streets into the one-time gardens of the flower children. In later years, the survivors of the summer of love were working under very difficult conditions indeed.

It would not be fair to end on so critical a note. We want to make it clear that we found it impossible not to admire some of the free clinics and the work they were doing—Boston's Project Place, to name one.

The conference of the National Free Clinic Council, held in Washington in 1972 and financed by Pfizer Laboratories and the Department of Health, Education, and Welfare, seems to have tolled the death knell for the free clinic movement. The 1972 meeting was concerned mainly with how to obtain a million-dollar loan for use in the war against drugs. David Smith, founder of the Haight–Ashbury Medical Clinic in San Francisco, the first free clinic, observed at this meeting that "free clinics are a part of the total health delivery system and want to be recognized as such."[19]

A vigorous debate took place at this conference, because the majority of the thousand delegates present were unwilling simply to be integrated into the medical establishment. Some representatives of "third world" clinics supported the conference organizers as a matter of realistic politics. But there was opposition, and it seemed that the conference might even reject the compromise. The ensuing scene is symptomatic of the ambiguities of the American counterculture. In the midst of the uproar, Jim Oss, the chairman of the meeting, asked for "a couple of seconds to pull myself together."

> He then began to weep and was greeted with much encouragement from the audience. "Go to it, Jim." "Let it all hang out. Do it." "That's what you're here for." Oss, back in tune with the meeting, extended his arms in the crucifix position, with two supporters on either side.

A third, in a fashion unknown in the Biblical version, held the microphone for Oss who revived his rap: "I've never met anybody working in a free clinic who I didn't like. We just thought we could pull this conference off to help you people. We didn't want to run a political trip on you; we just want to help. But it hasn't come together yet, and I don't think I can go on tonight. Maybe we should come back tomorrow morning at 9:30 and try to get it together." The audience was turned on; and a third of the assembly linked arms, ringed Oss and the Regency Ballroom and swung from side to side in silence. With that grand finale, further discussion of the need for and role of a National Free Clinic Council was also silenced.[20]

The next conference of the National Free Clinic Council was devoted exclusively to problems of financing and quality of care. By 1974 most of the remaining alternative institutions had been integrated into the medical establishment.

Cooptation of this sort inevitably had some impact on the official system, however. For one thing, the free clinics had shown that medical care need not be costly. It has been estimated that the cost of a free clinic session is no more than a few dollars—a twentieth of what a session with a psychoanalyst costs. Such an estimate was not without importance at a time when the insurance companies and the American Medical Association were justifying their opposition to national health insurance, particularly in the area of psychiatry, on the grounds of excessive cost. The free clinics probably added to the pressure for some democratization of the American mental health care system.

It seems likely, moreover, that in spite of the process of "reprofessionalization" described earlier, people who had worked in alternative clinics retained some of the values of the counterculture in their later practice. The free clinics that remain in operation today do offer services to specific fringe groups, even though they have generally become more middle class. Clinics now service college-educated young people of middle-class background who are dissatisfied with the formality of traditional institutions and who cannot afford individual psychotherapy or who hope to find answers to their problems in a more convivial atmosphere. For people of this sort, the clinics provide services they would not seek elsewhere if the clinics did not exist. Ideas spawned in the clinics have also helped to "liberalize" psychiatric practice. Some psychiatrists now explain to the patient what is going on, hierarchical distinctions between staff members have often been lessened, and the relationship between client and therapist has been placed on a more equal footing in some mental health settings. Many of the ideas of Szasz, Laing, and Cooper have thus influenced the establishment, owing to the work of the anti-institutional movement. It is still forbidden to question the efficacy of therapy itself, but criticism of rigidity and authoritarianism in the administration of therapy has been heeded.

In a similar vein, the free clinic movement and lawsuits brought in behalf of patients in mental hospitals (see chapter 4 as well as below) have helped to increase patients' rights and led to the installation of patient advocates (ombudsmen) in the hospitals. Some of the innovations introduced by the free clinics have been adopted by public institutions. The recent report of the Carter Commission even recommends full integration of the free clinics into the public mental health care system.

Even the army found ways to profit from the free clinic experience. In 1973, for example, an anti-drug-abuse center serving American forces in Europe was opened in Frankfurt: it was based on the example of the free clinics. In some ways, this example is typical of what happened to many alternative experiments: the principles that inspired the creation of counterinstitutions have frequently been put to work to improve the functioning of institutions fostering values the exact opposite of those that the dissident groups wished to promote. Often it is the ex-dissidents themselves who are the practitioners of the new methods.

FEMINIST THERAPIES

At the 1970 annual meeting of the American Psychological Association, women members of the radical caucus asked for a million dollars in reparations for the damage done to women by psychiatry. The money was to be used to get women out of mental hospitals and to develop new types of therapy. These radicals felt that research and therapy ought to focus on women's mental health problems that were the result of the domination of one sex by the other and of the position of women in a society that exploits them both in the family and in the workplace. Psychiatry should not label women neurotics: neurotic symptoms in women are merely normal defenses against the oppression to which they are subject.

This moment in history may be taken as the beginning of feminist therapy as such, a therapy born of a marriage between the search for alternatives to psychiatry and the women's liberation movement. Its roots may be traced back to a much earlier period, however. On the theoretical level, an early feminist critique of psychoanalysis was elaborated in the twenties and thirties, later to be revitalized and radicalized in the sixties and seventies. American feminists have been far less timid than their French counterparts in this area; the Americans began criticizing psychoanalysis much earlier, and carried their criticisms much farther, not stopping at spineless attacks on the "cooptation" of Freud. The feminist critique contributed importantly to ending the hegemony that psychoanalysis had enjoyed in the United States during the fifties. The efforts of American women to "reappropriate" their sexuality led to their challenging the psychoanalytic description of relations between the sexes. The debate was more than academic. The rejection of psychoanalysis and traditional psychotherapy was backed by a political movement and publicized widely in pamphlets, brochures, and books printed by alternative presses and distributed at political meetings, rock festivals, and on college campuses.

The history of the problem goes back to the debate in the twenties and thirties known as the Freud–Jones debate, even though Melanie Klein and Karen Horney played the decisive roles. Out of this debate came the earliest critiques of what French feminists call Freud's phallocratism. Karen Horney and Clara Thompson interpreted what Freud considered to be a primary factor in the development of female sexuality as a secondary reaction. In 1924 Horney wrote that if women looked upon their own genitals as inferior to the male organ, they did so in reaction to male narcissism. Penis envy no doubt exists, she argued, but as the consequence of male dominance. Using the work of Simmel, Horney developed an interpretation of prevailing ideas in psychiatry as products of a male civilization. Accordingly, if one abandons the exclusively masculine vantage and looks upon psychology from a feminine standpoint, one finds that little boys envy the female reproductive functions. The biological division between the sexes is reflected in the way the psyche is organized, and penis envy is merely envy of a symbol of power.[21]

Today, some American feminists see this debate as a precursor of the women's liberation movement. The twenties, when the debate took place, saw the first glimmerings of liberation for American women. Similarly, the more recent psychoanalytic controversy coincided with the second wave of American feminism.[22] In the words of Kate Millett, whose book *Sexual Politics* had a profound impact on the movement.

> The effect of Freud's work, that of his followers, and still more that of his popularizers, was to rationalize the invidious relationship between the sexes, to ratify traditional roles, and to validate temperamental differences. . . .
>
> [His discoveries were] invoked to sponsor a point of view essentially conservative. And as regards the sexual revolution's goal of liberating female humanity from its traditional subordination, the Freudian position came to be pressed into the service of a strongly counterrevolutionary attitude.[23]

Three or four important tenets of psychoanalysis were criticized openly by feminists in the seventies: the theory of penis envy; the concept of a "normal" feminine role and the supposition that women who deviate from this role suffer from a masculinity complex; the attribution to women of specific character traits such as masochism, passivity, narcissism, and the like; and, finally, the "myth of the vaginal orgasm." We cannot here enter into the details of these controversies, which have given rise to an abundant literature.[24]

Why has psychoanalysis aroused such hostility? At issue are both psychoanalysis itself and its role as a model for various kinds of therapy. Among the charges against psychoanalysis is that its authority has been used to promote an image of women as neurotic in which women's problems are dismissed as pathological symptoms, when in fact

> all so-called symptoms [should] be seen in a new light—no longer merely as defenses, maneuvers, or other such tactics, but as struggles to preserve or express some deeply needed aspects of personal integrity in a milieu that will not allow for their direct expression.[25]

Therapy should therefore be conceived in a totally new way. Diagnosis should not be a matter of pinpointing the areas in which a woman fails to live up to the models held out to her, but rather "the therapeutic exploration becomes centered on how woman's attempt to transform herself into something inappropriate has led to her problems. The crucial issue here is that the inappropriate transformation has been the prescribed one."[26] The aim of therapy, moreover, should not be to help women to accept their traditional role; rather "feminism means . . . the freeing of all people from the restrictions of their culturally defined sexual roles and the focus on balancing out the centuries of negation of female energy by the positive assertion and development of it in the world of today."[27] In short, the task of therapy is to help the patient find her own way. "Some women may be better off trying to make changes in their lives, such as getting a job, refusing to do all the housework, finding a new home, getting a divorce, etc., rather than attempting to adapt themselves to an unsatisfactory (but conventionally accepted) way of life."[28]

Behind the many different ideas of what feminist therapy is about, we repeatedly find the two concepts of transition and growth: "We call ourselves feminists because we are available to help with all the life choices that women make in order to grow and to learn."[29] Some might argue that the only point of feminist therapy is to validate feminist values. While this may seem circular, it has proved fruitful in practice. Feminist therapy has made contributions in two areas. First, it has developed critiques of standard therapies, professionalism, and traditional concepts of mental health. Second, it has contributed to the spread of self-help approaches.

In regard to the first point, the American feminist movement has made important contributions to criticism of the professional monopoly of health issues. Militant feminists believe that the therapeutic order is a social order and that standard forms of therapy have always contributed to masculine domination of that order. A study still regarded as authoritative was carried out in 1970 showing that the majority of therapists (men and women) correlated masculine behavior with "normality." By contrast, the behavior of women, even of women in good mental health, was associated with "infantile" personality traits: emotionality, lack of independence, desire to make an impression, sensitivity.[30] In a similar vein, Phyllis Chesler has suggested that

> many American women enter individual psychoanalysis just as they enter marriage: with a sense of urgency and desperation, and without questioning their own motives. . . . Psychotherapy and marriage are the two major socially approved institutions for women. . . . Both institutions are based on women's helplessness and dependence on a "stronger" male or female authority figure—as husband or psychotherapist.[31]

Thus psychotherapy reinforces the institution of marriage by forcing women with problems to see their difficulty as one of personal adjustment, as a question of individual psychology rather than of political conflict.

This assertion can be generalized to the medical order as a whole. Not long after writing the article just cited, Phyllis Chesler herself undertook to make such a generalization by reinterpreting the history and methods of psychiatry in a feminist light: she found that the number of women committed to mental institutions has been increasing relative to the number of men, that more women than men suffer from neurotic symptoms, that madness in women is usually self-destructive, and so forth—and that all this is because the women singled out by psychiatry are usually neither mad nor ill but rather victims of the requirements of a masculine society. The medical model that underlies psychotherapy, moreover, makes use of and reinforces the inequality in the patient–therapist relationship, an inquality that is psychologically destructive.[32]

There is ample reason to question the thoroughness and objectivity of Chesler's analysis as far as the collection of data and interpretation of statistics are concerned. But the book's success can be explained by the fact that it summed up feminist thinking on the subject and provided ammunition for an attack on the medical establishment. Traditional therapy depends on a fundamental mystification, in which the actual order of values is reversed. Once the true perspective had been restored by a feminist interpretation of the conditions to which women had been subjected, it became possible to see that to some extent the need for therapy created by the difficulties of accepting the role assigned to women was not at all a pathological symptom but rather an indication of good mental health. In 1971 one feminist asked if the well-adjusted housewife did not betoken "poor mental health."[33] Elizabeth Williams went even further in 1976 when she stated that, for women who found it difficult to adjust to their position in life,

> their psychological health is demonstrated by their courage in seeking what they believe might be radical changes in personality and life-style; by their open-mindedness in attempting a new, unorthodox, politically relevant psychotherapy; and by their willingness to examine and reevaluate their most intimate relationships as possible sources of their pain.[34]

The paradox, then, is clear: although the standard therapeutic relationship is fundamentally biased, some kind of therapy is still necessary. Different from the therapies proposed by the medical and psychoanalytic establishments, this new therapy has had to be invented. The first course chosen was to take the lesser of two evils and call upon the services of professionals less compromised than their colleagues by the traditional system. Often these were women who, to one degree or another, were at odds with the official agencies that employed them, which they reproached for discriminating against women and for using sexist methods. Feminist newspapers and organizations published directories listing names of trustworthy therapists together with such information as whether or not they had degrees and whether they were homosexual or heterosexual. Generally, however, these publications also indicated that this type of therapy, because it too closely resembled traditional therapies, promised no more than limited improvement:

> A therapist can be a good alternative for a woman in transition if she has the time and money (and if, of course, the therapist is sympathetic and understanding). . . . Keep in mind that therapists and other women are human, with human limitations. It is not likely that anyone but you can solve all the problems faced by a woman in transition, although some people can help.[35]

Accordingly, the main thrust of feminist therapy was to try to establish support services that can take the place of skilled professionals: self-help and consciousness-raising groups. Consciousness-raising sessions helped women to see that their problems were not unique and should not be seen as a form of illness. Therapy thus became part of a process of growing political awareness, directed toward effective political action.[36] Because most women's problems were of social origin, women could better help each other than be helped by professional therapists: "Not having experienced what it is to be poor, black, or a woman, their theories tend not to take the realities of poverty, racism, or sexism into account."[37]

This ideal of women's action was probably approached most closely by the medical self-help collectives. The movement grew as a reaction against the medicalization of the everyday problems of a woman's existence: pregnancy, abortion, body care, hygiene. In this context the principle, "our bodies, our selves" took on concrete significance when women reappropriated what traditionally had been methods practiced by women themselves, but which lately had been confiscated by medicine.[38] It was in these areas that the medical establishment reacted most strongly, for what was involved was not of peripheral concern, as in the case of the free clinics, but the monopoly of the medical profession over key questions of health. Several self-help collectives were forced to shut down. The danger for official medicine lay not so much in the direct competition of the clinics as in the way they were organized, without hierarchy (relying instead on peer review and counseling), for this demonstrated in a practical way that the technical skills of the specialists were not indispensable in many areas they had claimed as their exclusive domain.

Besides self-help groups, feminist clinics offered a wide range of services that partly overlapped those offered by the free clinics: hot lines, individual and collective counseling of one sort or another, consciousness-raising groups, etc. Some fifteen such organizations existed in the city of Boston and its suburbs alone. Most of them participated in the National Feminist Therapy Association. The 1976 conference of the Institute of Alternative Therapy was attended by several hundred feminists. There was also a feminist therapeutic community, the Elizabeth Stone House in Boston. Founded in 1974 by former mental patients and feminists, this collectively run self-help community offered living space for periods ranging from six months to a year; the governing spirit was that the problems of women should be approached politically.

The methods used by feminist therapists are as diverse as the feminist organizations themselves. Besides consciousness-raising groups, other groups attempted to adapt various techniques including postanalytic psychotherapy, Gestalt therapy, transactional analysis, Reichian bioenergetic treatment, sex counseling, and even "soft" forms of behavior modification (see chapter 8). There were, of course, many problems. As we shall see, these techniques chiefly emphasize experience and subjectivity, and it may be asked how far they are compatible with the idea of raising the consciousness of women as to the social causes of their alienation. One feminist therapist wrote that for women, the road to liberation and political power does not lead in the direction of the primal scream or the emotional excesses of religious experience. If women want equality, they must call upon their minds and their will as much as their emotions.[39]

Taking this admonition to heart, feminist therapy collectives have worked diligently to adapt their methods to the purposes of militant feminism.[40] It is doubtful, however, that techniques are malleable enough to be adapted to any and all purposes. If counterinstitutions use methods similar to those used in traditional institutions, there is likely to be less difference between the two than the advocates of change are wont to believe. Consider the problem of transference, for example. Most feminist therapies begin with a critique of the psychoanalytic theory of transference, which is either rejected outright or reinterpreted in a new light. The therapist is neutral, but is also a woman who, in her life, has faced the same problems and experiences as her patient and who has found a healthy way of resolving them.[41] Behind this conception, it is easy to detect the presence of a role model, with whom the patient can identify for ego-reinforcement. But this becomes a throwback to the psychoanalytic emphasis on "adjustment."

Accordingly, there is reason to wonder if feminist therapy in practice has always measured up to its avowed aim of subverting the standard therapeutic relationship. If feminist therapy has succeeded in going beyond psychotherapy, its success is attributable primarily to the type of client it has attracted. Generally clients are young, middle-class white women, college educated at the very least, not very happy in life, and, in at least half the cases, active in the feminist movement. As a group, then, these clients are quite different from the users of more traditional mental health services. Women who turn to feminist therapy do not see themselves as sick, and refuse to accept the usual disease classifications.[42] In other words, the group that accepts the contention that the medical model is outmoded consists of women who are not really sick and who are convinced in advance that the ideology being held out to them as a remedy for their malaise is well founded.

Once people begin to question whether there is really a sharp contrast between mental health and mental illness and to ask what "normality" really means, the medical model in any narrow sense of the term undoubtedly ceases to be adequate. At the same time, however, that model has been extended into new areas and sold to new clients. Once it becomes accepted that women today must undergo changes in order to be healthy, an enormous group of potential clients is opened up to the purveyors of new services. These clients are supposed to need help in coping with everyday problems, and some of the ways in which that help is likely to be offered are certain to be less democratic in their organization than the self-help groups. Thus there is a deeply rooted ambiguity in the ideology of personal growth that is prevalent among American feminists. We shall have more to say about this ambiguity later on, when we come to discuss "therapy for the normal" in the next chapter.

It is hardly cause for surprise, then, that traditional psychiatry has taken up some of the innovations of feminist therapy, just as it took up some of the innovations of the free clinics. For example, the psychological problems associated with rape, pregnancy, menopause, battered women, depression in women, and so forth have all been translated into medical idiom. Community mental health centers have frequently offered training courses to sensitize their staff members to women's issues. Enlightened psychiatrists no longer speak of frigidity but rather of the problems of "preorgasmic women." Family and couples-counseling now exists for lesbian and homosexual couples as well as heterosexual ones. Some psychiatrists have rejected certain disease categories sanctioned by the American Psychiatric Association in favor of such novel classifications as "persons in transition." Transitions affecting women in particular have thus spawned new sorts of groups: groups for widows, divorcees, lesbian mothers, rape victims, etc. Big business, too, has succumbed to the fashion, and nowadays we find many best sellers and how-to manuals with titles like *How to Say No* and *The Assertive Woman*. Assertiveness-training groups designed to develop the self-confidence of women and to enable them to get on in sexist society have spread widely, sometimes earning a good deal of money for their organizers.

Feminist therapies (as well as the gay therapies that we shall be discussing in the next section), like most products of the American counterculture, have had consequences of two distinct kinds. On the one hand, they have led to a politicization of certain areas of private life, raised consciousness about certain problems, and stimulated new forms of collective action and new institutional approaches. On the other hand, they have helped to enlarge the market for parapsychiatric services and to extend the coverage of new and more subtle forms of social control.

GAY THERAPIES

"Gay" does not mean precisely the same thing as "ho.nosexual."[43] "Gay" implies that homosexuality is not a fate that is passively endured but rather an orientation chosen by an individual for positive and conscious reasons. Gay therapy accepts the notion that homosexuality is a positive choice and is therefore to be distinguished from psychological and psychotherapeutic approaches for which homosexual activity is abnormal.

Although gay therapy has taken much of its inspiration from feminist therapy, the two focus their criticism on different aspects of traditional psychiatry and psychotherapy. The gay critique is based on the contention that standard psychiatric and psychoanalytic techniques are inhumane and dangerous for homosexuals. It is therefore argued that homosexuals need special services designed to help them deal with the peculiar problems they face in a society that is still dominated by heterosexual values. The different forms of gay therapy that we shall be discussing involve, for the most part, male homosexuals, since lesbians generally seek help from feminist therapists (discussed in the preceding section).

It must be said, first of all, that when the gay movement first began criticizing the sort of therapy offered homosexuals in the United States, that therapy left plenty of room for improvement. Homosexuals were subjected to such treatments as receiving electric shocks through electrodes attached to their heads in order to convert their "repugnant feelings toward the opposite sex into pleasurable feelings."[44] Other forms of so-called aversion therapy relied on the injection of chemical substances. In no other area have behavior modificationists shown themselves more imaginative than in the treatment of homosexuality.

These types of "therapy" were used comparatively little, however, and their significance was immediately apparent, so that they were perhaps not as dangerous as other, subtler techniques inspired by psychology. These do not "cure" the homosexual but rather add to his problems by preying on his feelings of guilt. A book published in 1970 defended the use of such techniques. It stated that when he encounters the psychotherapist, the homosexual is generally in a period of self-doubt and therefore particularly vulnerable. This is an opportunity that must be seized. The therapist can manipulate the crisis situation to convince the subject that his homosexual relations are necessarily of short duration, that they are but a pale imitation of genuine interpersonal relations, that they express his dependence, his masochism, his inability to achieve satisfaction, etc. In this way the therapist may hope to set the subject back on the "right path."[45]

The most insidious aspect of American attitudes toward homosexuality is the way they are socially conditioned: antihomosexual attitudes are commonly taken as a mark of virility, and faith in the possibilities of therapy (as the heyday of psychoanalysis attests) is virtually unlimited. Thus the homosexual, even before he has seen a therapist, is convinced that his case is pathological, and he is prepared to accept a disparaging interpretation of his sexuality. There is abundant evidence suggesting that in such a social context psychotherapy is in fact dangerous for homosexuals. One author has presented data indicating that the standard therapies lead to higher rates of commitment, imprisonment, and suicide.[46] Another states that it has been proven that homosexuality and psychotherapy are incompatible. Many homosexuals who have taken their problems to a therapist have had every reason in the world to be sorry they did. According to this author, the price paid by patients for not having had the presence of mind or intuition to run immediately has almost always been to be subjected to a picture of their "pathology" even more devastating than the one they had to begin with. The loss of time and money is nothing compared with the aggravation of guilt feelings, loss of initiative, and other consequences of a misguided cure.[47]

If gay therapy rejects the standard methods, both "hard" and "soft," what does it recommend in their place? An exhaustive description of the various types of gay therapy is as difficult to give as an exhaustive description of feminist therapies. A better approach is to indicate a few of the major problem areas to which gay or "gay-oriented" therapists have addressed themselves in reacting against traditional therapies: low self-esteem and self-doubt, internalization of negative judgments of homosexuality, depressive tendencies, passivity, and self-destructive behavior such as alcoholism and drug abuse, to name a few.[48] As in the case of feminist therapy, the usual method is to change the negative evaluation of homosexual behavior to a positive one. Thus Clark defends "gay paranoia" as self-protection, "an early warning system that helps us to make social adjustments that smooth social interactions."[49] Homosexual paranoia, we are told, does not give rise to hostility and tension like ordinary paranoia, but rather makes it possible for the homosexual to be more open to others. "Coming out," that is, announcing to others that one is a homosexual, has been analyzed in a similar vein. The coming out period is a time of anxiety and conflict, and the gay-oriented therapist tries to help his client let his feelings surface and make decisions clearly, unlike the traditional therapist, who attempts to capitalize on the crisis in order to "destabilize" the homosexual's drives.[50]

Thus gay therapy tries to develop the homosexual's confidence and strength by changing his negative self-image into a positive one. Gay therapists claim that these "ego reinforcing" techniques are not intended to achieve conformity with general social values, as traditional therapy is supposed to do. Like feminist therapies, gay therapy relies on consciousness raising, which is supposed to help the client see his sexual choice in its sociopolitical context. Ideally, then, the homosexual is supposed to adjust to his condition without necessarily adjusting to society at large:

> Most of us are not yet ready for full integration. We must build more strength in our Gay identity first. Legal battles for full civil rights must be fought and won. We must learn to enjoy and be proud of some of the differences we have been told are shameful—like our ability to love while others compete, or our incisive camp humor. We must build our own ceremonies; weddings may be on their way out of style, but we need some sort of ceremony to give public dignity and support to our loving relationships and we need to be able to mourn openly as Gay people when someone Gay dies. We need to develop our own psychology, sociology, and anthropology—our study of ourselves and our culture—and then present it proudly to the rest of the world so that they can join us in celebration. We are Gay. We are growing. And we are learning how to be glad.[51]

Gay therapy, then, is intended to open the way to political action by emphasizing the value of those characteristics for which homosexuals have been persecuted. Just as "black is beautiful," so "gay is beautiful." The most radical gays view such self-assertiveness as a way of provoking outrage, which is seen as a revolutionary weapon. To quote Don Clark once more: "This violation to one's nature, along with the myriad of insults that accumulate during the years of growing up invisibly Gay, create enormous anger which never seems justified."[52]

Anger can help foster group solidarity and in some instances can lead to coordinated activities with other oppressed groups. Thus the radical therapies sponsored by the most highly politicized groups emphasize the importance of anger: this is true of women, homosexuals, former mental patients, racial minorities, and political radicals. The association that is sometimes made among these groups is probably not entirely spurious, and even if the unity evoked is largely mythical, it helps to raise consciousnesses. The Black Panthers' newspaper reprinted an analysis of anger by a leading radical therapist which gave some indication of the attitude of the politicized groups. The therapist wrote that anger is the normal response to oppression. When oppression is not met with anger, psychiatry may consider this a symptom that something is wrong. Radical psychiatrists believe that people turn to psychiatry because they are oppressed and suffer from mystification of their oppression. Anger, when it is directed against the oppressor, is a sign of a healthy reaction and not of mental imbalance. The people who need psychiatry are oppressed people who have come to believe the lies they are told about their oppression. Their justified anger becomes confused and often turns to violence or against themselves.[53]

Many in the gay community would like to think of gay therapy centers as rallying places where gays can come together in order to fight for their liberation. A description of the Liberation House Gay Collective stated that the services could lead to actions leading toward liberation, thanks both to the support the Collective gives to its members and to the community and to the way it is organized. As a gay community, the Collective is familiar with the oppressive attitudes of professional therapists. Facilities that use traditional methods of analysis and assistance do not stimulate homosexuals to create a liberated community. At the Collective, psychological assistance implied helping people to organize for change and liberation.[54] Many gay service centers are operated as self-managed collectives. They offer not only psychological support but also practical information regarding legal aid, social counseling, and events of concern to the gay community. Most staff members are nonprofessionals and are chosen for qualities other than technical competence: "Caring about others and being able to relate to their experiences, both joyful and painful, seemed to be the only valid human basis for choosing people with whom we wished to work."[55] Some of these centers, such as Gay Counseling of New York, refused to be integrated into the human services system.

Only a minority within the gay movement shares this sort of concern for radical purity, however. The temptation to become a part of the system is reinforced by the fact that much gay therapy—unlike feminist therapy—tries to involve heterosexuals who play an important part in the client's life in the therapeutic process. When family therapy techniques are used, for example, the therapist will often bring in the gay client's spouse, children, parents, etc. There is also a national organization of parents of homosexuals. It is difficult to reconcile practices of this sort with radical gay politics. The same is true of collaboration between homosexual groups and religious organizations or social service agencies, which generally seek the assistance of gay groups when they have to solve some thorny problem pertaining to homosexuals.

Initially run by homosexuals, the Santa Clara County Service in California has been held up as an example of the successful integration of gay services into a fairly traditional organization. Pressures on other gay centers to make similar kinds of changes have contributed to professionalization of the staff, as in the case of the free clinics. Boston's Homophile Community Health Service, for example, was opened in 1971 as a collective of nonprofessionals. Today its program for alcoholics is financed by public funds. As one participant in the project wrote, the main focus of the center now is "to provide high-grade professional services in a warm gay setting."

Gay therapists have had to face the same kinds of problems as feminist and other "radical" therapists in adapting techniques that were developed for use in quite different contexts. The psychological cost of bearing up under oppression or of trying to work free of so-called normal social roles is heavy and sometimes requires emergency support. This leads to a paradoxical situation, the consequences of which are manifold. The acceptance of homosexuality—or lesbianism—as normal in certain quarters of American society has involved depathologization of homosexual behavior. When the homosexual tries to rid himself of the image of abnormality, however, it is as though he had no choice but to regard himself as sick before he can begin to heal the wounds caused by his condition. Herein lies the irony: often it is the therapist who is called upon to demystify the psychiatric interpretation of homosexual behavior.

Thus there is tension—common to all the alternative movements we have examined, and sometimes existing even within the experience of a single individual—between the rejection of medicine in favor of politics, on the one hand, and the desire to reform the psychiatric profession and enlist professional allies, on the other hand. And reform, apparently, yields the more impressive results. In December 1973, the congress of the American Psychiatric Association decided to remove homosexuality from its list of mental illnesses. It was replaced by a new category: "sexual orientation disturbance." This category concerned individuals whose sexual interests are directed mainly to persons of the same sex and who are disturbed by this or who want to change their sexual orientation. This diagnostic category was to be distinguished from homosexuality, which in itself now need not constitute a psychiatric disorder.

At the same meeting a motion was passed in favor of granting full civil rights to homosexuals.[56] In 1975 the National Association of Social Workers ratified the same positions. In that year also, under pressure from the Association of Gay Psychologists, the American Psychological Association declared that:

> Homosexuality per se implies no impairment in judgment, stability, reliability, or general social or vocational capabilities. Further, the American Psychological Association urges all mental health professionals to take the lead in removing the stigma of mental illness that has long been associated with homosexual orientation.[57]

Thus the clearest consequence of the gay movement is that homosexuals who seek psychiatric help can henceforth expect to be treated in a less discriminatory fashion. This is not an inconsiderable result. But a change of this sort leaves open the question of the qualities of such treatment, whether the recipient is gay or a member of some other group.

EMBATTLED MENTAL PATIENTS

Since most attempts to set up alternative forms of treatment have been connected in one way or another with the countercultural movement, there is no reason to make too sharp a distinction between one sort of experiment and another. As we have just seen, the free clinics, feminist therapies, and gay therapies have much in common. The various movements begun by former mental patients are something else again. Patient groups have been less interested in seeking practical alternatives to existing forms of care than in questioning the value of the entire traditional system of mental health care. The people who join these groups believe they have something to say about psychiatric oppression because they have lived through it. These movements have been strengthened by successes in lawsuits against mental hospitals charged with maintaining intolerable conditions (see chapter 4).

As we have seen, the notion that individuals have a right to treatment, which gained prominence in lawsuits over patients' rights, was something that the psychiatric establishment had no difficulty accommodating itself to. Certain factions within the establishment even managed to capitalize on the notion in their efforts to modernize the mental health care system. In other law-suits, however, the divergence with psychiatric ideology was more pronounced. In the same year as the Wyatt trial, for example, another class action suit, which was brought in behalf of the crim-inally insane held in a Pennsylvania prison hospital, challenged the use of psychotropic drugs. According to the court, "invol-untary administration of drugs which have a painful or frightening effect can amount to cruel and unusual punishment in violation of the Eighth Amendment."[58]

Another suit brought by seven patients and former patients of Boston State Hospital accused fifteen doctors of having forced patients to take drugs and of having kept them in isolation for no reason in 1974 and 1975. The plaintiffs asked $1,200,000 in dam-ages.[59] This case marked a step in the direction of a right to *refuse* treatment, which, if upheld, would lead to a thorough overhaul of the way psychiatry is practiced. In principle, each step in a course of treatment would have to be justified before being taken, and the patient would be allowed to question the reasons for the treatments administered.

Another case that caused much ink to flow went to court at about the same time. This case revolved around yet another prin-ciple marking a step beyond the reformist notion of a right to treatment. A patient by the name of Kenneth Donaldson was held for fifteen years in a mental hospital, even though he went to court nineteen times during that period to ask for his release, arguing that he would be capable of finding housing and work on the outside. After lengthy delays, in 1975 his case finally reached the Supreme Court, which awarded him $400,000 in dam-ages. In the opinion of the Court, a patient cannot be held against his will without treatment, particularly if he is capable of living outside and not dangerous. One of the justices asked whether a state could confine harmless individuals simply to get them out of the sight of other citizens who find them different.[60] As the first case of its kind to reach the Supreme Court, the Donaldson case has had tremendous influence,[61] and many liberals have been quick to see it as the beginning of the end of psychiatric repression. What would become of the repressive function of psychiatry if psychiatrists had to prove that every person committed was in fact dangerous and that every treatment administered was in fact justified? If every decision is subject to scrutiny by the courts, psychiatrists will lose their autonomy and the mental hospitals will become subject to the judicial authorities. As one critic of court-legislated reform has argued, now some judges have become the administrators of the institutions they were trying to reform.[62]

Still, many court decisions are likely to have a superficial effect at best. Progressive lawyers have called the judgments in these cases mere paper victories. To enforce them would require the installation of permanent surveillance within the mental institutions. Attempts to set up human rights committees composed of concerned citizens and specialists to oversee the hospitals have not produced very promising results. Contrary to the mythology that has grown up in the wake of Watergate, hospital administrators and state governors are not sent to prison for failing to enforce court orders in the mental hospitals. Some of those who brought suits hoped to use the courts to close the hospitals down, but few closings have actually resulted, even though many hospitals are manifestly in violation of many of the standards laid down by the courts.[63]

Patient groups intially set out to fill the gap between the principles established by the courts and actual practice in mental institutions. They were not alone. At about the same time, progressive lawyers and law students began organizing groups to provide legal advice and to go to court in efforts to halt abuses of power by psychiatrists (among these groups were the Center for the Study of Legal Authority and Mental Patient Status, or LAMP, at Berkeley, and the Mental Patient Civil Liberties Project in Philadelphia). The movement was spearheaded, however, by former mental patients, who mobilized their experience and perhaps also their resentment to help inpatients assert their rights and fight against abuses such as arbitrary commitments. In Massachusetts, for example, the Mental Patients Liberation Front published and distributed in the state mental hospitals a patient guide entitled "Your Rights as a Mental Patient in Massachusetts," which explained existing laws, reminded patients of their rights within the institution, and listed various possible legal remedies.[64] As many of these groups were quick to discover, however,

> . . . the legal approach alone is a limited one—it is often predicated on the assumption that large-scale mental incarceration is valid if patients are generally treated humanely and fairly, given all their rights. Even people legally challenging involuntary commitment don't necessarily accept responsibility for the deeper problems of how to prevent commitment in the first place, how to support those who have problems in living once they're out of the institutions. . . .[65]

Patient groups have therefore tried to move beyond the limitations of legal remedies, on the principle that "the liberation of mental patients is up to the patients themselves." As a first step in this direction, they launched an attack on some of the methods and facilities of the psychiatric establishment. The Network Against Psychiatric Oppression in San Francisco, for instance, occupied the offices of the governor of California in 1976. Among the group's demands were recognition of the right to refuse treatment, an end to forced labor in mental hospitals, and payment of a minimum wage for voluntary labor by inpatients. In 1977 the same group organized a demonstration against psychosurgery and occupied a hospital accused of administering electroshock treatments. Such actions went beyond the limits of the law, since these psychiatric methods were officially accepted as legal. In its journal, *Madness Network News*, the Network Against Psychiatric Oppression has published information about psychiatric methods it deems destructive, attacked doctors who used such methods by name, and so on.

The movement has also set up a self-help network for mental patients and encouraged the formation of consciousness-raising groups. In this regard it is similar to the free clinic movement. A New York group, Project Release, ran a community for former mental patients. In all these activities the accent has been placed not so much on therapy as on raising consciousnesses as to the socioeconomic status of mental patients. The Lincoln Detox Program in the Bronx, though for drug addicts, has probably gone farther than any other patient-run experiment, even though it continues to use the services of professionals. The program at Lincoln is based on a rejection of the medical model and the use of medication (methadone). Instead, acupuncture has been tried, and there is political analysis of the meaning of drug use in the ghetto, interpreted as complicity by racial minorities in their own cultural genocide. Once the medical model had been thrown out, patients and staff were free to work together on a new basis. Because the drug problem in the ghetto was so serious, the Lincoln Program, which was founded in 1971, was able to continue to receive federal funding even though it pursued an independent course.[66]

Mental patient groups in various cities have made attempts to organize themselves and to work toward a comprehensive critique of the mental health care system. The Fourth Annual North American Conference on Human Rights and Psychiatric Oppression, which was held in Boston in May 1976, adopted the following general program:

> We reject *compulsory commitments* to mental hospitals, not only by the courts, but, in general, all involuntary admissions procedures and even "voluntary" commitments where the patient gives his consent without full knowledge of the case. . . . We reject psychiatric treatments imposed on the patient, such as drugs, electric shocks, psychosurgery, isolation, aversion techniques, and behavior modification therapy. . . . We reject the mental health care system, because it is by nature despotic and acts as an extra-legal parallel police force for the suppression of cultural and political dissidence. . . . We reject the concept of "mental illness," because it is used to justify involuntary commitment, and in particular we reject the imprisonment of people who have committed no crime. . . . We reject the use of psychiatric terminology, because it is intrinsically stigmatizing and degrading, nonscientific and magical, and we propose replacing it with good English words, "recluse," for example, instead of "mental patient." . . . We believe . . . that the mental health care system is essentially a pacification program controlled by psychiatrists and designed to force people to adjust to prevailing social norms. In all strata of society, more and more people are currently working free of those norms. More and more people are demanding autonomy and popular control. More and more people are becoming aware that economic and political power are concentrated

in the hands of a few, who are determined to hold on to it by whatever means, including involuntary commitment to mental hospitals. We maintain, however, that commitment as an instrument of social control is a thing of the past. We demand the abolition of involuntary commitment, and we demand freedom and social justice. We intend to make these words a reality, and we shall not rest until we have done so.[67]

The patients' movement thus laid down a challenge to the medical establishment, and those who experienced the brunt of the attack generally perceived it as a challenge. To cite one example, the Pennsylvania Mental Patients Civil Liberties Project received authorization from the governor of that state in 1972 to set up a legal assistance program at the Haverford State Mental Hospital. At first the hospital was willing to accept the program as a convenient way of dealing with troublesome patients who insisted on their rights. But the patients who organized under the program's auspices drafted a tract against psychosurgery, and some of them took advantage of a weekend furlough to demonstrate at an international conference of neurosurgeons. The hospital's lawyer then accused the program of using "slogans" and "of having based its work on political rather than legal objectives." In April 1973, patients published a newsletter, but all whose articles appeared in it were released from the hospital as soon as the first issue came out. The organization then brought a class action suit to put an end to forced labor at the hospital. The hospital administration fought the idea, taking advantage of hostility against the proposal on the part of the least trained members of the staff, mostly black aides. In July 1973, the program was suspended.[68]

As this example shows, the battle waged by patient groups against the psychiatric establishment was a battle of David against Goliath. In the first place, the patient groups were very loosely organized. The antipsychiatric newsletter *Rough Times* estimated their number at forty-five in 1977, with a total membership of just a few thousand throughout the United States. Like all small groups, they were subject to factional disputes. Among the most hotly debated issues was the question of whether an alliance with some members of the psychiatric profession was possible or whether mental patients must take charge of their own liberation. Finally, given the imbalance that existed between the power of the groups and the power of the institution they were attacking, there is room to wonder whether the radicalism of most of the groups was enough to keep them from being swallowed up by the establishment. Their main role seems to have been to contribute to the general ferment, following up lawsuits on behalf of mental patients by helping to establish legal assistance services in many hospitals. Crowning the movement's efforts, the Carter administration instituted a national mental health advocacy program. By 1977 fifteen states had adopted one. At the International Congress of Psychiatry held in Honolulu in August 1977, American psychiatrists were able to polish up their tarnished liberal escutcheon at the expense of their Soviet counterparts; an official of the National Institute of Mental Health congratulated himself on the growth of the mental patient movement:

> For the first time in history, large numbers of former patients have been speaking out about the poor treatment they received in American mental institutions, and they have not gone unheeded. They have been heard both by the public, which is concerned by the quality and value of mental health care, and by lawyers, who have taken up the cause of patients' rights with diligence and zeal.

This psychiatrist found cause for regret, however, in the fact that some of his colleagues had reacted with disappointment and resentment over the way mental health practice had been modified as a result of court decisions and new laws. He condemned the defensiveness of psychiatrists and their inability to recognize past and present abuses committed by their colleagues, an attitude that, he claimed, helps make them excellent scapegoats.[69] The implication was that psychiatrists ought to accept the criticisms of their patients in order to become better psychiatrists. The whole process reached its culmination in 1978, when experts working for the Carter Commission approved nearly all the demands for patients' rights and legal guarantees that had been won in the courts after prodigious efforts.

Once again we encounter a dialectic we have seen at work on

several previous occasions. How did outside challenges to the mental health system, even would-be radical challenges, come to be taken up by the system itself and used to make it work more smoothly and efficiently?

The problem that psychiatry confronts today, and not only in America, is one of achieving a balance between the legacy of the past and up-to-date innovation, between continuity in its inspiration and change or adaptation of its methods. The issue is to meet the challenge of the times, to bring about a modernization. This crisis of modernization has given rise to tensions within the establishment, where, roughly speaking, we find two factions, one traditionalist, the other modernist, with a range of more moderate positions in between. While the traditionalists stand for continuity and want to keep faith with the past, the modernists hold out the possibility of spreading the faith into virgin territories through missionary work. Such expansionism carries with its risks of heterodoxy and even heresy. But there may be something to be gained by flirting with the devil, provided it is for a good cause, in particular to bring lost sheep back into the fold.

In this chapter we have examined a number of experiments—the free clinics, feminist therapies, gay therapies, and patients' movements—which, as they see themselves, are not only peripheral to the psychiatric establishment but generally defined in opposition to its brand of psychiatry. We have also tried to keep the establishment's counterstrategy in view throughout our discussion, or, at any rate, to keep an eye on the strategy adopted by the most dynamic segments of the establishment, which, rather than condemn the innovations of the antagonists outright, have tried instead to take advantage of them in order to further their own expansionist, modernizing aims. The best way to enlarge the scope of the system is to welcome whatever looms up on its boundaries, translating each innovation, as far as possible, into the idiom of the system.

It is probably impossible to eliminate this kind of ambiguity. While we have emphasized its omnipresence in this chapter, our intention has not in any way been to disparage the efforts of men and women who have committed themselves to working against the system. Nor do we intend to deny that these efforts may have improved the lot of many patients who otherwise would have been much more severely oppressed. Nor do we mean to imply that any search for alternatives will ultimately end in cooptation. Our aim has been simply to explain the process by which psychiatric models are diffused and modernized. All too often, "psychiatric imperialism" is pictured as an irresistible tide, which little by little comes to inundate an ever broader expanse of the landscape. In fact the process by which psychiatry expands is more dialectical. Medicalization encounters obstacles and must fight off counteroffensives. Still, the medical model has seldom lost ground. Wherever psychiatrization meets with resistance, it is transformed, and what emerges in each instance is a novel and more flexible psychiatric model. The most recent illustration of this process may be found in those recommendations of the Carter Commission whose purpose was to mobilize alternative forms of mental health care so as to extend and diversify the public mental health system (see chapter 5). When we come to study the present proliferation of group therapies in the private sector, we shall have further confirmation of the essential characteristics of the process: merely to state that an activity is nonmedical does not guarantee that in practice its effects are altogether different from the effects of therapy. Psychiatry makes progress, in some cases, in the wake' of the progress of parapsychiatry and even of certain forms of antipsychiatry.

CHAPTER 8

Psy Services and Their New Consumers

Historically, western medicine has alternated between two extremes, in the United States as elsewhere: private medicine, based on an intimate relationship between patient and doctor, on the one hand, and institutionalized care, based on the hospital, on the other hand. In recent years, however, not only has there been diversification on the institutional side, there has also been a transformation of health care on the private side. In both areas, the United States has been in the forefront. While the mental hospital inpatient is the extreme case of complete and utter dependence on the psychiatric system (dependence that is also exhibited to a lesser degree in other institutions in the mental health care system), the private patient would seem to enjoy freedom of choice in contracting for services with a competent specialist. The client generally chooses a form of service compatible with a normal or near-normal existence. He is neither institutionalized nor completely incapacitated; he neither loses his rights nor his obligation to carry on with his ordinary activities. Therapy thus penetrates the client's everyday life and vice versa. The boundary between social life and the therapeutic relationship can therefore be crossed in either direction. The permeability of the boundary opens up the possibility of contamination. Behavioral models used in therapy extend their effects to daily life; the transfer is facilitated by the narrowing of the gap between the normal and the pathological. It has long been noticed that psychoanalysis turns ordinary life into a sort of prologue for the play enacted on the analyst's couch (patients have been known to dream for their analysts and even to fall in love so that they could later describe the experience on the couch). Conversely, interpretations worked out in the course of analysis are commonly projected into ordinary life; social life is thus deciphered in terms of private fantasy.

It is important to notice, however, that in the United States the main vehicle of exchange between the therapeutic situation and social life in general is no longer psychoanalysis (and therefore the quantitative limits on the effects of such an exchange, which were established by the relatively small number of patients in analysis, are no longer operative). Democracy has won out: new therapies are today within the reach of all, or nearly all. A survey of the various new methods in use in the United States thus affords a glimpse of a futuristic—and alarming—vision. One comes away with an impression that everyday life is utterly suffused with interpretations stemming from medical psychology; the methods are now so flexible that nothing further stands in the way of their unlimited proliferation. The political implications of this colonization of social life by psychology are enormous.

THE METAMORPHOSES OF THE PRIVATE-CARE MODEL

Private psychotherapy first developed on the fringes of the public hospital system. In the latter part of the nineteenth century, neurologists practicing in large cities were the first to build up a private clientele while continuing to work in hospitals (see chapter 2). The history of the spread of psychoanalysis in the United States during the second decade of the twentieth century also shows that it was hospital staff members from nonpsychiatric institutions (such as general hospitals and university teaching clinics) who first began seeing clients at home, in many cases before deciding to devote themselves exclusively to private practice. Until the end of the Second World War, however, these developments were of limited significance. In 1940 the American Psychoanalytic Association had only 192 members. By 1944 there were no more than

3,000 psychiatrists in public as well as private practice throughout the United States. As we have seen, it was around this time that the idea of a need for psychiatric intervention took hold, along with the idea that there was a dearth of trained personnel to meet that need (see chapter 3). The National Institute of Mental Health took charge of the private as well as the public aspect of the problem by financing a number of training programs in psychiatry, including some designed for general practitioners already in practice.

Thus the private sector developed at roughly the same pace as the public sector. What is more, each had a great influence on the other, because part-time work in public institutions is widespread in the United States. Today, out of a total of 30,000 American psychiatrists, about half work mainly or exclusively in the private sector. They treat between 1.5 and 2 million patients each year.[1] Even though it is possible for psychiatrists to work in both private and public sectors at the same time, the client recruitment networks are quite different. A recent study showed that 90 percent of private patients came directly to the doctor's private office for consultation, compared with only 10 percent who were referred through an institution.[2] The private sector, then, is concerned mainly with a different population from the one that frequents the public institutions.

What form does private practice most commonly take in the United States? Until recently, psychoanalysis dominated the private as well as the public sector. Not that psychoanalysts are in the majority: at present, one could estimate that there are some 4,000 of them, treating approximately 30,000 patients with more or less orthodox versions of Freudian technique. But the spectacular increase in the number of psychiatrists after the Second World War came at a moment when psychoanalysts held key positions in the field of medical education. Even today more than half of all medical school deans are psychoanalysts. In the late fifties two-thirds of the psychiatric students in leading universities took courses in analysis as an integral part of their training.[3] Thus Freudian concepts, watered down or adapted in one degree or another, formed the backbone of a psychiatrist's training. What is known as "dynamic psychology," a relational approach based on exploring the psychic makeup of each individual patient, has become the dominant mode of treatment—or at any rate the dominant point of reference—and serves as a rationale for a variety of practical methods, particularly those used in institutions.

This overwhelming fact has relegated questions of psychoanalytic orthodoxy to the second rank. In addition to the American Psychoanalytic Association, would-be guardian of the Freudian legacy, which has 2,500 members (plus 700 analysts in training), there are many dissident Freudian schools in the United States, such as the Karen Horney Institute in New York, characterized by "culturalist" leanings, and the William Alanson White Institute, which was founded by Sullivan and which emphasizes "interpersonal relations." Certain of the more eclectic schools are represented by a rival organization, the American Academy of Psychoanalysis, founded in 1967 by Frantz Alexander, Ray Grinker, and Frieda Fromm-Reichman, which sees itself as more dynamic and open-minded than its rivals and which today numbers some 850 members. Do these rival schools attest to the adaptability of the Freudian tradition or to a betrayal of that tradition? As in Europe, this question has given rise to theoretical disputes, personal polemics, and the expulsion of dissidents. It is nonetheless true that the rival factions, together with other groups even farther removed from strict Freudian orthodoxy (such as the followers of Rogers, Erikson, and others), have together produced a psychotherapeutic model that has dominated American mental medicine.

This model today seems to be in crisis. In the early sixties, when the community mental health centers were set up, the importance accorded to social models led first to a lessening of the influence of psychoanalysis. The antiprofessional predilections of the counterculture worked in the same direction. Psychoanalysis proved to be of little use in dealing with the problems that preoccupied both the psychiatric establishment and public opinion: drugs, youth unrest, poverty and deprivation. A campaign was launched that was critical of the elitism of psychoanalysis as well as of its high cost, useless technical complexity, and lack of efficacy in coping with the most important problems in the field of mental health. In 1964–66 the number of trainees in schools of psychoanalysis fell to half what it had been in 1958–60.[4] Today, behavior modification and other supposedly more effective and scientific methods, including those developed in various types of therapy groups (see below), are battling for supremacy. It is frequently said that psychoanalysis is now outmoded. Such a judgment is too sweeping and needs to be corrected in several respects.

The influence of psychoanalytically-inspired psychotherapy continues to make itself felt in practice, particularly in the private sector. A recent study found that the "dynamic approach" was invoked as the prime mode of therapeutic intervention not only by 90 percent of the psychoanalysts but also by 67 percent of all psychiatrists; 81 percent of private clients were still being treated in individual therapy in 1974 (though it is true that this figure includes behavior modification therapy). Hence the various forms of group therapy, family therapy, and so forth were still of secondary importance in psychiatric practice proper, even though these other therapies were growing rapidly in popularity. More traditional medical approaches were likewise of secondary significance: fewer than one-third of psychiatrists in private practice rated (or at any rate said that they rated) drugs and shock treatment as primary therapeutic options.[5]

Psychoanalysis, moreover, is still being chosen by large numbers of young psychiatrists, including many of the brightest and most ambitious of them, particularly in the leading medical schools along the East Coast. They are aware that psychoanalysis is still a royal road to wealth, prestige, and power in the medical profession—and that it has something to offer the intellectually curious and theoretically speculative, as opposed to newer forms of treatment, which tend to encourage a rather profound anti-intellectualism and an uncritical devotion to immediate efficacy. The Psychoanalytic Society of Boston, one of the leading centers of Freudian orthodoxy in the United States, has, for example, kept up its enrollment over the last few years.

Incontestable though the reaction against psychoanalysis is, its significance is nevertheless complex and ambiguous. In part, the reaction is indicative of a turn back to biological, pharmacological, and psychoexperimental views that are, or seem to be, in contradiction with the psychoanalytic model of interpretation. But it is of at least equal importance that many of the challenges to psychoanalysis have been mounted from positions still strongly subject to its influence. Most of the new methods that we shall be examining shortly differ from the standard psychoanalytic treatment in one or more respects: psychotherapy is said to be too long, too costly, or too intellectual, or to be monopolized by professionals, or to neglect the body, the present, spontaneity, the role of current events, of the social environment, and so on. Whatever the specific grounds for criticism, then, the aim in each case is to thoroughly rework the psychoanalytic method rather than to reject it out of hand. It might therefore be justifiable to refer to nearly all these new therapies (except behavior modification) as bastard forms of psychoanalysis, which itself may have been, when it dominated the scene, no more than a bastardized form of Freudian orthodoxy.

The relation between these recent innovations and psychoanalysis is therefore just as much one of continuity as of discontinuity, and therein lies the crux of the problem. Doubtless it is correct to say that psychoanalysis is outmoded in the United States in that it is no longer the most up-to-date form of therapy: most innovations nowadays are conceived in opposition to it. But in order to go beyond psychoanalysis they count on its existence. The real issue in the current debate over psychoanalysis in the United States is not so much the question of Freudian orthodoxy, which most American analysts have long since given up, as it is the future of a particular way of interpreting and manipulating human relations, a way that was initially justified by psychoanalysis but that is continuing to increase in popularity now that the prestige of psychoanalysis is on the decline. The same society that welcomed Freud as the messiah continues to celebrate his lesser epigones. Why? Because the role that psychoanalysis played in the United States was not limited to dominating, as it once did, the narrow field of mental medicine. Psychoanalysis was the main instrument for the reduction of social issues in general to questions of psychology. Psychoanalysm—to coin a word intended to convey the idea of an active effort to force the many dimensions of social history into the Procrustean bed of a theory focused exclusively on individual subjectivity[6]—found in the United States a fertile soil in which to flourish. The "psychoanalytic deluge" quickly inundated important areas of American social life (chapter 2). Later on, we shall attempt to indicate what structural features of liberal society made it possible for psychological reductionism to play a key role in the formulation of political strategy (in the sense intended by one American sociologist who said that, if Freud had not existed, it would have been necessary for Americans to have invented him).[7]

The special status that psychoanalysis has enjoyed in the United States has always been precarious, however. At first, there were no more than a few dozen psychoanalysts in the entire country, later a few hundred, and even today no more than a few thousand. Their clients number only in the tens of thousands (if we count only those treated in a strictly one-on-one client-analyst setting). The efficacy of psychoanalysis as a method, besides being controversial, is limited in the main to what can be accomplished in this kind of setting. Hence attempts to extrapolate the psychoanalytic model outside the domain of private psychotherapy are apt to be viewed as irresponsible, "ideological" in the pejorative sense. Psychoanalysis has never been shown to produce valid results in nonstandard settings. Even in institutions, notably mental hospitals, psychoanalysis has not so much contributed to genuine changes in hospital practice as served to justify modernization. Psychoanalysis is therefore caught in a dilemma. Its practical effects are limited, unpredictable, and obtainable only after long and costly treatment, applicable only to small numbers of carefully selected individuals. At the same time, however, it has been elevated to a position so august that it is supposed to furnish principles for the interpretaton of all social life. How can the gap between the narrow applicability of analytic methods and its broad sociopolitical function be overcome?

Postpsychoanalytic innovations can for the most part be interpreted as attempts to make analytic methods more widely applicable (while at the same time, no doubt, impoverishing their content). The following goals were seen as imperative: to reach more and more people with practical and effective new techniques; to intervene more quickly and effectively; and to extend the usefulness of the techniques beyond the client–analyst relationship into a broader social setting. The aim of all recently developed techniques has been to widen the applicability of the reductionist methodology first codified and invested with scientific prestige by the psychoanalysts, and at the same time to achieve greater efficacy.

These methods were first tried out on a group that has been called the Friends of Psychotherapy, people who, for one reason or another, were drawn to psychoanalysis in its early days. A sample of such people has been analyzed by Charles Kadushin, who found that they differ in striking ways from mental patients cut from a more traditional mold.[8] Early analysands tended to be wealthy, sophisticated, verbal, and so on—in short, they fit the common image of the analysand. What is more important, though, is that many of them occupied strategic positions in the intellectual world, the medical profession, the media, the entertainment business, and other key areas, which helped to make psychoanalysis widely known. It may be worth mentioning, in passing, that in 1970 Beverly Hills had seventy-seven practicing psychoanalysts, while six states in the American hinterland were without a single analyst. Last but not least, analysands as a group were people with special needs. Unlike the typical mental patient, who suffered from more serious maladies often related to organic damage or major shortcomings in family life or social relations, the Friends of Psychotherapy were mainly afflicted with "sexual problems, difficulties in interpersonal relations, and dissatisfaction with oneself."[9] To put it another way, these patients suffered not from a clear-cut pathology but rather from malaise, a malaise that seems to have been quite widespread, at least among the middle classes.

The number of patients who could be accepted for psychoanalysis was limited drastically, however, by the length and arduousness of the treatment and by the social criteria that had to be met. The Friends of Psychotherapy in the United States probably number in the millions, but those who actually became clients are counted in the tens of thousands. The reasons for this disparity have to do both with the nature of the Freudian method and with the lack of physical resources. With the new methods, it became possible to respond to the desire for help with nonpathological problems. These methods helped "democratize" access to a paratherapeutic type of relationship, the concept of which was dominated almost exclusively by psychoanalysis. The ensuing wave of new consumers of psychological services represented more than mere quantitative change. Traditionally, and more or less by definition, therapy was intended for those who were sick or presumed to be sick and identified as such. Psychoanalysis blurred the boundary line between the normal and the pathological, but only for a small, select clientele. With the arrival of the postpsychoanalytic era it has become possible to speak of "therapy for the normal" on a much wider scale. This is an important change, for it implies that anyone and everyone now falls within the purview of one of the new types of therapy.

THE NEW METHODS

Most of the new methods that we shall be looking at were developed during the fifties, though it was not until the sixties that they found a wide audience. Taken together, they do not necessarily mean that the one-on-one therapeutic relationship is now discredited, but rather that therapy has tended to focus more and more on techniques suitable for incorporation into more "democratic" types of practice. Most of the new methods were developed by professionals and hence have not undermined traditional professional standards. Because simplified procedures were adopted, however, the new methods lend themselves to use outside the professional setting.[10]

Behavior Modification

Behavior modification is the only one of the new methods that is not in some measure a bastard form of psychoanalysis. Behavior modification techniques are based on the principle that all behavior, no matter how complex, is learned and therefore that inappropriate behavior can be unlearned and replaced by behavior of a different kind, more in keeping with the desired norm. Behavior modification therapy was developed in psychology laboratories, and its success has brought a new kind of specialist into the field of mental medicine, men and women trained not as psychiatrists or clinicians but rather as "scientists": specifically, as experimental psychologists.[11] Psychologists in private practice as well as institutions found these new methods useful as a way of legitimating what they were doing; such legitimation was necessary because, in the United States, psychoanalysis is virtually the exclusive province of medical doctors. Behavior modification does not pretend to seek out the causes of pathological behavior or to understand its motives, but rather treats the symptoms as they manifest themselves to the observer.

In the eyes of its proponents, the modesty and common sense of the experimental method account for the efficacy of the new therapies. These features also explain the growing popularity of the new approaches.[12] Specialized treatment no longer has to rely on medical definitions of specific pathologies, or cases. Treatments are available for any kind of behavioral dysfunction or deviance, and, for that matter, for any detectable deviation from normal or average behavior. Witness the primary indications for the application of behavior modification as listed in an official report of the American Psychiatric Association: behavioral therapy is "highly effective" for "phobic reactions and anxiety, enuresis, and stammering and tics associated with Tourette's syndrome." It yields "frequent improvement" in cases of "obsessive and compulsive behavior, hysteria, incontinence, impotence due to psychological causes, homosexuality, fetishism, frigidity, transvestitism, exhibitionism, passion for gambling, obesity, anorexia, insomnia, and nightmares" as well as for "behavioral problems in near-normal children, such as fits, head banging, thumbsucking, refusal to eat, and frequent scratching." Finally, it has yielded "promising results" in dealing with "behavior that causes problems in the family, such as persistent questioning, hostility, sibling rivalry, and, outside the family, reclusiveness, voluntary dumbness, hyperactivity, and problems relating to classmates."[13]

To deal with so wide a range of "indications," the techniques themselves must be quite varied, ranging from the crudest forms of intervention (punishment, aversion therapy) to assertiveness training.[14] The techniques are not limited to handing out rewards and punishments, and they are applicable in a wide variety of situations, going far beyond the uses discussed earlier in our examination of behavior modification in prisons and mental hospitals (chapters 4 and 6). The techniques are probably most effective when the individual's environment can be subjected to total control. More flexible and wide-ranging programs can, however, be set up in noninstitutional settings, including private practice situations. The client's family and associates can also be enlisted as collaborators in the therapy. To cite one example, the parents of a "problem child" can be made responsible for administering "scientifically determined" doses of appropriate rewards and punishments in accordance with a timetable worked out in collaboration with the therapist (see chapter 6). These programs, which provide a scientific rationale for old-fashioned discipline and which are based on simple, rational, easy-to-follow procedures, are generally well received by parents and teachers. They have also met with favorable receptions from plant managers, clergymen, and other institutional officials. Sometimes, moreover, behavioral therapy is voluntarily sought out by people trying to deal with obesity, quit smoking, overcome shyness, and so forth. Thus, behavior modification has been used as a way of imposing scientifically designed controls on the daily routine of many people; it therefore lends itself to a virtually unlimited range of applications. With some exaggeration, perhaps, it might be said that behavior modification turns all of life into an educational and disciplinary institution.

Family Therapy

Family therapy is less a unified body of doctrine than a broad range of different approaches. In the fifties, for example, "conjoint family therapy" introduced the method of bringing two or more members of a family together in the presence of the therapist, the idea being that problems within the family itself were more important than individual pathology. In "multiple impact therapy," a team of therapists works intensively with several members of a family for several days, both individually and in groups.[15] "Network therapy" goes beyond the nuclear family and brings together "a group of people having permanent significance for one another in meeting certain specific human needs." The network "treated" in this way may consist of as many as forty persons.[16]

All these various approaches, too diverse to analyze here in detail, share two common characteristics that differentiate them from individual psychotherapies.[17] First, they take a systems approach that originates with social psychology and communications theory rather than with individual psychology, whether analytic or not. One of the fathers of family therapy, Nathan Ackerman, who was influenced by Kurt Lewin, uses the idea of a social role as one of his key concepts, on the basis of which he hopes to establish a "scientific" discipline.[18] The work of Haley and Jackson at the Palo Alto Mental Research Center in California is also fundamental. The concept of the "double bind," inspired by communications theory, sees the family "victim" as a person placed in an impossible situation by two contradictory demands. Such a situation is typical of the families of schizophrenics but is also found in "normal" families.[19] Ultimately, the emphasis on communication leads to an interest in cybernetics, to which Jackson turned toward the end of his life. Instead of contrasting sickness and health or looking at the dynamics of an individual personality, one focuses on interactions within a system, which are viewed in the same way as the "inputs" and "outputs" of an electronic device, without regard to what is going on inside the black box.

A second difference between family therapies and more traditional kinds of therapy has to do with the role assigned to the therapist. The family therapist does not pretend to be neutral but takes an active role in several ways. Ackerman, for example, holds that there must be an intense emotional interaction between the therapist and his clients, with the therapist's personality in a sense filling in the gaps in the family's interactions. Satir has developed a program of instruction to teach families how to communicate, offering himself as a model of clear and simple communication.[20] For Jackson, the therapist must act as a disruptive influence in order to break down pathological defensive systems.[21]

Family therapy thus represents a move away from the traditional conception of mental health as a kind of equilibrium of various forces within an individual's personality. The target of family therapy is the family system and the obstacles to communication that it raises. The focus is on change, on development of the system, rather than on curing a syndrome. Ackerman takes note of this shift when he asserts that "the goal of family therapy is not merely to remove symptoms or to adjust personality to environment, but more than that—to create a new way of living."[22]

Sex Therapy

The names most commonly associated with sex therapy are William H. Masters and Virginia E. Johnson, who have been studying sexuality in men and women under laboratory-controlled conditions for more than twenty years.[23] Steps have been taken to insure that the research carried out at the Reproductive Biology Research Foundation in Saint Louis, which they founded, will meet scientific standards of rigor. The policy of the Foundation requires that at least ten years of study be devoted to each area of human sexual behavior before the results are made known to the scientific community.[24] This great show of rigor carries over into the practical training programs, which are designed to teach sexual behavior through a carefully planned series of exercises. In actuality, however, sex therapy is a confused, nebulous field in which innumerable counselors, teachers, and clinicians use a bewildering variety of techniques, including sexual intercourse with their clients. In a 1976 lecture, Masters estimated that there were between 3,500 and 5,000 clinics offering "what they call sex therapy, but that probably fewer than 100 centers used professional techniques and properly trained professional therapists."[25]

Nevertheless, all sex therapies share certain features in common that make them more widely applicable than traditional forms of therapy. Sex therapists are generally critical of the length and ineffectiveness of the sort of "dynamic therapy" that is inspired by psychoanalysis. They argue that it is pointless to treat the subconscious or to try to cure deep-seated personality conflicts and disorders. Accordingly, sex therapy is brief—five or six sessions spread out over three to six weeks for the treatment of premature ejaculation, for example, and ten sessions over a six-week period for vaginismus.[26] The treatment is a form of crisis intervention directed at a precise objective and intended to "treat the symptom" using behavior modification techniques, nonverbal communication, and body-awareness training.

Sex therapy also represents a move away from the idea of one-on-one therapy. This accords with the notion that the client's problem stems from a system of relations involving at least one other person. Thus Masters and Johnson stress the importance not only of the "conjugal unit" but also of poor communications in general, of unrealistic social expectations, deception, and so on.[27] As a general rule, this means that no person can be treated individually. Two therapists of opposite sexes often collaborate in treatment sessions, in order to get away from the one-way transference to which conventional individual therapy is subject.

Bioenergetics

Alexander Lowen, the originator of bioenergetics, is a disciple of Wilhelm Reich. His criticisms of psychoanalysis resemble those of his mentor: verbalization may enable the patient to take cognizance of his condition, but not to experience or transform it.[28] Bioenergetic therapy is aimed at releasing the energy trapped within the body as a result of childhood sexual traumas. Essentially, it works directly on the body.

Bioenergetics employs techniques requiring professional training and usually treats patients one at a time. It has even been used in traditional mental institutions.[29] Lowen is critical of mysticism, of brief, superficial treatments that in his judgment have no lasting effect.[30] Effective bioenergetic therapy is lengthy and must follow precise rules. Despite this traditionalism, Lowen has affinities with the more modern types of "humanist" psychotherapy in that he accords great importance to the growth of the individual and sees tension between the needs deriving from growth and the need to adjust to society: most people go into therapy because their development has been arrested by a hostile, repressive world. Work on the body makes it possible to unblock the growth process, and each "peak experience" is integrated through self-awareness into the personality. Thus there is no longer any distinction between sickness and health. Everyone is to some extent unhealthy. The "cure" is therefore no longer something that can be perceived objectively but rather a process that can continue indefinitely.

Gestalt Therapy

Frederick S. Perls, the founder of Gestalt therapy, was, like Lowen, a disciple of Reich. Perls' criticism of psychoanalysis is similar to Lowen's: analysts place too much emphasis on verbalization and past experiences. But Perls, who was also influenced by Lewin, has carried the anti-intellectual character common to most of the new therapies to extreme lengths. The unconscious, he argues, does not exist, nor does repression. There is nothing to be interpreted, for everything occurs in the here and now: "Everything is grounded in *awareness*. *Awareness* is the only basis of knowledge, communication, and so on."[31] Gestalt therapy is based on a holistic view of the individual, whose personality lies hidden beneath a veil of neurotic fixations, social roles, and cultural alienation. The individual must get rid of these imperfect forms (gestalts) and take responsibility for his own life, while the therapist is reduced to playing a subordinate role in the process of individual self-awareness. Perls' famous "prayer," made popular by posters in the early seventies, is a good expression of the fundamentalist individualism that served as a rationalization for the retreat from commitment on the part of young people as the countercultural movement waned:

> I do my thing, and you do your thing
> I am not in this world to live up to your expectations
> And you are not in this world to live up to mine.
> You are you and I am I,
> And if by chance we find each other, it's beautiful
> If not, it can't be helped.[32]

This individualist philosophy calls for constant personality growth, a far more sweeping notion than the medical concept of a cure. According to Perls, the individual tries to move toward a self-regulated state of equilibrium in a continuous process demanding a full awareness of the present moment. Society as it exists today, however, thwarts this development. The individual in contemporary society is characteristically in "a chronic state of disequilibrium in which the gratifications we seek never come."[33] Everyone is constantly bombarded with negative stimuli that arouse fear, anxiety, and frustration. Hence everyone is dissatisfied, in search of a healthier existence, and thus a potential client for Gestalt therapy. Gestalt techniques are in fact used for more than just therapy, finding application in schools, social work, and elsewhere, and the vocabulary of Gestalt therapy ("do your own thing," etc.) has begun to replace such outmoded psychoanalytic concepts as complexes, projections, defense mechanisms, and so on in the common parlance of the middle classes.

Primal Scream

Arthur Janov, the originator of primal scream therapy, shares with other inventors of therapeutic techniques the belief that he has discovered the formula that will revolutionize therapy:

> Some years ago, I heard something that was to change the course of my professional life and the lives of my patients. What I heard may change the nature of psychotherapy as it is now known—an eerie scream welling up from the depths of a young man lying on the floor during a therapy session.[34]

The "primal scream," which is supposed to rise out of the depths of the individual, gives vent to the pain caused by frustrations that a person faced as a child when his or her basic needs were not met. These tensions have to be relived, thereby triggering a panic expressed in the scream but at the same time freeing the individual of his anxiety. For Janov, this method is the only way to cure neurosis, and he has tried to establish its value scientifically by making physiological measurements of the effects of the scream.[35] Janov is quite contemptuous of other types of therapy. Although psychoanalysis, he claims, had the merit of recognizing childhood experiences as the traumatic root of all neuroses, it confined its efforts to interpretation and symbolism and thereby missed the importance of actual experience of the traumatic situation, which alone has the power to cure.[36]

At first sight it would seem to be difficult to adapt primal scream techniques for large-scale use. The therapy is long and costly. The Janov Institute in Los Angeles accepts patients for a one-month course of treatment that costs $6,000 (which pays for seventy-five group sessions spread over a three-week period and a final week of individual therapy).[37] Janov imposes stringent professional standards on his disciples, whom he supervises closely. But his writings have been widely popular, and after reading Janov, many people tried primal scream on their own or in small groups because there were no primal scream therapists in the area.[38] Many primal scream centers opened in recent years are to one degree or another at odds with Janov and his followers. Former disciples like William Swartley have popularized similar but less strict methods such as "primal integration."[39] Probably because primal scream is a tough method that produces intense experiences, many of its adepts have founded communities or support networks.

Transactional Analysis

Transactional analysis, developed by Eric Berne during the fifties,[40] was the most popular and widely practiced of the "humanist" therapies. It is a sort of simplified plagiarism of psychoanalysis: an individual is a synthesis of three ego states, the parent, the adult, and the child. These states are almost real entities: although the different states do interact, an individaul "is" in only one state at a time. In social life, therefore, he takes part in "transactions" with others which are governed by demands determined by one of these states. For example, in a love relationship, the "child" in one individual often relates to the "child" in another individual. In a business transaction it is presumably the two "adult" parts that communicate. In any encounter, then, several different combinations are possible, and there are several ways in which the relationship can go wrong. The best relationships are of course those that form between adults, and the surest way to "be O.K." is to enter into a relationship as an adult.[41]

Transactional analysis is brief. Frequently the "contract" between the therapist and the client (formalizing their prior expectations) is for a limited period of time, and after a few weeks the objectives can be revised. According to Harris, "all persons can become Transactional Analysts."[42] The method can be used in a one-on-one setting, but it is more commonly employed in a group. The promoters of transactional analysis have an undeniable aptitude for teaching and business. The key ideas are simple, not to say demagogic, and Berne's 120 "games," that is, the "transactions" that most commonly structure social relations, have catchy titles like "sweetheart," "cops and robbers," "kick me," "peasant," "let's pull a fast one on Joey," etc.[43]

By Harris's own admission, the reason for this simplicity is related to the aim of "how to get Freud off the couch and to the masses."[44] And this wish seems to have been fulfilled. The method has been turned into a tool that anyone can use, and that nearly everyone does use, without the slightest reference to mental illness. Transactional analysis is employed in prisons, hospitals, schools, churches, businesses, and factories. Among the largest users are IBM, major airlines, and the U.S. Navy. It is supposed to be beneficial for psychotics, alcoholics, delinquents, the overweight, smokers, children, parents, housewives, salespeople, shop foremen, managers, and others. Even "radicals" use it, transforming the parent into the "pig parent," the cop—symbol of the authoritarian evil from which people must liberate themselves.

Claude Steiner, a leader of the "radical therapists," has written a book on treating alcoholics with transactional analysis that has been well received, and he is cited with approval in *The O.K. Boss*, a book written for business executives and people who would like to resemble them by the vice-president of the International Transactional Analysis Association, which has 8,000 members in the United States.[45]

Transactional analysis is undoubtedly, along with behavior modification, the technique best adapted to promoting social conformity among those in common use in the United States. It reduces social life to a few typical situations, or "games," which can be manipulated by rational, instrumental means. The way to be "O.K." is to be accepted by others. Who can resist the temptation to acquire at low cost and in a few easy lessons the recipe for achieving the ideal state of total conformity?

Unfortunately, it is impossible to give precise figures for the number of clients treated by each of these types of therapy. No official statistics exist, and our attempts to obtain figures from the proponents of each technique have generally ended in disappointment. Most partisans of the new therapies tend to be proselytizers, and they are therefore inclined to praise their own pet methods and claim superiority over all others rather than measure their effectiveness or gauge the actual size of the audience for them. Taken together, though, these new therapies have attracted a second circle of Friends of Psychotherapy that surely numbers in the hundreds of thousands. This group falls in between the first circle of clients involved in a professional relationship with certified mental health specialists and the third circle of people well disposed toward psychoanalysis but not in therapy themselves. The new techniques have found application in two different areas. On the one hand, they have helped to make traditional therapy more flexible, adding to its arsenal of techniques. Family therapy and even sex therapy, for example, are essentially extensions of "dynamic psychology." New techniques generate new symptoms which in turn generate new clients. But these innovations can also be fitted, after necessary adjustments, into a fairly standard sort of clinical relationship, in which one or two patients seeking treatment consult with one or two competent specialists. On the other hand, such techniques as transactional analysis not only meet this demand but go beyond it, finding applications in which not the slightest reference is made to mental illness. Although the originators of each method tend to glorify their own approach and run down the rest, it is worth noting that in many applications eclecticism is the rule. A practitioner may well do a little family therapy, a bit of behavior modification, some transactional analysis, and so on, using whatever technique he deems best suited to the "symptoms" of each patient. To European therapists this kind of eclecticism may seem surprising, but it is a basic feature of American practice. In the eyes of most practitioners, nearly all therapeutic approaches are compatible with one another. In particular, simultaneous use of psychoanalysis and behavior modification, which to the French observer seems absolutely astonishing, is not only commonly practiced but even justified theoretically by respected representatives of both schools.[46]

Thus, we can now begin to make out, alongside the area covered by psychoanalysis and neuropsychiatry, the outlines of another rapidly growing area in which medico-psychological techniques are influential. Whether integrated into older psychiatric practices or extended to new specialists and institutions, the more modern therapies have broadened the influence of the older ones, even where the former are conceived as criticisms of the latter.

One example of the way in which professionalism has been revitalized and adapted to changed circumstances is the Liberty Street Associates, a small private institution in the wealthy Boston suburb of Danvers. It was founded by two or three pschiatrists and psychologists fed up with the difficult working conditions in public institutions. New members were added to the initial group and brought with them both new skills and additional capital. The work is shared among colleagues and carried out in attractive offices amid pleasant surroundings. The Associates offer a wide range of services, from treatment of severe cases to basic counseling. Family therapy is the dominant approach, but other approaches are not ruled out. When we went to the offices for a visit, it was suggested that we undergo a "family checkup" at a cost of $100. Families generally are urged to undergo periodic examinations to evaluate how well balanced they are, just as they might go regularly to the dentist. Is heartache less serious than toothache? Family quarrels, divorces, suicides, alcoholism, drug abuse, runaway children, "and countless other chronic symptoms of life in our society"[47] might, according to the group's advertising, be prevented if disorders in the family were caught early.

There are at present in the United States hundreds upon hundreds of institutions similar to this one, frequently relying mainly on a particular one of the new therapeutic techniques, but willing to try others if necessary. They offer the middle classes diversified and often attractive services. While their cost is relatively high, on the order of a session with a psychoanalyst, the treatment does not last as long as analysis. Frequent recourse to group techniques, moreover, makes it possible to offer lower rates. Thus, parallel to the expansion of the public mental health system (chapter 5) and alternative forms of care (chapter 7), a growing number of patients, or at any rate "people with problems," mainly from the middle classes, have fallen under the influence of this refurbished mental health care system. Eschewing, more or less overtly, the psychodynamic clinical relationship made popular by psychoanalysis, the fashionable new technologies have in fact considerably extended the influence of mental medicine.

NORMALITY AS A SYMPTOM

The new technologies, perfected during the last fifteen years and designed to make therapy for the normal available to all, were prevented from gaining wide currency as long as they continued to require the services of professional therapists and/or institutions whose major purpose was therapeutic. The full potential implicit in these technologies could not be realized in everyday life until a new type of institution had been invented, whose sole function was to spread the new methods. This came in the late sixties, when a new type of group exploded into popularity. In many countries 1968 marked the high point of the student protest movement and the end of a revolutionary dream. In the United States 1968 was, according to *The New York Times*, "the year of the group." Groups flourished not only in the countless "growth centers" that were then being opened but also in universities, businesses, churches, social service agencies, and many kinds of training programs.[48]

An encounter group typically (though devotees of the subject say no two groups are alike) consists of a dozen or so persons, together with a group leader. The purpose of the group is to allow its members to express and share their true feelings, to discover themselves through others, and to liberate themselves from the constraints of society, thereby gaining insight into the true nature of their developing being. The accent is placed on "feeling," on the immediate emotional content of the encounter. The values that are held in high esteem—sincerity, authenticity, intimacy, candor, spontaneity, openness, and self-fulfillment—are the opposite of those said to be dominant in the outside society.

For the participants, the encounter group has an intrinsic value and is an end in itself. It lasts only as long as its members are assembled, unless another group is brought together to relive the undying happy moments of group experience on a still higher plane. The groups foster an almost religious zeal that has led some adepts to speak of "conversion experiences" or "peak experiences" and consequently to scorn the compromises of everyday life with all the contemptuousness of newly-initiated fanatics. On the other hand, these group experiences are invariably aided by the latest techniques and use methods that are often arduous, gadgets of one sort or another, well-known books bent out of shape to serve alien purposes, and pretentious theorizing, in order to reach their goal of instant ecstasy. The encounter groups are built around a paradox. On the one hand they represent an idealistic and utopian social movement with roots in the counterculture and probably beyond that in American religious tradition. On the other hand, however, they constantly invoke rational procedures, claim to be applying the latest discoveries of the social sciences, and often resort in their arguments to a level of petty detail that they justify as experimental methodology. The group

> seeks to court spontaneity and authenticity by artifice; to combat instrumentalism instrumentally; to provide access to experience by reducing it to a packaged commodity; to engineer autonomy by group pressure; to liberate individuality by group shaping.[49]

Before we turn to an examination of the many different kinds of groups, special mention must be made of a phenomenon that is like the encounter group phenomenon in some respects, in particular in wanting to move beyond therapy and in competing for the same group of clients, but that differs from the encounter groups in other respects: namely, "cocounseling" or "reevaluation counseling," a form of self-help based on research done by a former Seattle union leader, Harvey Jackins. Disappointed by Marxism, Jackins worked out a theory of spontaneous interpersonal assistance: one untrained person offers his "free attention" to another, thereby enabling the latter to unburden himself of his emotions and gain access to happiness of a rational, efficacious, and constructive sort.[50]

Cocounseling brings together (for a session of approximately two hours) two people interested in bringing painful emotional states to the surface (an obvious vulgarization of the psychoanalytic notion of "abreaction"). Simple techniques are used to relieve stress: holding hands, talking about the emotion-charged situation to the point of tears and trembling, and so on. The expression of emotion is supposed to unblock the subject's constructive capacities, thereby enabling him to approach new situations in a rational and emotionally positive way. This type of self-help is supposed to be completely reversible. The "client" becomes the "counselor" and can immediately offer the same service to another person. The training is simple, short, and not very expensive: to become a cocounselor one need only attend class along with fifteen or twenty other students once a week for sixteen weeks. During these sessions the principles of the technique are explained and cocounseling procedures are discussed and taught. If a member of the class has any special difficulties in learning how to arrive at the state of "free attention," he receives special help from an experienced practitioner. After the initial training, however, graduates become part of the great family of cocounselors, people who have received help themselves and are qualified to help others. Any place, any time of day or night, any graduate can call upon the services of any other; all must be ready to render service to other cocounseling participants.

Cocounseling thus forms a sort of community, not to say a church, which spreads by proselytism. Beyond any possible therapeutic effect, the method aims to provide a real alternative to oppressive social institutions. The open emotional expression it encourages has been contrasted with "the bureaucratically-oriented personality style and interpersonal organization prevalent in advanced industrial societies."[51] Learning to be responsible for one's own life leads to the acceptance of social responsibilities. Jackins seems to have invested this microtechnique with the Marxist messianism that had inspired him in earlier years. He felt that each of us must take full responsibility for the "most distant atom in the most far off star in the remotest galaxy," because if we limit our responsibility in any way that would mean we are abandoning all responsibility.[52]

Hundreds of thousands of people in the United States today (along with others around the world in countries to which the cocounseling doctrine has already spread) share the goal of revolutionizing society, and are working to win others to the cause. Underlying the scheme is a sort of vulgar Rousseauism: man, say its adherents, is spontaneously a rational and emotionally constructive being; society is oppressive, but its structure has no autonomous character, is subject to no deterministic forces, and therefore can be transformed if, first, individuals are transformed one by one. Still, there is something novel and paradoxical in the way cocounseling is organized: a technique that enables one individual to manipulate the emotions of another has been shaped into an instrument for forging a community with a self-proclaimed universal mission, a political goal that is as integral a part of the movement as the procedures for instrumental manipulation. The enthusiasm of cocounseling's adepts is reminiscent of that of the chosen few, who harbor no doubts that ultimately they will succeed in persuading the entire world to join them. In practice, cocounseling seems to be the most democratic of the methods we have examined: the roles of the person giving and the person receiving help are indeed interchangeable, and while leaders do undeniably play a role in initiating others and maintaining doctrinal purity, that role is reduced to a minimum and is aimed at helping others achieve independence.

Cocounseling has thus spread widely as a sect of committed initiates, who, having solved their personal problems and invented a mode of interpersonal communication, now proclaim themselves ready to take on the problems of mankind. Compared with a prophetic vision of this sort, therapy is indeed outmoded.

The encounter group movement (which has recently come to France under the name "human potential" movement) offers another example of the same surprising combination of instrumentalism and messianism. It is more complex in its origins, however, and more diverse in its manifestations. Considerations of space allow us only to mention here the major influences that the movement has unified into a coherent whole.[53] One precursor was the work of Moreno, who was the first to emphasize the importance of the "here and now" and the "encounter," and who used his work in New Deal social programs to apply his discoveries in a nontherapeutic setting.[54] Another influence was the work done at the National Training Laboratory, continuing Kurt Lewin's research on groups. Still another was the "scientific management" tradition, which focused on internal group processes in abstraction from the group's explicit objectives (T-groups).[55] Also important was the "client-centered therapy" developed by Carl Rogers, which used nondirective techniques. Rogers was critical of irrelevant intellectual and professional concerns in therapy and emphasized the creative potential of the client. His influence was enhanced by his role as a prophet of the movement while working at the Western Behavioral Science Institute at La Jolla, California, and later at the Center for the Study of the Person.[56] Finally, there were the self-help groups, which are deeply rooted in American cultural and religious tradition. Ever since the foundation of Alcoholics Anonymous in 1935, such groups have promoted the values of self-awareness, individual responsibility, mutual solidarity, distrust of institutionalized authority and purely technical competence, and so on—values that provided a fertile soil in which "growth" groups were able to feverish.[57]

These multifarious influences were finally combined at the Esalen Institute into the novel synthesis characteristic of the encounter group movement. Founded in 1962 by a former philosophy and theology student upon his return from a long stay in India, the Esalen Institute is perched on a rocky promontory on the California coast. It has welcomed representatives of the various aspects of the counterculture, as well as adepts of a newly fashionable psychological culture hostile to the academicism of the psychiatric and psychoanalytic tradition. Among those who visited the institute were Aldous Huxley; Alan Watts, the popularizer of Oriental religions; leading figures in "human psychology" such as Abraham Kaplan and Abraham Maslow; Frederick Perls, the founder of Gestalt therapy; Alexander Lowen, the founder of bioenergetics; feminists; ex-leftists; and even behaviorists such as B. F. Skinner.

Oriental techniques such as yoga, Tai Chi Chan, and aikido were successfully transplanted at Esalen. Sensory awareness and body expression techniques were also developed, along with massages ("rolfing," Ida Rolf's method for integrating mind and body through vigorous massage, was born at Esalen), spontaneous dancing, breathing techniques, and so on. Above all, Esalen is devoted to spontaneous interpersonal relations, good vibrations, and unhindered growth and self-realization. Michael Murphy, Esalen's founder, explains that "our primary concern is the affective domain—the senses and feelings."[58] Esalen promulgated an up-to-the-minute ideology (incorporating proven marketable aspects of the counterculture) which became fashionable and exerted a certain snob-appeal. Dozens of other "growth centers" (Kairos, Oasis, Orizon, Anthos, etc.) were set up first in California and then throughout the United States. Esalen training became the calling card of a new breed of tanned, effusive, and superficial therapists, who carried the new gospel of free spontaneity to every corner of the country. Many people were drawn to Esalen not because they thought they were sick but because they were looking for personal growth.[59]

"Therapy for the normal," then, uses an array of mental and, particularly, physical techniques to maximize the "human yield" of each individual; it is not aimed at healing, as standard therapies presumably are. The goal is not to get well, but to become healthier (that is to experience more pleasure, to "get in touch with one's feelings," to become more aware of one's body, etc.). Medical healing gives way to personality growth: Encounter groups are designed for people who are functioning normally but who wish to improve their relationships with others. They "have been used extensively with industrial executives, government administrators, professional groups, and laymen—groups considered to be normal and well-functioning."[60] An even better account of the significance of the shift away from clinically-oriented psychotherapy has been given by Arthur Burton:

> Psychotherapy is no longer for the diseased. Some form of it is demanded by large numbers of students, management and supervisorial personnel, religious people, the formerly married, the unmarried, the sadly married, the literate, and the artistic and creatively inclined. . . . Its tenets are being offered as a new method of general education—of emotional rather than cognitive learning. It is freedom's approach to growth—and the possibility of being in a world which now severely curtails existence.[61]

Does this change represent a shift in emphasis or a reordering of priorities? Normality has not become the symptom to be treated. So-called normal individuals are in fact in a bind because "their alienation, loneliness, despair, and anxiety are ignored precisely because they are normal." To earn the right to treatment (as psychoanalysis had suspected), the normal individual must exhibit neurotic symptoms. But what is a symptom? "A psychic symptom today is no longer a symptom but a sign that life lacks joy."[62] Normal life—social life—is sick. It requires therapy, therapy for normality, and techniques to develop human potential and foster autonomy and enhance pleasure in a sad and alienated world. Adjustment, then, has been supplanted by a normative notion of normality—normality seen, in this new light, as the product of "working on" one's own personality.

Several features of American life have helped to spread this ideology to the social strata in which the bulk of its audience is to be found, namely, the white middle classes, particularly young people with a smattering of academic culture and susceptible to the modern values popularized by the marketing of the counter-culture. The movement exploded into popularity in California, whose population is highly mobile and includes a high proportion of individuals born in other states and belonging to the middle classes. Back has observed that encounter groups are a sort of respectable singles' club in which the enduring characteristics of American sociability—openness, warmth, and superficiality—are reproduced. Group participation facilitates social integration or, if need be, takes its place. Because the emotional ties formed are intense but short-lived, the groups make it easy both to enjoy social contact and to break it off.[63]

Deeper socioeconomic factors also play a role. In *Future Shock*, a well-known book widely read among the members of the counterculture, Alvin Toffler predicted the advent of "experiential industries . . . whose sole output consists not of manufactured goods, nor even of ordinary services, but of pre-programmed 'experiences'."[64] New aspirations of this sort can emerge when the basic needs have been satisfied, which was the case for the American middle classes in the late sixties, a period of economic growth. But this growth left those whose material well-being it assured dissatisfied and frustrated with their surroundings and interpersonal relations. Capitalism has probably gone further in America than anywhere else in imposing profitability, efficiency, and technological rationality as the pitiless criteria of success, with consequences for individual life and interpersonal relations that have often been described.[65] The desperate search for spontaneity, for authentic relations with others, and for free expression of feelings is surely a reaction against the coldness of bureaucracy and joyless labor. Group symbiosis and the interchangeable relationships of cocounseling are the authentic experiences toward which the lost members of the "lonely crowd" are groping.

Those who sing the praises of this sort of liberation apparently do not see how far it is conditioned by the very structure of what it is fighting against—to the point of internalizing it. The productive body, the machine for manufacturing desire or pleasure, and the instrumentalization of technically manipulated "authentic" relations are all merely transpositions into the realm of "liberated" subjectivity of the mechanisms that are being rejected in social life. The antithesis is pathetic but not dialectical, a flat contradiction of the platitude of human relations in a society where genuine relations have been destroyed by the imperatives of industrial rationality: this cult of the body, the moment, and the feelings uses its ridiculous techniques to imitate the alienation that it rejects. This pretentious dream of transparent communication is exposed as a mirage the minute one sets foot inside a "growth center." It is immediately apparent that what is really going on in these places is the promotion and marketing of a new consumer product. The "experience industries" have become part of big business, with their prostituted pitchmen, their upwardly mobile professionals, and their avid consumers, who once again are dropping their coins into the collection plate of the latest salvation-selling huckster.

The few noteworthy studies of this social phenomenon that have been done recently confirm these impressions, which are based on attending the meetings of a number of groups. These studies highlight the ambiguities in the attempt to "go beyond therapy."

In regard to the motives of group participants, it has been found that many of them first received more standard forms of psychotherapy before turning to group experiences.[66] Furthermore, the time and money saved by using groups rather than more medical forms of treatment may not be as great as first appeared. As a general rule, of course, group participation does not last as long as psychotherapy and is less costly for the client. But many individuals move from one group to another, and as soon as one experience is over begin looking for the latest new one to plunge into. Sometimes, moreover, traditional practitioners send clients to encounter groups to complement their own therapy; nor is it unheard of for professionals and ex-professionals to convert to the group ideology, starting and leading groups of their own (in many cases quite lucratively).

The practical consequences of participation in groups may be questioned in two respects. Certain studies are beginning to show worrisome rates of mishap, with as many as 9 percent of group participants becoming involved in acute crisis situations, psychotic episodes, or suicides. To understand how group sessions might well have a traumatic and destabilizing effect on precarious personalities, one has only to attend a few. Furthermore, the long-term beneficial effects seem almost nil. Participation in a group certainly does produce elation, temporary relief, and a sharing of warm feelings (as well as violence and hostility). But the effect soon fades, and the formulas learned appear to be of little use in coping with life's serious problems.[67] This would have been evident from the first had the mythology of change and the enthusiastic, fantastic reports of proselytes not caused many people to forget that changing one's desires is not enough to change the world.

Probably the most important change brought about by the groups is in the social and demographic characteristics of the clients as compared with the characteristics of clients of more conventional therapies. According to an American Psychiatric Association report, the majority of group clients is made up of young people, predominantly mental health workers, managers, and housewives.[68] Based on our own observations, we would say that many clients are also people with tenuous connections to professional careers, including both college students and, more commonly, dropouts living a precarious existence in what remains of the counterculture. Compared with psychoanalysis, then, recruitment is more "democratic," in the sense that clients are less well off, less cultivated, and less securely established. On the other hand, this democratization does not extend to the elderly, to low income groups, to ethnic minorities, or even to the working class. Rarely did we see a person older than forty-five, a black, or a Puerto Rican at any of the group sessions we attended (which does not mean that there were no exceptions to the rule). When a worker did show up at one meeting, his presence provided the occasion for a telling "ethnological" observation: the man, who had clearly wandered in by mistake, vehemently defended himself against the alien values foisted on him by the group, calling upon all the cultural resources at his command.

It is therefore necessary to modify somewhat the assertion that therapy for the normal is extending manipulative psychological techniques to the entire population. In the first place, the number of individuals attracted to the groups has been estimated at about one million.[69] In itself this is a large number, but it is small in relation to the total population of the United States. Second, the "universal" values being popularized by the groups are in fact the values of only a segment of the middle classes (as with other forms of psychotherapy). The social impact of a technology is not limited, however, to the clients actually treated (a remark illustrated by the case of psychoanalysis in an earlier period). Group techniques, together with other technologies developed over the last fifteen years (see above), have greatly increased the number of individuals subjected to one form or another of medico-psychological manipulation of the newer and more subtle variety. Accordingly, new Friends of Psychotherapy are being recruited among people who would have been turned away by psychoanalysts had they not been deterred from seeking analysis for economic, social, and ideological reasons. Last but not least, regardless of the direct impact of the new methods, they have come to be widely used throughout society. In this we find the most persuasive proof that they offer no real alternative to the alienating social life from which they claim to be liberated. Once introduced into everyday life, they serve to make oppressive practices more effective and contribute to the operation of institutions that, to say the least, are not out to insure the free growth of the personality.

POSTPSYCHOANALYTIC SOCIETY

One of the latest avatars of the group ideology has been the opening in California of an outfit known as Prosperity Training. This group's message is aimed at people who have money problems, either because they haven't enough of it or because they have too much of it. Adapting techniques popularized by Esalen, Prosperity Training organizes four-day marathon sessions, during which the participants play with money, dance to songs that talk about money, fantasize about mountains of money piled on their knees, and even chew dollar bills. At the end of the session, participants felt it had helped change their perception of money; now they feel less guilty when they spend it.[70] The philosophy of the undertaking has been spelled out by its originator: "Money is spiritual. . . . It represents universal energy and exists only in the mind." Does this philosophy represent a distortion of the original spiritual thrust of the encounter groups or an awareness of the real "spiritual principle" of American society?

Whatever ambiguities may have remained during the growth phase of the human potential movement (which coincided with the death throes of the counterculture) are now being dispelled. The central agencies in the spread of the new techniques no longer hide their commercial character: Esalen, for example, is now selling golfing workshops and gadgets of one sort or another along with its balms for the soul. The groups that have grown most rapidly in recent years are more realistic and cynical, such as the Erhard Seminars Training (est), named for its originator, a former businessman and self-taught psychologist.

Est centers have already trained a hundred thousand disciples. The seminars are aimed at people who want to be "winners."[71] The rule is simple: accept the world as it is and maximize your own awareness and ability to adjust by using an array of new techniques. According to Erhard, the fact is that the world makes no distinction between the victim and the victimizer, the rape victim and the rapist, the murder victim and the murderer, the bomber pilot and the child killed by his bombs. What is, is. A deft reminder of American atrocities during the war in Vietnam:

the most important thing is not to feel guilt but rather to learn to be a winner in this world, where, among other things, the devastating effects of American imperialism "are" what they "are." Accordingly, Erhard continues, "If God told you exactly what it was you were to do, you would be happy doing it no matter what it was. What you're doing is what God wants you to do. Be happy."[72] For an investment of sixty hours spread over two weekends and $250, est adepts learn how to "choose to be what they are," i.e., how to be efficient cogs in the social machine with the blessings of God and the psychological sciences: "The est scenario duplicates and intensifies the hierarchical, bounded structure of corporations and other institutions that employ most of est's trainees."[73]

Thus the pathos of individual liberation has given way to the language of efficiency and cynicism. Est programs in the prisons have succeeded in making convicts believe that their sentences are deserved: "This replaced their earlier views that someone else had been responsible of that they had been the innocent victims of circumstances."[74] The virtues of the new techniques are obvious: what long years of moral conditioning and constant pressure failed to achieve is obtained in a few hours of intensive psychological manipulation.

Erhard Seminars Training is no doubt the extreme example of total identification with the prevalent American values of efficiency, profitability, and conformity. But the other techniques share the same logic and, though more subtle, work toward a similar end in applications to many aspects of social life, helping to conceal if not to resolve all social contradictions. Nor are these significant differences between the areas to which the ostensibly "hard" techniques such as behavior modification are applied and those in which the softer techniques stemming from the "human relations" tradition are used.

As we have seen, the prisons make use of transcendental meditation, transactional analysis, and est, as well as behavior modification. Behaviorism is widely used in the schools, because it is easy to translate into terms suitable for classroom use. Behaviorist methods can be used in "programmed training," for example, in which the different phases of learning a subject are planned by computer; the machine also hands out rewards and punishments. More often, though, the program focuses on the student's motivation, which the behaviorist tries to influence either by handing out rewards and punishments directly or by using a system of tokens. Discipline is of greater concern than learning, however: the behavior that is modified has to do with sitting up straight, standing up, walking, running, jumping, failure to sit still, rocking back and forth, foot tapping, paper crumpling, talking, crying, singing, whistling, laughing, turning to face another child, looking at a friend.[75] Group techniques, various forms of counseling inspired by the methods of human relations psychology, and work on feelings are also widely practiced in the schools, though this does not mean that drugs are not also in common use (see chapter 6).[76]

Since Elton Mayo's well-known experiment at Western Electric in the thirties, American industrial psychology has amassed considerable experience in manipulating human relations in the workplace.[77] Similar work was carried on by Kurt Lewin and his followers in "action research," the original source of many of the new group techniques. The invention of the T-group and the idea of "stages of awareness" gave this old approach a new lease on life, focusing more on supervisory personnel than on workers. In the late fifties, for example, all middle management personnel at Esso received T-group training. When the National Training Laboratory began its "President's Lab Program" for company management, its budget swelled tenfold[78] (which indicates that it attracted not only top management but also middle- and lower-level managers eager to show that they shared the ideology of their leaders). Carl Rogers, the "prophet" of the encounter group movement, has obligingly listed the nine benefits to be expected from the use of encounter methods in industry, ostensibly to benefit employers, employees, and firm alike—the three are presumed inseparable. Rogers also mentions the usefulness of encounter groups in churches, government agencies, schools, and families.[79]

Serious racial tension in the United States has provided another prime area for the application of so-called comprehensive methods aimed at reducing racial and ethnic conflicts to problems of communication, self-perception, or prejudice. This accounts for the importance of role playing techniques, which enable an individual to "understand" what members of another community are feeling: in New York, white foremen and supervisors were asked to wear black masks in order to experience how their black employees felt "from within"[80] (nothing is said, however, about what they felt when they removed the masks). Awareness training was also used in the development of community policy in the War on Poverty during the sixties, in order to increase participation by ghetto residents and identify viable leaders,[81] i.e., leaders who would share the ideology of cooperation and "democratic" conflict-resolution backed by the policy's promoters. One stark example will give a better illustration of the political function of these initiatives than will a lengthy disquisition. In January 1972 a group of Black Muslims arrived in Baton Rouge, Louisiana, for the purpose—so they said—of "giving the city back to the black people." Shooting broke out and two black militants were killed, along with two policemen. The city was extremely tense and a curfew was declared. Social service officials and leaders of both the black and white communities responded by organizing a sensitivity-training group. What the whites asked the blacks was this: "How does your anger *feel?*"

This pacifying approach to tension has even found application in the field of international relations. In August 1969, in order to resolve the border conflict between Somalia, Ethiopia, and Kenya (subsequent developments in the region need no comment from us), six representatives of each country were invited to participate in a two-week encounter session. Apparent consensus was achieved in the small group encounters, but it broke down as soon as attempts were made to identify points of agreement on a common policy. The result was no doubt predictable. This did not prevent the American organizers of the session from evaluating it positively, while the Africans concluded that it was a failure.[82]

The last example suggests that these efforts often involve much naiveté. This should not lead to the conclusion that they are harmless, however. Undoubtedly, most of these approaches—except for behavior modification—are vitiated by an apparent major flaw: their effects are dubious, to say the least, outside the narrow sphere in which they were worked out experimentally. Nearly all the evaluations now being made of encounter groups emphasize, as we saw earlier, that their influence is tenuous and short-lived once the participants return to their normal situations.[83] In 1969 a front page article in the *Wall Street Journal* gave a pessimistic assessment of the results of using awareness training to increase the productivity of managers, and many large firms have since given up on such doubtful investments.[84]

As soon as one formula is cast aside, however, it is replaced by another. Yankee ingenuity in coming up with new manipulative technologies is inexhaustible. The endless stream of innovations merely masks a constant strategy, however: namely, to shift the focus of attention from sociopolitical issues to technological manipulations. Each technique is of dubious effect in itself, but together they enforce one particular approach to the problems of American society, an approach that hampers the search for possible political alternatives. After all, psychoanalysis never proved its effectiveness outside the one-on-one therapeutic relationship either—if it ever so much as proved its effectiveness within that context. It nevertheless enjoyed a thirty-year reign as the dominant ideology, not only in psychiatry but in social work generally as well as in large areas of daily life. It was the first stage of a process that has now culminated in the new technologies. For some fifty years now a model of social action has gradually taken shape in the United States, a model that has served to drain the life out of political and social issues and to invalidate collective forms of action, the better to replace them, in the name of realism and scientific objectivity, with a system of individualized treatment, the target of which has been specific individuals and groups, presumably the only available objects of action for social change. This has entailed certain consequences for American society as a whole.

For several reasons, the United States today is not only the richest country in the world but also one of the poorest from the standpoint of providing health care to those of its citizens who happen not to be rich—whether we measure wealth in terms of material possessions, health, youth, or promise. It is a society in which there is not even a unified system of social insurance to cover the costs of illness and old age; a welfare state in which help can only be obtained by subjecting oneself to humiliating scrutiny; a society in which the rhetoric of human rights and individual self-fulfillment goes hand in hand with reservations for American Indians and desperate ghettos to which the affluent society consigns masses of unfortunates afflicted with chronic poverty, unemployment, violence, and drugs. The point is not to blame psychological manipulation for these aspects of American life, much less to argue that psychologists are somehow responsible for the deplorable conditions just outlined. Rather, it is merely to observe that manipulative psychological techniques have come into their own along with a particular political system, a system that uses those techniques to help maintain and reproduce a specific set of social relations.

For reasons intrinsic to the history of the United States and to the structure of class relations in America, moral, psychological, individualistic, and meritocratic interpretations have always had priority over social and political interpretations. We cannot possibly undertake a thorough analysis of these reasons here. Among the most important of them, as our second chapter has suggested, is the fact that the labor force was built up gradually as wave after wave of immigrants came to America and replenished the lowest strata of society, allowing a fair number of those who arrived earlier to move up in status. Those who did move up felt that their success was due to their enterprising spirit and personal qualities, while they looked upon the exploited lower classes as uncultured, stupid, and limited in their vision, poor because they were inherently mediocre. Out of this situation arose the contrasting but complementary myths that underlie the mental image Americans have formed of the structure of their society: success rewards merit, and failure is the fault of the individual who fails. The same basic mentality also accounts for the belief that unsatisfactory states of affairs can be transformed by altering the emotional makeup of individuals. If a man's social status is merely a product of the way he lives his life, then it is possible to use technical means to manipulate the factors that enter into his choices. With regard to relations between social groups, this outlook has led unions, for example, to take a particular line, namely, to make demands aimed at enabling the category of worker they represent to "play the game" successfully within the system, i.e., to compete successfully in the struggle for advancement. With regard to the lowest strata in the society, it has led to a welfare policy that seeks to minister to individual shortcomings without touching the structural conditions that may be responsible for them.[85]

In the twenties, this background produced an early strategy for psychological intervention in social and political issues, which the combined resources of the mental hygiene movement and psychoanalysis made possible. The purpose of this strategy was to interpret, and wherever possible to treat, social failure according to a code that reduced all problems to psychological terms (emotional immaturity, weak ego, broken family, etc.—see chapter 2). This strategy was limited in two respects, however: first, it treated only individuals on the fringes of society—the poor, the sick, and the handicapped—of whom it could plausibly be said that they carried the seeds of their shortcomings within themselves; and second, it dealt only with social problems, i.e., with situations that created specific problems for the "social order," such as illness, disease, violence, and so on. The last few years have seen the birth of a new and much more extensive version of the same strategy. The new strategy is concerned with more than just "unintegrated" members of society, identified as such by themselves or others. Furthermore, it envisions intervention in conditions other than those associated with social instability. Aimed at the normal or near-normal individual, the new strategy attempts to manipulate the environment of the healthy as well as the sick. It deals positively with the problem of adjustment and does not limit its concern to cases of "maladjustment." Concerned with

social questions as well, the new strategy aims not only to eliminate dysfunctionality but also to maximize the yield of the socialization process.

The shift from the old to the new strategy has been accomplished mainly by applying behavior modification and group techniques on a large scale. The application of behaviorism to large
groups does not rely on a definition of health or on general norms
of any sort. The negative behaviors that are to be eliminated are
distinguished by their incompatibility with the norms of the specific milieu in which the method is applied (school, family, etc.).
Group techniques have also yielded operational models for social
manipulation. No longer is it necessary to reduce social problems
to individual cases, as the medical model used to require, even in
its psychoanalytic form. Using the new group technologies, the
environment itself can be manipulated, quantified, and engineered
via "feedback," "self-regulation," "input," "output," and other
techniques borrowed from the lexicon of engineering. In effecting
this transformation of the very concept of the "social," Kurt
Lewin's work has been crucial; everything was excluded from the
concept that could not be manipulated by the "social engineer,"
using his special knowhow and methods. The apparently more
utopian and less mechanical human potential movement and other
humanistic approaches have done no more than contribute a somewhat more colorful vocabulary, add a few methods of their own,
and extend the instruments of the social engineers to the domain
of emotions and feelings.

These new technologies have become the only officially sanctioned mode of social action, the only one worth taking seriously,
i.e., the only one that is scientific and rational. "Planned change,"
"community development," and other, similar projects are based
on these methods, which have supplanted earlier approaches to
social change—approaches now discredited as utopian artifacts of
the "old" politics or as irresponsible whims of militant activists.
Social action is now seen as a matter of technical manipulation of
dynamic variables in order to improve communication, rationalize
the decision-making process, and so on. Everything else is meta-
physics, i.e., ideology or politics.

Some will see this approach as progressive and liberating, because change is its watchword. To change is to live authentically, to develop the potential of individuals and of society to the full, to eliminate outmoded practices, to dispel illusions, to liberate mankind from alienation. But how? According to the currently fashionable view, the only way is to focus action on the group, the individual's immediate environment, because this is where the new technologies are applicable, and to enlist the support of individuals as "agents of social change"—in other words, as component parts in this carefully planned apparatus. The scope of individual and social action is henceforth to be limited to the area circumscribed by the technological–scientific model. Is there anyone old-fashioned enough to dream of justice, politics, or happiness—save perhaps as the target of manipulative strategies, or as their underlying principle? What is being worked out, in short, is a completely rational concept of man, a concept perfectly attuned to the dominant notion of what is rational. The problem then ceases to be one of healing the sick, reeducating the guilty, or controlling deviant behavior (these goals remain, of course, but as objectives allied with new techniques). Instead, "normal" man has come to the fore as the center of attention in a society whose only passion is to produce earnestly and efficiently.

To heal is good, to prevent is better, but to maximize output by adjusting each individual to his social role and by calibrating change to the social dynamic as required by the necessity to reproduce the social order is surely the ideal of policy without politics.

CONCLUSION

————•∎•————

The Psy World

We have analyzed both practices within American mental medicine and practices judged, at least by their proponents, to be independent of that system. What conclusions should be drawn from our work by people outside the sphere of influence of the American model? Our results should be of interest to anyone willing to step back a bit from the European scene, to gain some perspective on the "immediate data" of European consciousness (*pace* Bergson). We have deliberately avoided treating the American situation in terms of questions currently in the air in Europe. Space did not permit a truly rigorous comparative study. Still, neither our choice of material nor the order in which we have presented our argument can be regarded as innocent. For we began with certain assumptions, which we regard as fundamental. These had to do with the significance of the changes now occurring in mental medicine systems in both the United States and Europe, which have together embarked on the same journey. They also had to do with the role played by the state in establishing public welfare programs and mechanisms of social control. Thus two problems must be considered: (1) What is the probable course of development of therapeutic practices legitimized and supported by psychological science? and (2) What is the relationship between the evolution of these practices and the power structure of a "liberal" society? Study of the American situation yields some surprising answers to both these questions.

THE MYTH OF DEINSTITUTIONALIZATION

For some years now it has been common to interpret changes in the mental health system in terms of deinstitutionalization. On this there has been general agreement, both among those who applaud the development, seeing it as a way for psychiatry to bring itself up to date, and among those who attack it as the first step in extending the powers of the new technicians of the soul beyond all bounds. This agreement has been the result of the obvious fact that the center of gravity of the mental health care system has been shifting away from the mental hospital and toward what is called the "community" in the United States, the "secteur" in France, the "territory" in Italy, and so forth. This switch to modes of treatment more directly related to social life may seem to require no explanation. But appearances are deceptive, as the analysis of the most recent developments in the United States has shown. Not that the United States was the first country to experiment with liberating psychiatry from its old bastion in the asylums.[1] But the process began abruptly in the United States and, once begun, proceeded rapidly, so that we can best evaluate its significance today by examining the American scene, which offers the best vantage point on the future.

Looking back at the various analyses attempted throughout this book with an eye to their cumulative import, it seems clear that developments over the past thirty years have wavered dialectically. What has been called, too sweepingly, "deinstitutionalization" describes and in part conceals processes of three kinds, which have profoundly altered the mental health institutions, professions, and practices, and yet have not done away with either the fact of institutionalization, the recognition of professional competence, or the predominance of technique. Once this triple mechanism is recognized, it becomes clear that, rather than a widespread unlocking of hospital gates, what has actually happened is far more complex, and its implications for the future—in Europe as well as in the United States—are quite different from what has been thought.

1. Institutionalization is far from obsolete as a solution to the problems of mental health and other forms of deviance; rather, custodial treatment programs have been rationalized and in certain respects reinforced. This has been the result of a twofold process: the functions of the mental hospital and criteria for commitment have been redefined and tightened, and a new range of "total" institutions (as defined by Erving Goffman) has been created.

Let us begin by considering the first aspect of this process. It seems clear that the emotions aroused by the supposed decline of the mental hospitals stemmed mainly from the belief that the patients removed from the hospitals did not belong there in the first place. In other words, as the patient population swelled, the traditional mental hospital came more and more to resemble the old general hospital, serving as an "asylum" for an ill-assorted collection of residents: old people without families, poor people with no place to go, chronic patients who did not respond to therapy, or in any case did not respond to the therapy dispensed by the hospitals, and so forth. All these patients either found places elsewhere or, more commonly, were abandoned to their fate. Their expulsion from the mental hospitals trimmed the fat—as the technocrats like to say— from those institutions and left them in a better position to perform certain specific functions, in particular the treatment or control of individuals most disruptive of the social order.

Turning now to the second aspect of the process, we find people discovering that chronic patients need not be locked up in gigantic hospitals surrounded by walls and moats. Less imposing institutions with a more rapid turnover of inpatients are now available to take over some of the functions once performed by mental hospitals. These newer institutions can also deal with social problems which were unheard of in the golden age of alienism but which are the crux of the matter today. Consequently, tens of thousands of patients "freed" from mental hospitals have been sent to one of the growing number of smaller-scale closed institutions sometimes referred to as "mini snake pits," such as nursing homes, board-and-care facilities, and private proprietary homes for adults.

The future most likely belongs not so much to these institutions, however, as to others less directly associated with mental illness, whether real or alleged. The "therapeutic communities" for drug addicts, for example, have invented a new rationale to justify the confinement of patients and the imposition of strict discipline: the object is said to be to completely reprogram the lives of participants. Other examples are provided by the various institutions that occupy an ambiguous position on the borderline between psychiatry and the courts, both adult and juvenile. Not only are the prisons themselves becoming psychiatric institutions (though they have yet to be deinstitutionalized), but many individuals classed as "criminally insane," "abnormal delinquents," and "sexual psychopaths" would find it difficult to say whether they are being "treated" in hospitals or prisons; they frequently shuttle back and forth between one sort of institution and the other. In any case, as they are well aware, they have hardly been deinstitutionalized.

Since the days when asylums and prisons more or less dominated the scene, the network of secure institutions has grown much more diverse. Confinement now covers a rather confused landscape, which is difficult to map accurately. But it would be extremely naive to take literally the progressive rhetoric that focuses exclusively on innovations, or else acknowledges continuity only by admitting the existence of atavistic practices and survivals of outmoded ideas. Naive, and dangerous—for one of the political functions of the ideology of change is to divert attention from the state of a social system and to focus instead only on the most spectacular changes, even though they may have no effect on the most basic aspects of the system. All the new initiatives, novel departures, radical experiments, and "advanced" technologies are based on the custodial institutions and their endemic brutality. What has changed is not that fewer people are being committed but that more and more individuals and groups within the society are being taken in charge by an increasingly flexible and wide-ranging network of institutions. This lesson holds true outside the United States as well.

2. There is in the United States an abundant and ill-assorted literature concerning the "medical model": its structure, variants, evolution, and crisis. One thing is clear, however: for the past fifteen years, serious challenges have been mounted to the practice of psychiatry as traditionally defined by the medical schools. This has led to a crisis, which is related to factors of two kinds, the effects of which have become increasingly severe.

First, the establishment of community mental health centers, particularly in the poorest areas, brought psychiatrists into contact with a host of problems that were as much social and political as medical in nature, for which their training left them unprepared. Second, even in other respects, American society confronted psychiatrists with challenges that they were apparently ill-equipped to meet. Drugs, the counterculture, feminism, and gay liberation all caught off-guard a medical establishment used to working inside sterilized institutions where it could carefully control the relationship between doctor and patient.

There were various reactions to this situation. Some professionals worked to undermine their traditional role. Other psychiatrists, because they subscribed to progressive ideologies or had to adapt in order to survive, particularly if they practiced in the ghetto, attempted to add a new social and political dimension to their work, to eschew therapies that relied on elaborate techniques, and to take note of the needs of the most deprived groups in the society. In doing so they "deprofessionalized" themselves—i.e., increasingly removed themselves from the traditional role of the doctor, as defined by the medical schools. They also brought in "indigenous workers" to assist the professionals, as a way of making community needs felt directly. If these outsiders were heeded, however, the medical principles on which community treatment facilities were premised were inevitably called into question. Thus the staff in some community mental health centers came to doubt truths of which they had previously been certain and were steered in the direction of political activism.

Nonprofessionals broke even more sharply with the medical model. In some areas, in which the incompetence of psychiatry to deal with the new problems was particularly glaring, or in which there existed neither established traditions, proven techniques, nor recognized institutions, laymen came forth to take up the challenge. They improvised free clinics for young dropouts, therapeutic communities for drug addicts, counseling and self-help centers for the alienated of one sort or another, and encounter groups tailored to the new demand for services.

At first, these newcomers wanted nothing to do with the specialists and did not see themselves in the role of auxiliaries. Most of them came from the groups they wished to serve and were critical of the rigidity and narrowness of psychiatric training as well as its conformist outlook and its basic inability to meet the vital needs of people in distress. Thus an openly antiprofessional ideology became popular in the sixties and for a time seemed to threaten the hegemony of established medicine. "Reprofessionalization" is now in the ascendant, however, for a number of reasons.

In the first place, the establishment, which at first had been disconcerted by so many problems it could not deal with, and which was relieved, in some instances, to unload them, was not long in mounting a counteroffensive. After the peak of the crisis had passed, the establishment regained control of the situation by seeing to it that laws governing institutional and professional standards in the paramedical field were tightened; by making grants of aid contingent on proof of professional competence (presumably monopolized by the medical establishment itself); and by criticizing and disavowing members of the profession who had compromised themselves by getting too deeply involved in activities presumed subversive. Doctors are now in general agreement that the "abuses" of the sixties are to be regretted and that psychiatry must remain secure in its medical niche.[2]

Most of those who set themselves up as competitors of the official mental health care system have now returned to the fold, in part because of the pressures we have described, in part because of changes in their outlook over the years. This statement applies both to the "indigenous workers" from the ghettos and to the countercultural personalities who set up alternative institutions. The most radical of the indigenous workers were defeated, while the majority found subordinate positions in the health care system and thereby opened the way to some measure of social advancement for themselves. Most of the free clinics and other self-help groups either had to give up the fight or meet the standards imposed by the establishment. Reprofessionalization is so pervasive that it has affected even encounter groups and awareness training, the ambiguities of which were discussed in the previous chapter. The encounter group movement was launched by professionals who had renounced orthodoxy and who vigorously questioned the value of standard forms of training. Many laymen rushed into the breach thus opened. Since then, however, even the groups that are most critical of the medical establishment have come to devote much attention to the training of personnel, weeding out undesirables and presenting an image of respectability to the public.

Reprofessionalization obviously does not mean that the system is headed back to the situation it was in before the sixties. There has been both quantitative and qualitative change in the health professions. A new labor market has opened up: growth in this area of the service sector has been among the most spectacular in recent years. Staffs have been enlarged, new categories of skills have emerged, and middle-level jobs have proliferated. The disparity between the top and the bottom—the exclusive authority psychiatrists once enjoyed and the menial jobs once left to the lowliest workers—has been reduced. The system is now based on mutual support, sharing of skills, delegation of power, and multiple functions. Jobs that psychiatrists cannot do are done by paraprofessionals. As professionals have become more adaptable, new types of institutions have proliferated. With more flexibility in treatment, there is more room for people with new and different kinds of skills. In the absence of proof to the contrary, however, we continue to maintain that professionals still dominate the job pyramid in the psy sector, in which they enjoy a monopoly on prestige and power, even though antiprofessional rhetoric is common (while professional positions are coveted). Each person in the system contributes in his own way to reproducing its main features. Since the system was largely successful in warding off the great protests of the sixties, it is hard to see how it could possibly collapse now. On the contrary, all signs indicate that we are now in a phase of normalization: the profession is settling accounts with dissidents in its ranks, regularizing relations with its satellites, and establishing uniform standards covering the entire field, now considerably broader than it was, over which it enjoys hegemony.

3. Changes in technique have paralleled changes in professional standards. Techniques are the instrumental aspect, if you will, of professional change. The medical model is based on a clinical conception of treatment, in which a distinction is made between the somatic and the psychic dimensions of disease. The body is examined to disclose possible organic etiologies of mental illnesses, and the mind is examined, using one form or another of psychotherapy, to disclose any possible psychic etiology. The necessary skills for both kinds of examination are monopolized by specialists. Similarly, available treatments range from drugs to tools for psychological understanding; specialists, guided by their knowledge and clinical instincts, are supposed to be adept at using all these implements.

It has become increasingly difficult to maintain the clinical relationship envisioned by the medical model as the focus of the practice of mental medicine has shifted to clients unlike either the institutionalized psychotic or the private outpatient. As has long been recognized, psychotherapy demands too much in the way of capacity for verbalization and introspection to be suitable for use with a broad public. In the ghettos, moreover, the demand for services was heavy, communal, and centered on vital needs, so that the psychotherapeutic model was not merely hard to apply but literally useless. In the middle classes, on the other hand, the search for ways to promote personal growth rather than merely to repair personality dysfunctions tended to discredit the standard psychotherapeutic approach. Worshippers of immediacy, feeling, spontaneity, and so forth had little use for the roundabout manipulations of the scientific specialists. The rise of antiprofessionalism, which reached a peak in the late sixties, brought with it rhetorical denunciation of methods requiring technical training in psychiatry and related disciplines. But the dust has now settled in this area, too. A decade later, the most clear-cut consequence of antiprofessional critiques seems to be that the number of different kinds of therapy increased, as did the number of cases in which one specialist or another—old style or new—feels competent to intervene.

Community mental health has survived by developing such new techniques as crisis intervention, short-term psychotherapy, sophisticated forms of counseling for people in positions of responsibility, and so on. The problem was to redefine the relationship between the psychiatric profession and the population so as to make it possible to extend services to new groups within the society: what was needed was a series of techniques for specific, rapid intervention aimed more at symptoms than at underlying etiology and designed to work on the environment at least as much as on the internal equilibrium of the individual, techniques that could do without drawn-out interviews and that focused on defusing potentially explosive conflicts. This new emphasis represented a break with traditional notions of technique but not a rejection of technique as such. In fact, it has resulted in renewed insistence on the virtues of specialized knowhow rooted in basic knowledge taught by the medical schools and requiring a long professional apprenticeship.

A similar transformation took place in the alternative institutions, which developed new techniques for dealing with problems that traditionally trained psychiatrists were unequipped to handle: psychological counseling for people not suffering from standard maladies but nonetheless disturbed, a new approach to suicides and drug-related incidents, and feminist counseling, to name a few. These innovations were subsequently taken up by official institutions and have become a part of the standard arsenal of techniques.

The renewed emphasis on technique has been most striking in certain groups, which originally insisted that their purpose was not therapeutic. With the "human potential" movement, for example, spontaneity becomes a task, pleasure is preprogrammed, the body is an emotion-generating machine whose levers can be consciously manipulated. Criticism of standard psychological techniques has thus come full circle, culminating in a fascination with technique that is quite fantastic. Taylor was probably the first to treat human behavior as subject to technological manipulation. The applications of Taylorism were limited to the productive sphere, however. The ideology of "personal growth" and "personality development," which claims to be freedom-enhancing and wears a utopian garb, emphasizing spontaneity and the primacy of feeling, is in fact a Taylorism of the whole individual. The idea is that each individual is the engineer of his own moods, the manager of his own personal emotion-factory—properly programmed, ineffable sensations are within the reach of everyone. Within the reach of everyone, that is, provided they are willing to learn how to produce pleasure artificially, to manufacture freedom according to program, to entrust themselves to some guru equipped to perform alchemy on the soul, to release the exquisite individuality locked within. "Therapy for the normal" has brought the full range of human experience into the sphere of technological manipulation (which now ranges far beyond mere pathology).

There is a paradox in this spate of new techniques, in that they are products of a desire to move beyond psychotherapeutic instrumentalism. This desire is only an aspect of a more general phenomenon, however, and it may not be the aspect with the most important implications for the future. Other techniques, far more suitable for use in conjunction with the medical model, have also become widely popular in recent years. Never before has such high value been placed on biological research, not only into mental illness but also into the causes of behavioral anomalies of every variety (such as hereditary factors in delinquency, in behavior disruptive of family life, in discipline problems at school, and so on). Similarly, active research on new drugs is being financed both by drug companies and by official agencies responsible for the formulation of mental health policy, such as the National Institute of Mental Health. Progress on this front has made it possible to tighten chemical control over life in mental institutions and to extend the use of drugs outside the hospitals (for example, lithium is used to maintain patients who might otherwise require hospitalization, methadone is used to neutralize drug addicts, amphetamines are used to normalize maladjusted children, etc.). The only real "scientific" competitor to drug research is research on behavior modification techniques now being conducted in experimental psychology laboratories and government research facilities (some formerly sponsored by the Army or the CIA).[3] Ten years ago we would probably have given a different diagnosis. After the turmoil of the sixties, however, the pendulum has swung back in the other direction. The most important development in the area of social policy has been a renewal of emphasis on positivistic research, reflecting the ambition to use "scientific" means to overcome or transform undesirable behavior.

Deinstitutionalization, which should of course be viewed in relation to other changes in the system, is part of a larger process. Institutionalization, professionalization, and technicalization are the dialectically interrelated factors that together are determining the future of the mental health care system in America. What is happening in the United States is only the clearest example of a transformation now under way in other countries, still underdeveloped in comparison with the advanced psychiatric society that exists in America. By looking at these three factors, we can understand what we said in the introduction are the two most distinctive features of the present situation in psychiatry: the extension of the jurisdiction of mental medicine to cover a larger number and greater variety of social groups, and the continued viability of modes of treatment ranging from the most archaic to the most modern, all of them functioning together as parts of one comprehensive system.

In regard to the first point, the variety of institutions, skills, and techniques has made it possible to accept ever larger numbers of patients for treatment while targeting a growing range of demands and problems for specific attention. Everyone, or nearly everyone, can find his niche in the system, from psychosurgery to the latest balm for troubled souls. Overwhelming social pressure forces some people to seek services, while others come—or think they come—of their own free will, seeking a better way of life. In either case, the institutions are ready with appropriate techniques and qualified specialists to "treat the problem," regardless of whether the patient experiences it as a personal difficulty or as something he must confront because someone has defined him as a "social problem." Of course very little of this kind of treatment is psychiatric in the strict sense: we hope to have shown that this label hardly applies to all the different techniques we have described. In an advanced psychiatric society, psychiatric intervention is not "special" in the sense that nineteenth-century alienists used to speak of "special medicine" and "special establishments." In that case would it perhaps be better to use another term? Terminology is not the important thing, however—another term is likely to be just as ambiguous. The crucial point is to grasp the nature of the process.

Mental medicine began by instrumentalizing what might be called (to borrow Erving Goffman's term) a "servicing model," i.e., a set of techniques for restoring a small number of gravely ill patients to normal life, or, failing that, rendering them harmless via confinement. With the advent of the "prevention model," mental medicine set itself the further goal of modifying environmental conditions apt to endanger, preserve, or restore health. This shift in focus led to an increase in both the number of different methods in use and the size of the targeted population. The possible extent of these increases was still limited, however, by the reliance on medical norms, which meant that conditions that could not be classified in relation to sickness and health could not be treated. With the development of therapy for the normal and, more generally, of "scientific" techniques for manipulating individuals and their environment (such as behavior modification and group techniques), a new model has emerged, the "model of enhanced normality." Now the aim is no longer to heal the sick or even merely to maintain the health of the healthy; rather, it is to correct deviations from the norm and to maximize individual efficiency, by taking the view that human beings are open to technological manipulation and that the environment is amenable to scientific control.

This may spell the end, if not of medicine, then of the hegemony of the medical model. It is not an accident that the authority of medicine is no longer invoked by behavior modification and recent group therapies. Diminished though the authority of medicine may be, the change has come about only as the program inaugurated under the auspices of medicine has required it in order to be carried through: namely, the program of influencing the relation between "normal" man and the social environment through the use of scientific methods under the control of specialists. The difference between the new approach and the traditional one (and it is an enormous difference) is that the problem is no longer seen merely as a matter of correcting dysfunctions presumed (whether rightly or wrongly) to be of pathological origin. The new problem is how to strengthen the influence of social norms on deviance-prone individuals, a group that becomes larger and less well-defined as time goes by. Until quite recently most people could count on not being classified as "insane" as a matter of statistical certainty. As the jurisdiction of the mental health system has broadened, however, fewer and fewer people can be sure that they are not ripe for treatment by one of the new methods.

It is wrong, however, to think that archaic methods have been replaced by modern ones or that hard forms of intervention have been replaced by soft ones. The strength of the system—the law that governs its operation as a whole—lies in the fact that techniques at either end of the spectrum can be and are being emloyed simultaneously, along with other falling in between the two extremes. It is not difficult to establish a typology of techniques using these criteria. At the most conventional, repressive end of the spectrum, we find four prominent characteristics: greatest degree of institutionalization (e.g., the mental hospital), most traditional medical technology (e.g., electroshock and drugs), professionals in conventional specialties (e.g., psychiatrists), and the most seriously incapacited patients (e.g., psychotics, the mentally retarded). At the other end of the spectrum, all the characteristics are the reverse: less imposing institutions, relatively unsophisticated techniques, less specialized personnel, "normal" clients. Encounter groups and cocounseling programs typify this combination of characteristics. It is clear, however, that these different forms of treatment can overlap and mutually support one another. Some can come to the fore either temporarily or permanently while others recede into the background. Such shifts do not imply that the mental health system has moved irrevocably from one end of the spectrum to the other. In the United States, for example, encounter groups spread like wildfire in the early seventies but are now just holding their own. More standard medical treatments, on the other hand, are making a strong comeback. Is this "progress" or "regression?" Probably neither, but rather a change in the relative emphasis placed on one element or another in a system that functions as a unified whole in a given social and historical conjuncture.

THE LIBERALITIES OF LIBERALISM

Synthetic overviews are always somewhat schematic. The one we have just given suggests—perhaps a bit too dogmatically—that the system is so tightly knit that nothing can be done to change it. The die is cast, as it were, and every attempt to create an alternative or rebel against the status quo is doomed to be reintegrated into the all-embracing system. The problem is that, whenever one tries to identify the key elements in the structure of a system, one is forced implicitly to play up the coherence of that system and consequently to play down the obstacles that in reality make such coherence difficult to achieve. There is of course always "play in the gears," and sometimes the different parts get out of whack. There are holes—room for new initiatives. And, finally, there is friction, backlash, the possibility of a snag in the works. We have tried to take all this into account (chapter 7). As we have seen, though, the ultimate fate of many alternative ventures was ambiguous, and, to understand that ambiguity, we have had to investigate what it is that makes America's capacity for assimilation so extraordinary.

What is a "liberal" society? Among other things, a society in which protest against the system is controlled by the system itself. Mental medicine in the United States has withstood numerous attacks: lawsuits in which its dirty linen has been washed in public, revolts by patient groups, competition from the counterculture, political opposition led by such exemplary groups of intellectuals as Health P.A.C., etc. For a while it seemed as though the mental health care system in the United States had really been shaken by all these criticisms, but—as the Watergate affair shows in the political arena—it seems as if the criticism in the end merely provided the system with an opportunity to show how adaptable it was in meeting the new situation. This raises the following question: What is the relation between the mechanisms of social control in which psychiatry plays a part and the power structure, not only in the United States but, more generally, in so-called advanced industrial or advanced liberal societies?

One common criticism of the increasing control over social life exerted by medical psychology is aimed at the alleged collusion between the government and the mental health care system. According to this line of argument, mental medicine, along with such other "repressive" agencies as the courts, the bureaucracy, the police, and so on, has been bearing part of the burden of maintaining the social order by helping to control troublesome groups, enforce conformity, and eliminate deviance. Treat rather than punish, but only to enforce discipline: the "therapeutic state"[4] supposedly represents a new stage in the organization of governmental power, in which medicine assumes responsibility for functions that used to fall under the province of government. An extreme example is the Soviet Union, in which dissidence is identified with mental illness and the psychiatric authorities are directly affiliated with the government. Official psychiatrists brutally uproot dissidents and send them to repressive prison hospitals for "treatment." There is litte real difference between psychiatrists and agents of the KGB.

The collusion between psychiatry and government in the Soviet Union is so blatant that it arouses (or seems to arouse) the ire of everyone. The wrong is so obvious only because the system is so crude. It thus offers all too convenient a foil to play off against liberal psychiatry, which looks rather good by comparison. No doubt the most important lesson to be drawn from our investigation, however, is that the interplay between mental medicine and conservative social functions can be far more complex than in the Soviet Union, and, consequently, that the political implications may be quite different. And these political implications are of primary concern to the citizens of advanced liberal societies.

That the American liberal model is different from the Soviet model does not mean that the two are diametrically opposed in every respect: coercion continues to play a large part in the United States, as we have seen. Nor is the American system merely more complex or highly developed: even in the USSR, the mental health system is not limited solely to prison hospitals.[5] The differences between the two systems have to do mainly with the way they are organized locally and with the relations that exist between the government and the psychiatric establishment.

One prominent characteristic of the American medical profession is that individuals and organizations having no official function play an important role. Take, for example, the movement that has probably had a more important impact than any other on medical techniques, the mental hygiene movement. This was a typical product of the American system, with its enthusiastic reformers, its pioneers whose interests extended into the spiritual realm, its moralists bent on telling others what is best for them, its entrepreneurs eager to invest in the "soul sector," its generous philanthropists always vigilant to see how their gifts are being used, and its disinterested professionals convinced of the value-neutrality and efficacy of their techniques. To all these well-intentioned men and women, and certain others besides (for we had best not forget those who were hardly disinterested: stockholders in the major drug companies; shrewd managers of the "health empires" controlled by the nation's leading hospitals; the medical guilds such as the American Medical Association and American Psychiatric Association; and all the professionals, paraprofessionals, and even antiprofessionals who work for the free-enterprise health care system in jobs of less exalted rank), America owes the most highly diversified and tightly knit network of social control that exists anywhere in the world.

This is paradoxical only in appearance. So-called liberal society—American society par excellence—does not present a homogeneous aspect to government. Civil society has its knots and hard spots, which centralized supervisory agencies cannot altogether eliminate. Indeed, rather large segments of society are apparently left to their own devices, free to govern themselves, owing to the imperfect coordination of the various agencies responsible for the management of the citizenry and the maintenance of order at both the local and the federal level: welfare agencies, police, courts, and bureaucracy. Because of this loose structure, American society is extraordinarily innovative and capable of taking initiatives not promulgated from on high. The very survival of the system requires local regulatory mechanisms to fill in the gaps between the areas covered by the various official agencies— patching a social fabric stretched to the breaking point, to over-extend the metaphor a bit. Thus the system allows not only for obligatory vertical integration but also for voluntary horizontal integration, accomplished by negotiation. Participants in the social system can collaborate and help one another through an unofficial network of cooperation, which allows everyone to express distrust of the bureaucrats and politicians, the symbols of outside author-ity. Specific problems can therefore be dealt with on the local level: local authorities eliminate social disturbances, clamp down on unrest, and control deviance, relieving the outside authorities of the necessity to intervene. Admirers of this sort of "democracy" generally neglect to point out that the aim is usually to achieve consensus, peacefully if possible, by force if necessary. The ideal would be a self-regulated system based on internalized controls, with each individual assuming responsibility for his own behavior and for reproving deviant behavior in his fellows.

This, of course, is merely an ideal: in many areas, society func-tions only because the outside authorities wield considerable pow-ers of repression. But in an impressive number of areas, self-management is the rule: charitable foundations, self-help groups, religious sects, psychological counseling groups and other, similar organizations use shared beliefs, self-interest, and even emotional blackmail to manage themselves and, in so doing, to reinforce adherence to, and help to insure compliance with, the values of American society. Surveillance and prevention are accomplished by "scientists" and by members of the silent majority themselves at a much lower cost than if police were required to achieve the same results—neither the FBI nor the CIA does the job, much less government policymakers.

The most novel development revealed by our work is that prac-tices related to mental health and not supported by the federal government have assumed tremendous importance. In Europe and especially in France, because of the long ascendancy of the asylum system and the close relationship between mental hospitals, psychiatrists, and the government, the mental health system is commonly thought to be characterized by large-scale institutions and bureaucracy—a public service controlled by the central government. Protests against the mental health care system in Europe have also been directed chiefly against the "total institution" and the arrogance of psychiatry, which has disguised its political and administrative function beneath a cloak of therapy. These are the two main themes developed over the past ten years by a protest movement that quickly earned the label "antipsychiatric."

While this approach is not to be rejected in toto, it now seems inadequate for at least two reasons. In the first place, the movement is now securely established. At this point it needs to strike at its targets rather than go on repeating what they are ad nauseam. Even more important, this kind of criticism applies only to a smaller and smaller proportion of current psychiatric practice. In France, for example, the 1838 law providing for compulsory commitment, which established what for many years was the basis of the relationship between psychiatry and the government, accounted for almost 80 percent of the cases treated by psychiatrists as recently as fifty years ago. Today, however, the number of cases of this sort is insignificant compared with the total number of people receiving therapy. Thus, to continue to focus criticism on this one law is all too likely to make everything that has been done since 1838 look good by comparison. If the "arrogance" of psychiatric power continues to be defined in relation to the law of 1838, what can be said about so-called free services, home visits, and the use of psychoanalysis in the schools and courts—to say nothing of the general pervasiveness of psychoanalytic concepts?

This is not the worst of it. When it comes to attacking new methods, the critics content themselves with putting new wine in old bottles. By attacking the repressive uses of psychiatry by the government, they are repeating arguments that may have been cogent in other contexts but simply ricochet off the new targets without effect. Thus critics describe the *politique de secteur*, the French equivalent of the community mental health program, as a mere "police measure" taken by the central government, analogous to old-fashioned custodial care. As for the political role of the psychoanalyst, the critics see in the analyst no more than a representative of the ruling class and hence a representative, at least in an indirect sense, of governmental authority. It is easy to understand why these lame analogies have scarcely any effect on the people who are now working to make the new technologies available. They argue that their methods are untainted and that cooptation by the government is impossible: as long as they do not work directly for the government, they believe their political position to be neutral—and this argument is in fact widely accepted. Thus the statement commonly made in psychoanalytic circles (see Maud Mannoni, among others), that analysis has nothing to do with the social and political problems of power as long as the analyst does not succumb to the temptation to work for the government, is not seen for what it is: an incredible bit of naiveté. Leaving aside polemics among professionals of different specialties, it is hard to see why the same argument could not be made by the behaviorists now busily making the latest behavior modification gadgets ready for use in France—if behaviorists did not prefer the productive silence of research to the analysts' predilection for pompous self-celebration.

To go beyond these irrelevant matters, what is needed is a more elaborate description of the relationship between social practice and its political functions than the Manichaean opposition between state and civil society or public and private sectors permits. One must stop looking for a policeman behind every curtain and a conspiracy of the government behind every new initiative (at the same time, of course, one must dispel the complementary illusion that if police and conspiracies are not found, the research is necessarily objective and neutral). In this regard the American case can be highly instructive, by suggesting the main outlines of a more satisfactory theory of the relation between modern control technologies and the power structures of society.

Indeed, in the United States more than in Europe, one would have to be blind not to see. Neither Dorothea Dix nor Clifford Beers nor Adolf Meyer nor Sigmund Freud via his American disciples nor Kurt Lewin nor B. F. Skinner were or are representatives of the government. Yet they have probably contributed as much to the reproduction of American society as the employees of the State Department or the Pentagon, insulting though it may be to mention their names in the same breath. To the question of who controls (and what), however, it is clear that the answer must be this: even those who don't care in the slightest about the social control function contribute to carrying it out. We can thus begin to identify several groups of actors, motivated by different interests and proceeding according to strategies that conflict on certain points and coincide on others.

Financial motives, for example are largely independent of the political aims of supervision and conformity. The mental health system, whatever else it may be, is also—and for many people, primarily—a market governed by the law of supply and demand under conditions of free competition. Capitalism dominates: large sums of money, public and private, can be mobilized, especially when it becomes necessary to attack problems viewed at a particular moment in history as especially urgent or worrisome: drugs, violence, a high scholastic failure rate, etc. Subsidies make possible research, experimentation, and marketing of new products and techniques. New careers emerge, jobs open up, and judicious investments yield huge profits. Though not disinterested, these motives generally have nothing politically cynical about them. Still, to give only one example, the result is that hundreds of thousands of problem children are declared hyperactive, bombarded with drugs, and surrounded by well-meaning counselors. One may wish to say that they are being made more "normal," but by whom?

Then there are the philanthropists and other humanist reformers. Doubtless they are as fond of order as the next person, but this does not mean that their activities form part of some political conspiracy. They are private individuals, often of considerable prestige, religious leaders, or industrialists who have found that by setting up charitable foundations they can do good and pay less income tax at the same time. These people act in their own behalf and are accountable only to their own consciences. Nevertheless, they are responsible for having taken initiatives that played a fundamental role in broadening the sphere of influence of mental medicine, such as the mental hygiene movement. More generally, philanthropy of this sort has been a constant influence in the formulation of all welfare policy since the mineteenth century; it has appeared time and again in one guise after another and served the bourgeois class interest by helping to shape much social legislation and social work.

Also playing an important role in the system are austere scientists and professionals convinced that their techniques are politically neutral. Some of them are paid by the government (and even by the CIA),[6] while others are paid by drug companies and still others by organizations with the most impeccable scientific credentials. There is no reason not to believe, however, that most of them are mainly interested in scientific research and its potential benefits to mankind, as well as in the opportunity that science offers to plan and rationalize human behavior. The list of scientific discoveries to date is impressive, and in all probability the future belongs to these people. Underlying the boldest attempts to standardize behavior is a conception of a sort of "scientific" utopia: to achieve happiness for both the individual and the community by means of rational planning carried out by technical experts.

Important roles are also played both by professionals working on the periphery of the system and by certain individuals working in protest against it. These people helped to set up alternative institutions and try out new techniques, hoping to catch the establishment off guard. When some innovations first tried as alternatives later turned up as parts of the dominant system, however, was there any justice to the charges that someone must have sold out or gone over to the enemy? As the sociology of religion has shown in another context, it may be that social practice goes through a developmental process beginning with an innovative phase and evolving toward general acceptance. Sometimes innovations occur with little or no warning in areas that had seemed highly structured. At first their impact is subversive, but before long the system tends to accommodate, as latent possibilities for reform emerge. This is what happened after the advent of psychoanalysis as well as with more recent developments. Because of such innovations, basic transformations of the system became necessary. Ultimately, new methods were extended to individuals whose normality was in doubt in one way or another.

Accordingly, the practices associated with mental medicine in the United States should be seen as the result of a balance of various forces, none of which can operate independently of the others. Competition, conflict, exchange, and reinterpretation produce a dynamic equilibrium. The role, or, rather, roles of the state in the system should be seen against this background. Our intention is not to deny that the central authorities play a key role, but to grasp the complexity of the process by which they do so. To begin with, it is taken for granted that certain spheres of action are more or less exclusively reserved to the state. This is true of matters directly pertaining to the maintenance and expansion of American imperialism, a rubric that covers both foreign policy and the major outlines of domestic economic policy. Except in times of crisis, however, the state rarely tries to develop its own social control mechanisms and impose them on society from above. Instead, it interprets methods developed by others in its own way, settles conflicts and, if necessary, enters into alliances with certain groups to influence the way problems are solved (e.g., the role of the state in collaboration with the psychiatric establishment in imposing standards on alternative institutions). The state manages, rationalizes, and standardizes (e.g., the role of the Democratic administration in the sixties in setting up the community mental health care centers). It provides a central source of information, coordinates diverse initiatives, and plans long-term projects (e.g., its role in creating prevention programs for children). The action of the state, moreover, has two distinct aspects, one managerial, the other more properly political. Thus officials of federal agencies have often worked together with psychiatrists to find better ways of administering the segments of the populace for which they share responsibility. In contrast, the federal government has in some cases acted directly to uphold order, as in inaugurating psychiatric examinations for the selection of immigrants and setting up programs designed to intimidate drug addicts.

Even when the central government does intervene directly, it is rarely to set up wholly new government-run institutions. In the entire history of American psychiatry, the federal government's most far-reaching attempt to intervene in the operation of the system was surely the establishment of the community mental health centers, which we examined in chapter 5. From the first, however, this project relied on existing community institutions and looked forward to close collaboration with the private mental health care system. Even in cases where institutions were being created from the ground up, federal financial incentives were handled in a manner typical of the way the American government works, at once aggressive and restrained. The federal government provided "seed money" to pay staff and operating costs for a limited period of time, with the amount of federal participation progressively decreasing. Even when the federal government plays its most active role, local sources of financing must eventually be found, thus shifting responsibility from the federal to the local level and insuring that the local agencies will become independent of the central government, to which they owe their existence.

The best evidence for the validity of this description of the complex relations between the federal authorities and other agencies may be found in the recommendations put forward some years ago by the commission named by President Carter to study the overall structure of the mental health care system in the United States. The purpose of this project was to integrate and unify the operations of all existing institutions and resources, public and private, whether created by federal or local initiative, professional organizations, groups of leading citizens, or even protest groups challenging the established powers. Thus official recognition was granted at the very highest level to the diversity so characteristic of the organization of the system, a diversity that was in fact taken as the basis for recommendations aimed at maximizing the efficiency of the system as a whole. Yankee empiricism, if you will—but, make no mistake about it, the commission's recommendations also show that it was aware of the basic dialectic that has informed mental medicine from the beginning and that ranges far beyond the antithesis between the public and private sectors.

We hope to have made contributions in two main areas. First we have attempted to underscore the complexity of the relationships between the various competing views within the mental medicine establishment on the one hand and the power structures of a "liberal" society on the other. Second, we have tried to explain the logic of mutual exchange and reinforcement that structures the mental health system internally and governs its transformations. This has led us to question the naiveté of those antitotalitarians for whom state power is the sole enemy of freedom and the presumptuousness of those who, in a sense, profit by taking a stance outside the system and its rules, even though they are in fact helping to extend its influence.

To raise the specter of a Leviathan state enveloping all of civil society in its tentacles is to blind oneself to the processes by which a different form of totalitarian control is being introduced into liberal societies. The choice to be made is not a strict alternative between, say, the use of psychiatry by the state for repressive purposes as in the Soviet Union on the one hand, and, on the other hand, a free enterprise system that allows the technicians of the mind to peddle their services in accordance with the laws of the market. The choice is not between coercion and contract: the health commodities now being dispensed by innumerable public and private agencies have become a new form of salvation, and people have little by little come to identify with the image put forward by the technocrats and behavioral programmers.

To understand how this has happened, we must recognize the role played by those who thunder against the medical establishment and medical methods of social integration—usually in the name of the latest techniques of their own devising. If the study of recent changes in psychiatry proves anything, it is how much the present expansion of psychiatry's sphere of influence owes to those who have come one after another to work on the fringes of the profession, pushing back its boundaries by "moving beyond" the old models, which they describe as archaic, coercive, prescriptive, and so forth. To anyone who regards this analysis as pessimistic, we can only answer that it is better to understand how a mechanism operates than to endure its effects in ignorance. One must know that nobody is exempt from the growing importance of social controls before one can prepare to work against them by mapping out and hopefully adding to the last remaining territory not yet fallen under the sway of the old guardians of law and order and the new engineers of the mind.

In confining our discussion mainly to the United States, our intention was not to beguile our French readers with an exotic tune. France, we are told, will also one day be an advanced liberal society. What does this mean? Among other things, an advanced psychiatric society. No longer a society in which psychiatry takes care of a few patients, whether really ill or merely purported to be, in any case defined by a stark contrast between the normal and the pathological; but rather an organization of everyday life in which manipulative techniques, more often than not developed and popularized by mental medicine, become coextensive with all aspects of social life. No longer the manifestation of naked power exerted directly to repress social and political differences; but rather diffuse pressures of many kinds, which invalidate such differences by interpreting them as so many symptoms to be treated. Not the country of gray dawns in which state commissars drag dissidents out of bed at the crow of the cock; but rather a padded world watched over night and day by squads of skilled specialists, many of them well-meaning. Skilled at what? At manipulating people to accept the constraints of society.

This picture already fits American society, to the extent that it is "liberal." A limited extent—because the existence of manipulative techniques has never prevented the use of other, more forceful measures. These, as we have seen, are always complemented and often reinforced by the new devices, but rarely are they withdrawn from the arsenal. We may as well know, then, if it isn't already too late, that there's not much to be gained from that kind of liberalism. On the contrary, there may be a good deal yet to lose of what we shall go on calling, begging the reader's indulgence if we seem somewhat old-fashioned, freedom.

Notes

PREFACE TO THE ENGLISH EDITION

1. Michel Foucault, *Madness and Civilization: A History of Insanity in the Age of Reason,* abridged (London: Tavistock, 1970). It must be noted that the original (unabridged) French version, different from the abridged paperback published by 10/18, first appeared in 1961. One cannot claim Foucault as a product of either 1968 or of antipsychiatry, although both movements discovered him around that time.

2. Robin Herman, "New York State Psychiatric Wards Overflow as Albany Changes its Mental Health Role," *New York Times,* December 8, 1980, p. B1.

3. In 1977, for example, 15 of the nation's 300 hospitals were closed, 11 new hospitals were opened, and one was "newly identified," leaving a net change of only 3. Unpublished data, Division of Biometry and Epidemiology, National Institute of Mental Health, 1981.

4. American Psychiatric Association, *Diagnostic and Statistical Manual of Mental Disorders* DSM III, 3d ed., February 1980.

CHAPTER 1: THE SUCCESS OF THE WORST

1. Albert Deutsch, *The Mentally Ill in America* (New York: Doubleday, 1938). These figures and a number of others have been taken from Deutsch, who gives a good description of the situation in the nineteenth century. The reader may also wish to consult Norman Dain, *Concepts of Insanity in the United States, 1789–1865* (New Brunswick, N.J.: Rutgers University Press, 1964); Gerald N. Grob, *The State and the Mentally Ill: A History of Worcester State Hospital* (Chapel Hill, N.C.: University of North Carolina Press, 1965); David J. Rothman, *The Discovery of the Asylum* (Boston: Little, Brown, 1971). For an illustration of the tendency to interpret history with the sole purpose of justifying current policy, see Ruth B. Caplan and Gerald Caplan, *Psychiatry and the Community in Nineteenth-Century America* (New York: Basic Books, 1969).

2. How to divide power among the local and central authorities remains a fundamental issue of American politics and a basic bone of contention between Republicans and Democrats. This has implications for welfare policy in general and for mental health policy in particular: broadly speaking, Democratic administrations have favored giving a preponderance of power to the federal government, except in the South; while the Republicans have defended the power of local units and clientele relationships.

3. J. R. Poynter, *Society and Pauperism: English Ideas on Poor Relief, 1795–1834* (London: Routledge and K. Paul, 1969). The basic poor law of 1835 replaced the workhouse as the centerpiece of the relief system in England. This, however, was a Malthusian reaction against the earlier Speenhamland Act of 1795, which provided an allocation for all domiciled indigents. In France, too, the Napoleonic administration tried for a while to restore to a place of honor the "dépôts de mendicité," but had precious little success in doing so. In regard to the way the problems of relief were reformulated in France at the beginning of the nineteenth century, see Robert Castel, *L'Ordre psychiatrique* (Paris: Editions de Minuit, 1976), ch. 3.

4. For a description of relief practices at this time, see two important documents that both sum up the situation and introduce the reformist ideas that would later inspire the establishment of the almshouse system: Joseph Quincy, *Report of the Massachusetts General Court Committee on Paupers Laws* (Albany, 1821); and John V. N. Yates, *Report of the Relief and Settlement of the Poor in the State of New York* (New York, 1824).

5. Rothman, *The Discovery of the Asylum*, ch. 8.

6. New York Almshouse Commissioner, *Annual Report for 1847* (New York, 1848), p. 6.

7. New York Association for Improving the Condition of the Poor, *Thirteenth Annual Report* (New York: John F. Trow, 1856), pp. 36–37.

8. Quincy, *Report*, p. 30.

9. Rothman, *The Discovery of the Asylum*, ch. 8.

10. Levi L. Barbour, "Argument Against Public Outdoor Relief," *Proceedings of the 18th National Conference of Charity and Correction* (Indianapolis, 1871), p. 42.

11. Deutsch, *The Mentally Ill*, p. 126. The city of Ghent responded to an invitation to build a home for its poor in the following terms: "We are completely opposed to this measure. . . . We wish to preserve our present privilege, to care for our poor in our own way, and not to be associated with other cities or the county."

12. C. R. Henders, "Public Outdoor Relief," *Proceedings of the 18th National Conference of Charity and Correction*.

13. Josephine C. Brown, *Public Relief, 1929–1939* (New York: H. Holt and Co., 1940).

14. See Robert Castel, "La guerre à la pauvreté aux Etats-Unis: le statut de

la misère dans une société d'abondance," *Actes de la Recherche en Sciences Sociales* (January 19, 1978), concerning welfare policy in the United States.

15. A somewhat different formula known as the "Wisconsin system" was used in a few states until recently: chronic patients were cared for in county hospitals, while the state set up hospitals to take care of acute cases. It should be noted that the Association of Superintendents, like its French counterpart, the staff organizations of the mental hospitals, always steadfastly opposed the separation of "acute" from "chronic" patients. An attempt to do so in New York, the Williard Act of 1865, which set up the Williard Asylum for chronic patients who were taken out of the almshouses, had to be repealed under pressure from the superintendents.

16. Deutsch, *The Mentally Ill*, p. 205.

17. *Ibid.*, p. 179.

18. See Castel, *L'Ordre psychiatrique*, concerning the origins of the French system.

19. Samuel J. Brakel and Ronald S. Rock, *The Mentally Disabled and the Law*, rev. ed. (Chicago: University of Chicago Press, 1971), p. 7.

20. Deutsch, *The Mentally Ill*, p. 421.

21. See Brakel and Rock, *The Mentally Disabled*, for a historical analysis of the evolution of this legislation. See Edward P. Scott, "Civil Commitment Status in the Courts Today," *Paper Victories and Hard Realities* (Washington, D.C.: Health Policy Center, 1976), concerning the present state of the question.

22. "Developments in the Law: Civil Commitment of the Mentally Ill," *Harvard Law Review* (1974), 87:1190–1406.

23. Rothman, *The Discovery of the Asylum*, p. 284.

24. *Ibid.*, p. 285.

25. *Ibid.*, p. 268.

26. William A. Hammond, *The Non-Asylum Treatment of the Insane* (New York, 1879), p. 14.

27. *Ibid.*, p. 227.

28. Weir S. Mitchell, "Fiftieth Anniversary Address," *Transactions of the American Medico-Psychological Association* (1894), p. 116. (The quotation is a re-translation from the French.)

29. Horatio M. Pollock, "Development of Statistics on Mental Disease in the United States in the Past Century," *American Journal of Psychiatry* (July 1, 1945), vol. 102.

30. Meyer Harvey Brenner, *Mental Illness and the Economy* (Cambridge, Mass.: Harvard University Press, 1973). Based on statistics for New York state asylums between 1841 and 1967, the study shows that the inmate population grows during periods of depression and shrinks during periods of recovery, independent of whatever may be going on within psychiatry itself. These periodic swings do not contradict the fact that, until 1956, the number of inmates tended on the whole to increase. Concerning the reasons for the reversal of this tendency after 1956, see chapter 4.

31. "The Wyatt Case: Implementation of a Judicial Decree Ordering Institutional Change," *Yale Law Journal* (1975), 84:1349.

32. Brakel and Rock, *The Mentally Disabled.*

33. Erving Goffman, *Asylums* (New York: Doubleday, 1961).

CHAPTER 2: THE PROGRESSIVE ERA

1. Nathan G. Hale, *Freud and the Americans: The Beginning of Psychoanalysis in the United States, 1976–1917* (New York: Oxford University Press, 1971). Besides discussing psychoanalysis as such, Hale gives a detailed analysis of the medical and social context for the period he covers, upon which we have drawn extensively.

2. Freud was practically unknown prior to his visit in 1909. The difference in prestige between Janet and Freud is indicated by the places to which they were invited: Freud received an invitation from Clark University, modern-minded but marginal, while Janet was invited to the dedication ceremonies for new buildings at the Harvard Medical School and to lecture at Cornell and Columbia—in other words, to the three major eastern medical schools.

3. Abraham Myerson, "Some Trends of Psychiatry," *American Journal of Psychiatry* (April 1944), vol. 100.

4. Hale, *Freud and the Americans*, p. 232.

5. Morton Prince, *Clinical and Experimental Studies in Personality* (Cambridge, Mass.: Sci-Art Publishers, 1929).

6. Ernest Jones, who emigrated to Canada in 1908 (as professor of psychiatry at the University of Toronto), played a role of the first importance in establishing psychoanalysis in the United States. Allergic to the ways of the New World, he was to return to Great Britain, however, in 1912.

7. See C. P. Obendorf, *An History of Psychoanalysis in America* (New York, 1953), in addition to Hale, *Freud and the Americans*. Obendorf, an early convert to psychoanalysis, was analyzed by Freud in Vienna before becoming one of the leaders of the American movement.

8. William A. White, "Psychoanalytic Tendencies," *American Journal of Insanity* (April 1917).

9. Erving Goffman, *Asylums* (New York: Doubleday, 1961).

10. Floyd Dell, "Speaking of Psycho-analysis: The New Boon for Dinner-Table Conversationalists," *Vanity Fair* (December 1915), 5(4)53.

11. Charles Kadushin, *Why People Go to Psychiatrists* (New York: Atherton Press, 1969).

12. Morton Prince, "Roosevelt as Analyzed by the New Psychology," *New York Times*, March 24, 1912, section 7, p. 1.

13. It would, however, be possible to say a great deal on this point, in view of the contemptuous attitude taken by many European and, especially, French psychiatrists toward their American colleagues. We had the opportunity to dis-

cover for ourselves, by contrast, that many American analysts are both lucid and modest about their role. In any case, two or three points need to be made. First of all, the way to various "deviations" in psychoanalysis was opened by Freud himself in his lectures at Clark University, including the tendencies to didacticism, moralism, optimism, and so forth that American psychoanalysis is often reproached for exhibiting. Second, it was under persistent pressure from Freud that the American psychoanalytic societies were created, despite the reservations of the American doctors, who did not want to compromise themselves to such an extent. It should also be recalled (or pointed out for the first time) that Freud himself was so keen to play the trump of New World modernism against the traditional opposition he was running up against in Europe that, during the autumn of 1921, he had five members of the New York Psychoanalytic Society in analysis simultaneously in Vienna (in other words, he was then spending about half of his hours in practice training American physicians).

14. Clifford Beers, *A Mind that Found Itself* (New York: Doubleday, 1908); citations are from the 1933 edition.

15. *Origin, Objects and Plans of the National Committee for Mental Hygiene*, Publication no. 1 of the National Committee for Mental Hygiene (New York, 1912), p. 2.

16. George S. Stevenson, "The Child Guidance Clinic: Its Aims, Growth and Methods," *Proceedings of the First International Congress on Mental Hygiene* (New York, 1932), 2:251.

17. V. V. Anderson, "The Contribution of Mental Hygiene to Industry," *Proceedings of the First International Congress of Mental Hygiene*, 1:698. Note that this text was applauded by members of the Congress of Mental Hygiene at Washington in 1930, the year of the great crisis.

18. Adolf Meyer, "The Organisation of Community Facilities for Prevention, Care and Treatment of Nervous and Mental Diseases," *Proceedings of the First International Congress of Mental Hygiene*. Note that this school of thought had direct and rapid influence in France and that it attracted the same modern-minded fringe of the psychiatric profession. The work of Edouard Toulouse and of Heuyer cannot be understood outside this context. The French Society of Mental Hygiene (of which Toulouse was president) was the second international affiliate of the American movement (preceded only by Canada); it was founded in 1921. The Second International Congress of Mental Hygiene was held in Paris in 1937, under the chairmanship of Edouard Toulouse.

19. William A. White, "The Origin, Growth and Significance of the Mental Hygiene Movement," *Proceedings of the First International Congress of Mental Hygiene*, 1:530.

20. William Healey, *Twenty-Five Years of Child Guidance: An Appraisal of Studies from the Institute for Juvenile Research* (Chicago, n.d.), series C, no. 256.

21. At the same time feeblemindedness associated with senility forged into the limelight as a crucial problem. In this form, however, the solution proposed was different: eugenics (see ch. 2).

22. Lawson G. Lowrey, "Psychiatry for Children, History of the Development," *American Journal of Psychiatry* (1944), 101:375–88.

23. William Healey, *The Individual Delinquent* (1915).

24. Lowrey, "Psychiatry for Children," p. 385.

25. Stevenson, "The Child Guidance Clinic," p. 251.

26. Reverend S. H. Gurteen, *A Handbook of Charity Organization* (Buffalo, N.Y., 1879), cited in W. I. Trattner, *From Poor Law to Welfare State* (New York: Free Press, 1974), p. 87.

27. Hannah Curtis, "Social Services in Retrospect and Outlook," *Bulletin of the Massachusetts Department of Mental Diseases* (1934), vol. 18.

28. Trattner, *From Poor Law to Welfare State*, ch. 8.

29. Mary E. Richmond, *Social Diagnosis* (New York: Russell Sage Foundation, 1917), p. 32.

30. Kathleen Woodroofe, *From Charity to Social Work in England and the United States* (London: Routledge & Kegan Paul, 1962). The phrase figures as the title of chapter six.

31. Jessie Taft, "Progress in Social Case Work in Mental Hygiene" *Proceedings of the 50th National Conference of Social Work* (Chicago: University of Chicago Press, 1923), p. 338. A special study would be necessary to analyze the relations between these two "vectors of psychologization": mental hygiene and the psychoanalytic "new psychology." In actuality, they worked together and were promoted by the same leaders. The more popular vocabulary of mental hygiene was the first to take root, however. The technical terminology of psychoanalysis began to become commonplace in the welfare literature for the most part from the late twenties onward.

32. Thomas W. Salmon, "Some of the Tasks of Organized Work in Mental Hygiene," *Proceedings of the 47th National Congress of Social Work* (Chicago: University of Chicago Press, 1920), p. 65.

33. Miriam Van Waters, "Presidential Address: Philosophical Trends in Modern Social Work," *Proceedings of the 57th National Congress of Social Work* (Chicago: University of Chicago Press, 1930), p. 19.

34. "Presidential Address," *Proceedings of the 25th Annual Meeting of the National Association of Manufacturers of the USA* (New York, 1930), cited in Woodroofe, *From Charity to Social Work*, p. 134.

35. Herbert Hoover, cited in H. S. Commager, ed., *Documents of American History*, (New York: Appleton-Century-Crofts, 1958), 2:405.

36. Agnes Murray, "Case Work above the Poverty Line," *Proceedings of the 45th National Congress of Social Work* (Chicago: University of Chicago Press, 1918).

37. William Ryan, *Blaming the Victim* (New York: Pantheon Books, 1971).

38. Robert Castel, "La guerre à la pauvreté aux Etats-Unis: le statut de la misère dans une société d'abondance," *Actes de la Recherche en Sciences sociales* (January 19, 1978).

39. See Stanley Davies, *Social Control of the Feebleminded* (New York: National Committee for Mental Hygiene, 1923); and Albert Deutsch, *The Mentally Ill in America* (New York: Doubleday, 1937), 16 and 17, on these matters.

40. Walter E. Fernald, "The Burden of Feeble-mindedness," *Journal of Psycho-Asthenics* (1913), 17:90–91.

41. Carlos F. MacDonald, "Presidential Address," *American Journal of Insanity* (July 1914), 71:9.

42. If sterilization for mere chicken theft seems particularly shocking, it is worth noting that this was an offense with which blacks were commonly charged.

43. Samuel J. Brakel and Ronald S. Rock, *The Mentally Disabled and the Law.* rev. ed. (Chicago: University of Chicago Press, 1971).

44. It is difficult to estimate the number of sterilizations that may have been carried out before laws were passed or independent of whatever laws were on the books, under the authority of the all-powerful asylum superintendents. We do know, for instance, that Dr. H. C. Sharp, a pioneer in sterilization and the "inventor" of the vasectomy, carried out several hundred illegal sterilizations at the Indiana State Reformatory in the late nineteenth century.

45. Clarence G. J. Gamble, "Sterilization Programs for the Prophylactic Control of Mental Diseases and Mental Deficiency," *American Journal of Psychiatry* (November 1945), 102(3).

46. The scientific justification for sterilization is in fact based on two assertions that have fallen increasingly under suspicion: (1) that diagnoses of incurable defects are scientifically certain, and (2) that the hereditary transmission of those defects is also a matter of certainty.

47. Brakel and Rock, *The Mentally Disabled.* On this subject, see the two versions (1961 and 1971) of this book published under the auspices of the American Bar Association. The 1961 version points out how difficult it is to apply the law "objectively," while the 1971 version takes a stand in opposition to the principle underlying the law. In 1963, it is said that 476 involuntary sterilizations were performed in the United Sates. See Nicholas N. Kittrie, *The Right to Be Different* (Baltimore, Md.: Johns Hopkins University Press, 1971), p. 360.

48. *The Journal of Abnormal Psychology and Social Psychology* (April 1921), 1:4. This journal was founded in April 1921. According to its Editorial Announcement in the first issue, it proposed to devote itself to "the problems of socialization, in a broad sense the fitting of the behavior of the individual and the social order."

49. John B. Watson, "Behavior and the Concept of Mental Disease," *Journal of Philosophy, Psychology and Scientific Methods* (1916), 13:590.

50. John B. Watson, "The Psychology of Wish-Fulfilment," *Scientific Monthly* (November 1916), vol. 3, cited in Hale, *Freud and the Americans*, p. 355.

51. Obviously, complicity between the two doctrines did not preclude po-

lemic and competition as well. Thus Watson carried out a conditioning experiment on an eleven-month-old child to "refute" the Freudian theory of phobia. See Jones Cover, "Elimination of Children's Fear," *Journal of Experimental Psychology* (1924), vol. 7. However, the purpose of the experiment was precisely to criticize hangovers of "endogenous" and "innatist" thinking in the psychoanalytic interpretation and to substitute an explanation in terms of pure external conditioning.

52. E. E. Southard, "Cross-sections of Mental Hygiene, 1844–1869–1894," *American Journal of Insanity* (October 1919), 76:110–11.

CHAPTER 3: THE THIRD PSYCHIATRIC REVOLUTION

1. Clara Bassett, *Mental Hygiene in the Community* (New York: Macmillan, 1934). See the table of contents, which shows how far psychiatric intervention had already gone beyond its traditional boundaries within the "special hospitals": medicine, social services, the adult and juvenile courts, parental education, preschool education, instruction of teachers and ministers, industry, recreation, psychiatric institutions and facilities, to name a few of the areas covered.

2. W. I. Trattner, *From Poor Law to Welfare State* (New York: Free Press, 1974).

3. Haven Emerson, "A Tribute to Dr. Thomas W. Salmon," *Proceedings of the First International Congress of Mental Hygiene* (New York, 1933).

4. Trattner, *From Poor Law to Welfare. State*, p. 173n6.

5. The Veterans Administration was set up after the war, however. It was responsible for general and mental hospitals devoted exclusively to the treatment of veterans. The VA mental hospitals differed little from state mental hospitals in structure, however (see chapter 4).

6. David Mechanic, *Mental Health and Social Policy* (Englewood Cliffs, N.J.: Prentice-Hall, 1969); Robert H. Felix, *Mental Illness, Progress and Prospects* (New York: Columbia University Press, 1967).

7. Henry A. Foley, *Community Mental Health Legislation* (Lexington, Mass.: Lexington Books, 1975); see also Robert H. Connery, ed., *Politics of Mental Health* (New York: Columbia University Press, 1968).

8. U.S. Senate, Committee on Education and Labor, *Hearings on S.1160, National Neuro-psychiatric Institute Act*, 79th Cong., 2d sess., 1946, p. 107.

9. It also explains the dependence of much of this sociology (with a few exceptions, such as Goffman's work) on the ideology underlying this reformist politics. The social scientist was called upon to support mental health professionals and administrators. The involvement of social scientists had consequences which, broadly speaking, can be characterized as progressive, insofar as they were concerned to criticize and reform an outmoded organizational structure and to seek ways to improve the practice of psychiatry. Social scientists had no authority to define the objectives, however, and they refrained from questioning

the ones handed to them. Only much later did more radical investigations of the professional monopoly of mental health care and the political significance of the strategies pursued by the profession begin to be undertaken.

10. Public Law 182, 84th Cong., 1st sess., July 28, 1955.

11. Thus the American Legion not only appears on the list but financed the publication of the final report, *Action for Mental Health*. This was a deliberate maneuver conceived by Jack Ewalt, the chairman of the Commission, to head off, as he himself explained to us, any possible charge that a "communist plot" was involved, a charge that is often raised in the United States against any attempt to increase public services, especially if they involve federal intervention. Such clever tactics are no substitute for democratic participation at the grass roots, such as Commission officials claim today to have achieved.

12. John F. Kennedy, "Message from the President of the United States relative to Mental Illness and Mental Retardation," 88th Cong., House of Representatives, February 5, 1963, document no. 58, p. 4.

13. Five other services were optional but recommended: specialized diagnostic services, preadmission services, readaptation services, postcure services for patients discharged from state mental hospitals, and research and training facilities. For a discussion of how these services actually worked, see chapter 5.

14. John F. Kennedy, "Remarks as He Signed into Law Mental Health Retardation Bill S.1576," *Presidential Papers* (New York: Putnam, 1963).

15. See, for example, Robert H. Felix, *Mental Illness, Progress and Prospects* (New York: Columbia University Press, 1967); Richard H. Williams, *Perspectives in the Field of Mental Health* (Washington, D.C., 1972).

16. Theodore R. Marmor, *The Politics of Medicare* (Chicago: Aldine Publishing Co., 1973). When the 95th Congress recessed in 1976, a dozen health insurace proposals were under discussion. See Marmor concerning the policy of the American Medical Association with regard to insurance bills. Besides Medicare and Medicaid, various prepaid health plans have been developed, offering health care services to the employees of some large firms, groups, etc. (health maintenance organizations). No comprehensive system now exists, however, even though the Carter Administration had started off in favor of one.

17. These figures are approximate, because it is common in the United States for doctors to practice both privately and in the hospital and to work part-time in a number of public or private institutions. Even in public facilities such as the community mental health care centers, only 42 percent of the psychiatrists work full-time, and private doctors can do work for the centers and be paid for the services they perform.

18. Health Policy Advisory Center (Health P.A.C.), *The American Health Empire* (New York, 1971), pp. 3–4. More generally, concerning the American health care system, see the remarkable critical analyses published in bimonthly bulletins by Health P.A.C. (17 Murray Street, New York N.Y.), as well as the work of the few sociologists who have not been content to accept the official

medical ideology: Egon Bittner, Marc Field, Elliot Freidson, Wolf V. Heyde-
brand, Elliot Mischler, Anselm Strauss, Eugen Zola, and others.

19. Harry C. Salomon, "The American Psychiatric Association in Relation
to American Psychiatry," *American Journal of Psychiatry* (July 1958). For France,
see Robert Castel, "Genèse et ambiguités de la notion de secteur," *Sociologie du
Travail* (January 1975). The one difference, which is crucial, however, is that
in France the movement to transform the system was headed by people who
worked on the staffs of mental hospitals.

20. Felix, *Mental Illness, Progress and Prospects*, p. 82.

21. Joint Commission on Mental Illness and Health, *Action for Mental Health*
(New York, 1961), p. xiv.

22. For this interpretation, see Foley, *Community Mental Health Legislation*
which, however, considers only the administrative and financial aspects of the
problem.

23. "Plank adopted in Platform of Democratic Party," cited in Foley, *Community Mental Health Legislation*, p. 31.

24. U.S. House, Committee on Interstate and Foreign Commerce, Hearings
on S.1576, 88th Cong., 1st sess., July 10, 11, 1963, p. 23. Testimony of Bois-
feuillet Jones.

25. Concerning the spirit of welfare, see Frances F. Piven and A. Cloward,
Regulating the Poor (New York: Pantheon, 1971); Robert Castel, "La Guerre à
la pauvreté aux Etats-Unis: le statut de la misère dans une société d'abondance,"
Actes de la Recherche en Sciences sociales (January 19, 1978). Fred Wiseman's film
Welfare (Zipporah Films, Boston 1975) depicts these practices remarkably well.

26. Piven and Cloward, *Regulating the Poor*; idem, *The Politics of Turmoil* (New
York: Pantheon, 1976).

27. Michael Harrington, *The Other America* (New York: Macmillan, 1962).

28. John Kenneth Galbraith, *The Affluent Society*, (Boston: Houghton Mifflin,
1958). He wrote that in the United States poverty "cannot be described as a
universal or common scourge," but that it was "more nearly an afterthought."

29. Piven and Cloward, *Regulating the Poor*, p. 261.

30. Code of Federal Regulations, Title 42, Public Health, Part 54204, January
1971, p. 110.

31. Franklin D. Chu and Sharland Trotter, *The Madness Establishment* (New
York: Grossman, 1974). For further information on these points, see chapter 5.

32. Erving Goffman, *Asylums* (New York: Doubleday, 1961), ch. 4.

33. "Primary prevention" is action to alter pathological or pathogenic factors
in the community. See Gerald Caplan, *Principles of Preventive Psychiatry* (New
York: Basic Books, 1964), and see also chapter 5 below.

34. Gerald Caplan, *An Approach to Community Mental Health* (London: Tavistock Publications, 1961), p. 238.

35. Leonard J. Duhl, ed., *The Urban Condition* (New York: Basic Books,
1963), p. 73.

36. Leonard J. Duhl, "Psychiatry and the Urban Poor," in W. Ryan, ed.,

Distress in the City (Cleveland, Ohio: Press of Case Western Reserve University, 1969), p. 118.

37. Caplan, *Principles*, p. 59.

38. *Ibid.*, p. 56.

39. Williams, *Perspectives*, p. 6.

40. Leonard J. Duhl and Robert L. Leopold, *Mental Health and Urban Social Policy*, (San Francisco: Jossey-Bass, 1968), p. 11.

PART TWO: AN AMERICAN DREAM

1. Benedict S. Alper, Foreword to Y. Bakal, ed., *Closing Correctional Institutions* (Lexington, Mass.: Lexington Books, 1973), pp. vii–viii.

2. The belief in general deinstitutionalization is not limited to the mental health field but is also commonplace in the literature concerning prisons and juvenile delinquency. See Andrew T. Scull, *Decarceration, Community Treatment, and the Deviant* (Engelwood Cliffs, N.J.: Prentice-Hall, 1977).

3. Milton Greenblatt and Erving Glazer, "The Phasing-out of Mental Hospitals in the United States," *American Journal of Psychiatry* (1975), vol. 132.

4. Bertram S. Brown and Harry P. Cain, "The Many Meanings of Comprehensive: Underlying Issues in Implementing the Community Mental Health Center Program," *American Journal of Orthopsychiatry* (October 1964), 34(5).

CHAPTER 4: PSYCHIATRIC HOSPITALS

1. Treatment episodes equals the number of patients in treatment as of January 1 plus the number of admissions during the year.

2. Franklin D. Chu and Sharland Trotter, *The Madness Establishment* (New York: Grossman, 1974), p. 29.

3. Mary J. Ward, *The Snake Pit* (New York: Random House, 1946); Albert Deutsch, *The Shame of the States* (New York: Harcourt, Bruce, 1948).

4. Erving Goffman, *Asylums* (New York: Doubleday, 1961).

5. Alfred H. Stanton and Morris S. Schwartz, *The Mental Hospital* (New York: Basic Books, 1954); Milton Greenblatt, R. H. York, E. L. Brown, in collaboration with R. W. Hyde, *From Custodial to Therapeutic Care* (New York: Russel Sage Foundation, 1955); I. Belknap, *Human Problems of a State Mental Hospital* (New York: Blakiston Division, McGraw-Hill, 1956); William Caudill, *The Psychiatric Hospital as a Small Society* (Cambridge, Mass.: Harvard University Press, 1958); H. Warren Dunham and S. Kirson Weinberg, *The Culture of the State Mental Hospital* (Detroit, Mich.: Wayne State University Press, 1960); A. F. Wessen, ed., *The Psychiatric Hospital as a Social System* (Springfield, Ill.: Charles C Thomas, 1964).

6. Greenblatt et al., *From Custodial to Therapeutic Care*.

7. "The Introduction of Chlorpromazine," *Hospital and Community Psychiatry* (July 1976) p. 505.

8. General Accounting Office, Report to the Congress by the Comptroller General of the United States, "Returning the Mentally Disabled to the Community: Government Needs to Do More," (Washington, D.C.,: Government Printing Office, 1977), HRD–76–152, p. 67.

9. From California Department of Mental Hygiene Data, Sacramento, 1971.

10. Andrew T. Scull, *Decarceration, Community Treatment, and the Deviant* (Englewood Cliffs, N.J.: Prentice-Hall, 1977), p. 146.

11. Senate, Special Committee on Aging, Subcommittee on Long-Term Care, *Nursing Home Care in the United States—Failure in Public Policy: Supporting Paper no. 7.* (Washington, D.C.: U.S. Government Printing Office, 1974). (The subtitle is more informative: "The role of nursing homes in caring for discharged mental patients and the birth of a for-profit boarding home industry.")

12. Kenneth Skivanck, Deputy Director for Mental Health Planning, cited in "The Discharged Chronic Mental Patient," *Medical World News* (April 12, 1974), p. 57.

13. Cited by Louise Lander, "The Mental Health Con Game," *Health Policy Advisory Center Bulletin* (July–August 1975), p. 1.

14. Cited in Chu and Trotter, *The Madness Establishment*, p. 39.

15. *Community Mental Health and the Mental Hospital* (Boston, November 1973), p. 34.

16. Dr. Robert Reich, former director of psychiatry for New York City's Department of Social Services, cited in Henry Santiestevan, *Deinstitutionalization: Out of their Beds and into the Streets* (Washington, D.C., December 1976), p. 44.

17. National Institute of Mental Health Statistical Note no. 107.

18. Report to the President, from the President's Commission on Mental Health (Washington, D.C.: Government Printing Office, 1978), p. 24.

19. "Position Statement on the Need to Maintain Long-term Mental Hospital Facilities," *American Journal of Psychiatry* (June 1974), 131(6):745.

20. *Holt* v. *Sarver*, 309 FSupp. 362 E. D. Arkansas, 1970.

21. Hunt Wiley, "Operation Baxstrom after One Year," *American Journal of Psychiatry* (1968), vol. 124.

22. Cited in Linda Matthews, "Supreme Court Mulls Mental Care Problems," *Sunday Advocate* (Baton Rouge, La.), May 25, 1975, p. 6.

23. "American Psychiatric Association Official Actions," *American Journal of Psychiatry* (May 1967), 123:1460.

24. Cited in Michael L. Perlin and Walter W. Siggers, "The Role of the Lawyer in Mental Health Advocacy," *The Bulletin of the American Academy of Psychiatry and Law* (1976), 4:208.

25. "The Wyatt Case: Implementation of a Judicial Decree Ordering Institutional Change," *Yale Law Journal* (1975), 84:1338–79.

26. *Ibid.*, p. 1348.

27. Cited in *Wyatt* v. *Aderholt*, U.S. Court of Appeals, 5th Circuit, no. 72–2634, November 1974, p. 721.

28. Harold W. Heller, "The Wyatt Standards: An Administrative Viewpoint," *Hospital and Community Psychiatry* (May 1977), 28(5):363.

29. Code of Federal Regulations 405–1022, 405–1023, 405–1027, 250–2023, Washington, 1973.

30. Layton B. Dorman, "Community Mental Health Services in Alabama after Wyatt," *Hospital and Community Psychiatry* (May 1977), 28(5).

31. "Note on the Wyatt Case," 84:1358n122.

32. *Souder* v. *Brennan*: 42 U.S.L.W. 2271, U.S. District Court, 1973.

33. "*Souder* v. *Brennan*: 'Impact in the Court,'" *Hospital and Community Psychiatry* (February 1976), 27(2):107.

34. Alan A. Stone, "Recent Mental Health Litigation: A Critical Perspective," *American Journal of Psychiatry* (March 1977), 134(3):277.

35. Alan A. Stone, "The Right to Treatment and the Psychiatric Establishment," *Psychiatric Annals* (September 1974), 4(9).

36. Milton Greenblatt, "The Need for Balancing the Right to Treatment and the Right to Treat," *Hospital and Community Psychiatry* (May 1977), 28(5):382–83.

37. Calculated from figures in National Institute of Mental Health Statistical Note no. 118, July 1975.

38. Based on National Institute of Mental Health Statistical Note no. 122, September 1975.

39. Based on National Institute of Mental Health Statistical Note no. 125, February 1976.

40. National Institute of Mental Health Statistical Note no. 91, September 1973, and no. 112, March 1975.

41. Lander, "The Mental Health Con-Game."

42. Based on National Institute of Mental Health Statistical Note no. 105, May 1974, between 53 and 72 percent of the patients falling under these nosographic categories entered the hospital voluntarily in 1972, compared with an overall rate of "voluntary" commitments of 48.6 percent for all categories.

43. National Institute of Mental Health Statistical Note no. 105, May 1974.

44. National Institute of Mental Health Statistical Note no. 129, May 1976. "Professionals" include psychiatrists and interns, physicians, dentists, psychologists, social workers, graduate nurses, pharmacists, dieticians, specialist therapists (work therapists, etc.), counselors, teachers, medical secretaries, etc. The rest of the staff consists of "attendants," without special training (nowadays officially called "mental health workers"), direct descendants of the asylum guards.

45. National Institute of Mental Health Statistical Note no. 115, April 1975.

46. National Institute·of Mental Health Statistical Note no. 129, May 1976.

47. See Goffman, *Asylums*, part 2.

48. Experience shows that, allowing for vacation time and for the need to

have three shifts working round the clock, 39 full-time attendants per 100 patients, or barely 10 per care unit of 25 patients, in fact amounts to 2 or 3 attendants actually present in the morning, an equal number in the afternoon, and 1 at night for each care unit.

49. "Note on the Wyatt Case," 84:1349–50n56.

50. The use of chemotherapy is of course not limited to mental hospitals. After a period in the early fifties when psychoanalytic models were paramount, and a period of prominence of social models in the sixties, lately we have been watching a comeback by chemical and biological models, which has affected psychiatric practice inside and outside the hospital.

51. National Commission for the Protection of Human Subjects of Biomedical and Behavioral Research, *Report and Recommendations: Psychosurgery*, Department of Health, Education, and Welfare, Publication no. OS 77-0001, Bethesda, Md., 1977. For an overview of the question, see Herbert J. Vaughn Jr., "Psychosurgery and Brain Stimulation in Historical Perspective," in Willard M. Gaylin, Joel S. Meister, and Robert C. Neville, eds., *Operating on the Mind: The Psychosurgery Conflict* (New York: Basic Books, 1975).

52. Greenblatt et al., *From Custodial to Therapeutic Care*.

53. R. C. Scheerenberger, "Public Residential Services for the Mentally Retarded" (Ph.D. diss., University of Wisconsin, Madison, 1976).

54. Cited in Alan A. Stone, *Mental Health and the Law: A System in Transition* (Rockville, Md.: National Institute of Mental Health, 1975), p. 128.

55. According to B. M. Rosen, M. Kramer, S. G. Willner, and R. W. Redick, "Utilization of Psychiatric Facilities by Children: Current Status, Trends, Implications," *Public Health Service Publication no. 1868*, 1968; and National Institute of Mental Health Statistical Note no. 130, April 1976.

56. Here we have considered only institutions figuring in the National Institute of Mental Health statistics (state mental hospitals, public institutions for the retarded, and private residential treatment centers). To get an overview of the number of young Americans institutionalized in penal as well as medical institutions, between which it is increasingly difficult to draw any hard and fast line, these figures need to be augmented by those given in chapter 6.

57. National Institute of Mental Health, series A, no. 18, *Private Psychiatric Hospitals 1974–1975* (Washington, D.C., 1977).

CHAPTER 5: THE ILLUSIONS OF COMMUNITY

1. Joint Commission on Mental Illness and Heatlh, *Action for Mental Health, Final Report, 1961* (New York: Basic Books, 1961), p. xvii.

2. Erich Lindeman, "Symptomatology and Management of Acute Grief," *American Journal of Psychiatry* (1944), vol. 101.

3. Gerald Caplan, *Principles of Preventive Psychiatry* (New York: Basic Books, 1964). Begun by Lindeman's work, the theory of prevention was put in system-

atic form primarily by Caplan, and extended and further developed in concrete applications by a group of authors, none other than the pioneers of community psychiatry in the sixties. For a bibliography of the major works of this school, see Bernard L. Bloom, *Community Mental Health: A Historical and Critical Analysis* (Morristown, 1973).

4. Health Policy Advisory Center, *Evaluation of Community Involvement in Community Mental Health Centers* (New York, 1972).

5. Public Law 88-164, Title II, *Community Mental Health Centers Act*, October 31, 1963.

6. Howard P. Rome, "Psychiatry and Foreign Affairs: The Expanding Competence of Psychiatry," *American Journal of Psychiatry* (December 1968), 125:729.

7. As of June 1972, 325 were in operation and 64 others had filed plans and obtained approval from Washington but were not yet open.

8. Report to the President from the President's Commission on Mental Health, Washington, 1978.

9. Franklin D. Chu and Sharland Trotter, *The Madness Establishment* (New York: Grossman, 1974), pp. 10–11.

10. Public Law 94–63, Title III, "Community Mental Health Centers," *94th Cong., S. 66*, July 29, 1975, pp. 5–31.

11. California Department of Mental Hygiene, *California Mental Health Progress*, Sacramento (January 1967).

12. Minnesota Department of Public Welfare, *Minnesota Mental Health-Mental Retardation Program in Perspective: A Comprehensive Summary* (January 1969).

13. Michigan *Public Act* 54, 1963.

14. Chaim Shatan, "Community Psychiatry—Stretcher Bearer of the Social Order?" *International Journal of Psychiatry* (May 1969), 7:318.

15. Antony M. Graziano, "Clinical Innovation and the Mental Health Power Structure: A Social Case History," *Congress of the Eastern Psychological Association*, Washington, D.C., (April 1968), p. 2.

16. Harris B. Peck, Melvin Roman, Seymour R. Kaplan, "Community Action Programs and the Comprehensive Mental Health Center," *Psychiatric Research Report*, American Psychiatric Association (April 1967), 21:103–4.

17. Matthew P. Dumont, *The Absurd Healer* (New York: Science House, 1968), p. 24.

18. Health Policy Advisory Center, *Evaluation of Community Involvement in Community Mental Health Centers,* (Rockville, Md.: National Institute of Mental Health, 1970), p. 20.

19. Interview with Martin Keeley, June 1972, cited in Chu and Trotter, *The Madness Establishment*, pp. 89–90.

20. Health Policy Advisory Center, *Evaluation of Community Involvement*, pp. 22, 80.

21. Chu and Trotter, *The Madness Establishment*, p. 33.

22. Health Policy Advisory Center, *Evaluation of Community Involvement*.

23. *Ibid.*, p. 22.

24. Warren T. Vaughan et al., "The Private Practice of Community Psychiatry," *American Journal of Psychiatry* (January 1973), 130(1):24–27.

25. *Ibid.*, p. 27.

26. Donald Daggett, "Planning a Community Mental Health Center in a Private Hospital Setting," *Consortium Proposal*, appendix 3.

27. Code of Federal Regulations, Title 42, Public Health, part 54210(2), January 1, 1971, p. 114.

28. H. G. Whittington, "Report of the Conference of Community Mental Health Centers," in Raymond M. Glasscote et al., eds., *The Community Mental Health Center: An Interim Appraisal* (Washington, D.C.: Joint-Information Service of the American Psychiatric Association and the National Association for Mental Health, 1969), p. 44.

29. Interview with Katharyn Fritz, June 1972, cited in Chu and Trotter, *The Madness Establishment*, p. 90.

30. Health Policy Advisory Center, *Evaluation of Community Involvement*, pp. 33–34.

31. *Ibid.*, p. 48.

32. *Ibid.*, p. 85.

33. Everett Hughes, "Profession," *Daedalus* (Fall 1963), 92(4):656.

34. Elliott Friedson, *Professional Dominance* (New York: Atherton Press, 1970).

35. Dr. Walter Barton, medical director of the American Psychiatric Association, cited in Chu and Trotter, *The Madness Establishment*, p. 73.

36. National Institute of Mental Health Statistical Note no. 108.

37. *Inside Westside* (newsletter of San Francisco's Westside Community Mental Health Center), September–October 1973.

38. According to Health Policy Advisory Center, *Evaluation of Community Involvement*, pp. 106–41.

39. *Ibid.*, pp. 60–105.

40. Conference organized in April 1978 by Horizon House Institute for Research and Development at Philadelphia on the theme, "The National Project on Improving Community/Facility Relations."

41. Based on Health Policy Advisory Center, *Evaluation of Community Involvement*, pp. 230–71.

42. F. Riessman, *New Careers: A Basic Strategy Against Poverty*, A. Philip Randolph Educational Fund, pamphlet no. 2, p. 1.

43. National Institute of Mental Health, *Staffing of Mental Health Facilities, United States, 1974*, publication no. 76308 (Washington, D.C., 1976).

44. Sam Alley and Judith Blanton, "A Study of Paraprofessionals in Mental Health," *Community Mental Health Journal* (1976), 12(2):154, table 2.

45. *Ibid.*, p. 153, table 1.

46. M. B. Smith and N. Hobbs, "The Community and the Community Mental Health Center," *American Psychologist* 21:506.

47. George Ritzer, "Indigenous Non-Profesionals in Community Mental

Health Centers: Boon or Boondoggle," in Paul Roman and H. H. Trice, eds., *The Sociology of Psychotherapy* (New York: J. Aronson, 1974), p. 225.

48. Riessman, *New Careers*, p. 69.

49. L. J. Crowne, "Approaches to the Mental Health Manpower Problems: A Review of the Literature," *Mental Hygiene* (1969), 53:182.

50. W. I. Halpern, "The Community Mental Health Aide," *Mental Hygiene* (1969), 53:82.

51. A. Gartner, "Organizing Paraprofessionals," *Social Policy* (September–October 1970), 1:61.

52. A. Haber, "Issues Beyond Consensus," *National Council for New Careers Organizing Conference* Detroit, 1968.

53. Cited in Ritzer, "Indigenous Non-Professionals," p. 229.

54. *Ibid.*, p. 231.

55. Concerning the walk-in clinics. See William C. Normand and Ann Pappi, "The Walk-in Clinic as Central Intake" (New York, n.d.). Mimeo.

56. Seymour R. Kaplan and Melvin Roman, *The Organization and Delivery of Mental Health Services in the Ghetto: The Lincoln Hospital Experience* (New York: Praeger, 1973).

57. "Tell It Like It is," June 9, 1968. Mimeo. (This quotation is a retranslation from the French.)

58. J. Christmas, H. Wallace, and J. Edwards, "New Careers and New Mental Health Services: Fantasy or Future?" *American Journal of Psychiatry* (1970), 126(10):1485.

59. Based on conversations with Merton Kahn, director of the facility, and Charlotte Schwartz.

60. In the spring of 1978, California voted in favor of Proposition 13, which reduced real estate taxes by nearly half. These taxes finance schools and social services in the state. If other states follow suit, the very existence of public services in the United States—already so mediocre—will be jeopardized.

61. Peter G. Bourne, "Human Resources: A New Approach to the Dilemmas of Community Psychiatry," *American Journal of Psychiatry* (June 1974), 131(6).

62. Report to the President from the President's Commission on Mental Health, 4 vols., Washington, 1978.

63. F. Riessman, "The President's Commission on Mental Health: The Self-Help Prospect," *Social Policy* (May–June 1978), p. 29.

64. See Robert Castel, "La guerre à la pauvreté aux Etats-Unis: le statut de la misère dans une société d'abondance," *Actes de la Recherche en Sciences sociales* (January 19, 1978) for a more complete analysis of the relationship between the operation of welfare services and psychology.

65. Françoise Boudreau-Lemieux, *Changes in the System for the Distribution of Psychiatric Care in Quebec, 1960–1974* (Montreal, 1977).

CHAPTER 6: THE PSYCHIATRIZATION OF DIFFERENCE

1. Gordon Pfister, "Outcomes of Laboratory Training for Police Officers," *Journal of Social Issues* (1975), 31(1):115.

2. John J. Hughes, "Training Police Recruits for Service in Urban Ghettos: A Social Worker's Approach," in John Monahan, ed., *Community Mental Health and the Criminal Justice System* (New York: Pergamon, 1974).

3. L. E. Newman and J. L. Steinberg, "Consultation with Police on Human Relations Training," *American Journal of Psychiatry* (April 1970), 126(10):1424.

4. Lindbergh S. Sata, "Laboratory Training for Police Officers," *Journal of Social Issues* (1975), 31(1).

5. Karl Schonborn, "Police and Social Workers as Members of New Crisis Management Teams," *Journal of Sociology and Social Welfare* (July 1976), 3(6):682.

6. Nicholas N. Kittrie, *The Right to Be Different* (Baltimore, Md.: Johns Hopkins University Press, 1971).

7. Cited in Anthony Platt, "The Triumph of Benevolence: The Origin of the Juvenile Justice System in the United States," in Abraham Blumberg, ed., *Introduction to Criminology* (New York, 1972).

8. "Massachusetts Annotated Laws," Ch. 123A, sec. 1 (1965), cited in Alan A. Stone, *Mental Health and the Law: A System in Transition* (Rockville, Md.: National Institute of Mental Health, 1975) p. 181.

9. Maryland, Annotated Code, article 31 B S 5 (1971), cited in Willard Gaylin and Ellen Blatte, "Behavior Modification in Prisons," *The American Criminal Law Review* (1975), 13(2):23.

10. David A. Rothman, "Behavior Modification in Total Institutions," *Hastings Center Report* (February 1975), 5:21.

11. Jessica Mitford, *Kind and Usual Punishment* (New York: Random House, 1973).

12. James Q. Wilson, "Changing Criminal Sentences," *Harper's* (November 1977).

13. Robert M. Force and Anne M. Lovell, "Diversion, Community Corrections and Other Alternative Incarcerations," *Selected Papers of the Subcommittee on the Criminal Justice System in Louisiana*, Baton Rouge, La., 1974.

14. Figures cited in Andrew T. Scull, *Decarceration, Community Treatment, and the Deviant* (Englewood Cliffs, N.J.: Prentice-Hall, 1977) ch. 3.

15. Nora Klapmutts, "Community Alternatives to Prisons," *Crime and Delinquency Literature* (June 1973), p. 5.

16. Scull, *Decarceration*, ch. 3.

17. Arnold Binder, John Monahan, and Martha Newkirk, "Diversion from the Juvenile Justice System and the Prevention of Delinquency," in John Monahan, ed., *Community Mental Health*.

18. Various studies have estimated the number of American youths involved with the police before they reach the age of eighteen at between 20 and 35 percent of the under-eighteen population (see Binder, et al., "Diversion").

19. The extreme case of deinstitutionalization in this area was the closing in 1972 of all Massachusetts institutions for delinquent children at the behest of Jerome Miller, an especially dynamic administrator. However, 35 to 40 percent of these juveniles, regarded as too dangerous to be set free, were turned over to a private institution. See Y. Bakal, ed., *Closing Correctional Institutions* (Lexington, Mass.: Lexington Books, 1973).

20. William Nagel, cited in Tony Platt and Paul Takagi, "Intellectuals for Law and Order: A Critic of the New Realists," *Crime and Social Justice* (Fall–Winter 1977), vol. 8.

21. Dr. Norman Fenton, cited in Erik Ohlin Wright, *The Politics of Punishment* (New York: Harper & Row, 1973), p. 43.

22. Kim I. C. Luke and T. L. Clanon, "Psychiatric Services Integrated into a Correctional System," *International Journal of Offender Therapy* (1971), 15(3).

23. Flora Haas, "Meditation and Production in Prison: T. Ming from Attica to Fomson," *State and Mind* (November–December 1976).

24. Don Jackson, "Gay Death at Vacaville," *Rough Times* (June 1972), 2(7).

25. Stephen L. Chorover, "Big Brother and Psychotechnology," *Psychology Today*, October 1973, p. 48.

26. American Friends Service Committee, *Struggle for Justice* (New York: Hill and Wang, 1971).

27. William R. Arnold and Bill Stiles, "A Summary of Increasing Use of Group Methods in Correctional Institutions," *International Journal of Group Psychotherapy* (January 1972), 22(1).

28. Wayne King, "Kansas Convicts Receive Awareness Training," *The New York Times*, January 26, 1975, p. 39.

29. This kind of self-mutilation was common in American prisons, particularly prison-farms in the South, where until 1973 prisoners often worked twelve hours per day in cane fields for wages of a few cents an hour.

30. Letter from a prisoner published in *Rough Times* (June 1972), 2(7):4.

31. King, "Kansas Convicts," p. 39.

32. Michael Serber and Claudia G. Keith, "The Atascadero Project: Model of a Sexual Retraining Program for Incarcerated Homosexual Pedophiles," *Journal of Homosexuality* (1974), 1(1).

33. Williard Gaylin and Helen Blake, "Behavior Modification in Prisons," *American Criminal Law Review* (1975), 13(11):26–27.

34. Joel S. Meiser, "Participation is Voluntary," *Hastings Center Report*, February 1975, p. 38.

35. Robert A. Burt, "Why We Should Keep Prisoners From Doctors," *Hastings Center Report*, (February 1975), pp. 25–34.

36. *The New York Times*, March 26, 1981, p. A17.

37. *National Commission on Criminal Justice Standards and Court Goals* (Washington, D.C., 1973), p. 375. (This quotation is a retranslation from the French.)

38. Richard R. Korn, "The California Brain Surgery Caper," *The Freeworld Time*, (February 1972).

39. Report to the President from the President's Commission on Mental Health, p. 201.

40. "Heroin Rate Rising, U.S. Official Says," *The New York Times*, March 8, 1976, p. 29.

41. *Federal Strategy, Drug Abuse Prevention* (Washington, D.C.: U.S. Government Printing Office, 1976).

42. Dorothy Nelkin, *Methadone Maintenance: The Technological Fix* (New York: G. Braziller, 1973).

43. Thomas Szasz, *Ceremonial Chemistry: The Ritual Persecution of Drugs, Addicts, and Pushers* (Garden City, N.Y.: Anchor Press, 1974).

44. Edward M. Bretcher and the editors of Consumer Reports, *Licit and Illicit Drugs* (Boston: Little, Brown, 1972), chs. 1, 2, and 3.

45. Arlene T. Lissner, John Jilmore, Kenneth J. Pompi, "The Dilemma of Coordinating Treatment with Criminal Justice," *American Journal of Drug and Alcohol Abuse* (1976), 3(4).

46. Robert A. Kadjan and Edward C. Senay, "Modified Therapeutic Communities for Youth," *Journal of Psychedelic Drugs* (July–September 1976), 8(3):209.

47. *Ibid.*, p. 209.

48. Dan Waldorf, "Social Control in Therapeutic Communities for the Treatment of Drug Addicts," *International Journal of Addictions* (March 1971), 6(1):35.

49. Kadjan and Senay, "Modified Therapeutic Communities," p. 213.

50. Arnold Schechter, "Consumer Acceptance of Drug Abuse Programs: A Provider's View," *Journal of Psychedelic Drugs* (1974) 6(2).

51. Barry S. Paner, "Methadone Maintenance for Narcotic Addiction," *Journal of Psychedelic Drugs* (Winter 1971), 4(2).

52. Vincent P. Dole and Marie E. Nyswander, "Rehabilitation of Heroin Addicts after Blockage with Methadone," *New York State Journal of Medicine*, August 1, 1966, p. 2012.

53. The fact that the majority of accidental drug addicts have been "cured" and "reinserted" into society with relative ease, while drugs continue to lay waste to the ghettos, shows that the drug problem is essentially a social and political problem.

54. Special Action Office for Drug Abuse Prevention, *Residential Methadone Treatment Manual* (Washington, D.C.: U.S. Government Printing Office, 1974), pp. 3–4.

55. P. G. Bourne and M. Deslade, "Methadone: The Merit of its Addictive Qualities," Office of Drug Abuse of Georgia, cited in *Residentials Methadone Treatment Manual* 54:5.

56. *Criminal Justice Newsletter* (June 20, 1977), 8(13):7.

57. Cited in Matthew P. Dumont, "Civil Commitment of Addicts: A Critical Analysis," *International Yearbook of Drug Addiction and Society* 1(19).

58. Schechter, "Consumer Acceptance," p. 219.

59. Nelkin, *Methadone Maintenance*, p. 65.

60. Ron Bayer, "Repression, Reform and Drug Abuse: An Analysis of Response to the Rockefeller Drug Law Proposals of 1973," *Journal of Psychedelic Drugs* (1974), 6(3).

61. Arthur Stickgold, "Medical Model or Medical Metaphor: The Impact of Third Party Payments on Drug Treatment Programs," *Journal of Psychedelic Drugs* (1976), 8(2):139.

62. Benjamin Rush, *Inquiry into the Effects of Ardent Spirits on the Human Body and Mind* (Philadelphia, 1791).

63. Bretcher et al., *Licit and Illicit Drugs.*

64. Jonas Robitscher, "Changing Concepts of Criminal Responsibility," in C. H. Wecht, ed., *Legal Medicine Annual: 1969* (New York: Appleton-Century-Crofts, 1969).

65. Robert A. More, "Ten Years of Inpatient Programs for Alcoholic Patients," *American Journal of Psychiatry* (May 1977), 134(5).

66. Szasz, *Ceremonial Chemistry.*

67. Cited in Larry Hart, "A Review of Treatment and Rehabilitation Legislation Regarding Alcohol Abuse and Alcoholics in the United States, 1920–1971," *International Journal of the Addictions* (1977), 12(5):669.

68. Bretcher et al., *Licit and Illicit Drugs.*

69. Alan Gartner, "Self-Help and Mental Health," *Social Policy* (September–October 1976), 1(7).

70. James L. Nichols and Vernon S. Ellingstad, "An Experimental Evaluation of the Effectiveness of Short Term Rehabilitation Programs for Convicted Drinking Drivers," *National Council on Alcoholism: Annual Forum*, St. Louis, May 1978.

71. Brief of American Psychiatric Association, American Association for Adolescent Psychiatry, American Academy of Child Psychiatry, and American Association of Psychiatric Services for Children, in *Kremens* v. *Bartley*, Brief of Appellees, Supreme Court of the United States, 4th quarter, 1976.

72. J. C. Borden, "Human Welfare Groups Concerned over Dispersal of Problem Children," *The New York Times*, August 14, 1977, p. 1 and 42.

73. *Ibid.*, p. 42.

74. Edith B. Back, "Can Children be Saved from Politicians?" *The Texas Observer*, November 28, 1975.

75. Cited in Peter Schrag and Diane Divoky, *The Myth of the Hyperactive Child and Other Means of Child Control* (New York: Pantheon, 1975), p. 18. The pages that follow owe much to this remarkably well-documented book.

76. Cited in *ibid.*, p. 19.

77. *Ibid.*, p. 20.

78. Report to the President, p. 149.

79. Harold Shane and Jane Shane, "Forecast for the '70s," *Today's Education* (January 1969).

80. Schrag and Divoky, *The Myth of the Hyperactive Child*, ch. 4.

81. *Ibid.*, p. 82.

82. Cited by Eli Messinger, "Ritalin and Minimal Brain Dysfunction: A Cure

in Search of a Disease," *Health Policy Advisory Center Bulletin* (November–December 1975), no. 67, 3.

83. The notions of hyperactivity, hyperkinesia, minimal brain damage, and minimal cerebral dysfunction are frequently used as near synonyms for minimal brain dysfunction. In treatment, dexedrine often competes with ritalin.

84. Paul H. Wender, *Minimal Brain Dysfunction in Children* (New York: John Wiley, 1971).

85. Barbara Fish, "Problems of Diagnosis and the Definition of Comparable Groups: A Neglected Issue in Drug Research with Children," *American Journal of Psychiatry* (January 1969), 125(7):902.

86. Sidney Katz et al., "Clinical Pharmacological Management of Hyperkinetic Children," *International Journal of Mental Health*.

87. Alan Sroufe and Mark A. Stewart, "Treating Problem Children with Stimulant Drugs," *The New England Journal of Medicine* (August 1973), 289(8).

88. Leon Oettinger, Jr., "Learning Disorders, Hyperkinesis and the Use of Drugs in Children," *Rehabilitation Literature* (June 1971), 32(6):165.

89. Schrag and Divoky, *The Myth of the Hyperactive Child*, p. 14.

90. William Ryan, *Blaming the Victim* (New York: Random House, 1972), p. 8.

91. William Redd and William Sleator, *Take Change: A Comprehensive Analysis of Behavior Modification* (New York: Random House, 1976).

92. Vernon Mark, William Sweet, and Frank Ervin, "The Role of Brain Disease in Riots and Urban Violence," *Journal of the American Medical Association* (September 1967, 201(11). See also V. Mark and Frank Ervin, *Violence and the Brain* (New York: Harper & Row, 1970).

93. Redd and Sleatov, *Take Change*.

CHAPTER 7: ALTERNATIVES TO PSYCHIATRY AND PSYCHIATRIZATION OF THE ALTERNATIVES

1, *State and Mind* (Winter 1977), 6(2); and (Spring 1978), 6(3). Concerning the situation in Europe, see Collectif international, *Réseau-Alternative à la psychiatrie* (Paris: Editions 10/18, 1977).

2. Walter H. Abrams and Gordon P. Holleb, *Alternatives to Community Mental Health* (Boston: Beacon Press, 1975), p. 2.

3. David E. Smith, "The Role of the Free Clinic in America's Changing Health Care Delivery System," *Journal of Psychedelic Drugs* (January–March 1975), 7(1):28.

4. Philip Brown and Nancy Henley, "Professionals: The Dialogue Continues . . . ," *Rough Times* (April 1972), 2(6):19.

5. Anita Friedman, Claude Steiner, Hogie Wyckoff, et al., "An Analysis of the Structure of Berkeley Radical Psychiatry Center," in Claude Steiner, ed., *Readings in Radical Psychiatry* (New York: Grove Press, 1977), p. 150.

6. Cited in Abrams and Holleb, *Alternatives*, p. 41.

7. Kristin Glaser, Eugene Gendlin, "Main Themes in Changes, A Therapeutic Community," *Rough Times* (June–July 1973), 3(6):2.

8. Project Place, *A Report on Our Progress in 1973* (Boston, 1973), p. 2. Mimeo.

9. Claude Steiner, "Manifesto," in Steiner, ed., *Readings in Radical Psychiatry*, p. 1.

10. *Rough Times* today goes by the name *State and Mind* (P. O. Box 89, Somerville, Mass. 02144). Along with *Madness Network News*, published in San Francisco, it is one of the two journals critical of mental medicine with the largest current circulation.

11. Herbert J. and Arlene F. Freudenberger, "1973—The Free Clinics Picture Today: A Survey," *Catalog of Selected Documents in Psychology* (Winter 1974), 4:41.

12. William M. Harvey, "The Special Problems of Free Clinics Serving Minority Groups," *Journal of Social Issues* 30(1):66. There was, however, a more radical tendency within minority groups themselves, which rejected cooptation by official agencies and wanted totally self-managed community facilities. See Rona M. Fields, "The Politics of Community Mental Health," *Social Policy* (September–October 1970), relating an experiment of this type in Los Angeles, which ran into opposition from the police and local government.

13. Claude Steiner, "Radical Psychiatry History," in Steiner, ed., *Readings in Radical Psychiatry*, p. 146.

14. Smith, "The Role of the Free Clinics," p. 37.

15. Cited in Abrams and Holleb, *Alternatives*, p. 55.

16. Rosemary Taylor, "Consumers Control and Professional Accountability in the Free Clinic," (Ph.D. diss., University of California, Berkeley, 1974), p. 15.

17. Abrams and Holleb, *Alternatives*, p. 39.

18. Smith, "The Role of the Free Clinics," p. 29.

19. Cited in Constance Bloomfield and Howard Levy, "The Selling of the Free Clinics," *Health Policy Advisory Center Bulletin* (February 1972), no. 38, p. 2.

20. *Ibid.*, p. 6.

21. Karen Horney, "The Flight from Womanhood: The Masculinity Complex in Women as Viewed by Men and Women," *International Journal of Psycho-Analysis* (1926), 7:324–39.

22. Jean Baker Miller, *Psychoanalysis and Women* (Baltimore, Md.: Penguin, 1973).

23. Kate Millett, *Sexual Politics* (New York: Doubleday, 1970), p. 178.

24. Besides Miller and Millett, see also, for example, Juliet Mitchell, *Psychoanalysis and Feminism* Baltimore, Md.: Penguin, 1976); Ruth Moulton, "A Survey and Re-evaluation of the Concept of Penis Envy," in Miller, *Psychoanalysis and Women*; Anne Koedt, "The Myth of the Vaginal Orgasm," in Shulamith Firestone and Anne Koedt, *Notes from the Second Year: Women's Liberation* (New York,

1970); Jean Strouse, ed., *Women and Analysis* (New York: Grossman, 1974). A recent, commercially exploited continuation of this line of criticism may be found in Shere Hite, *The Hite Report* (New York: Macmillan, 1976).

25. Miller, *Psychoanalysis and Women*, p. 381.

26. *Ibid.*, p. 379.

27. Anica Vesel Mander and Anne Kent Rush, *Feminism as Therapy* (New York: Random House, 1974), p. 39.

28. Women in Transition, Inc., *Women in Transition: A Feminist Handbook on Separation and Divorce* (New York: Scribner's, 1975), p. 404.

29. "Counseling for Women and their Friends." Mimeo. (This quotation is a retranslation from the French.)

30. Inge K. Broverman et al., "Sex-Roles Stereotypes and Clinical Judgements of Mental Health," *Journal of Counseling and Clinical Psychology* (February 1970), 34:6.

31. Phyllis Chesler, "Marriage and Psychotherapy," *The Radical Therapist* (1971), p. 175.

32. Phyllis Chesler, *Women and Madness* (New York: Doubleday, 1972).

33. Jesse Bernard, "The Paradox of the Happy Marriage," in Vivian Gornick and Barbara K. Moran, *Women in Sexist Society* (New York: New American Library, 1971).

34. Elizabeth Friar Williams, *Notes of a Feminist Therapist* (New York: Praeger, 1976), p. xiii-xiv.

35. *Women in Transition*, p. 402.

36. Mander and Rush, *Feminism as Therapy*.

37. Alice Krakauer, "Woman's Body/Woman's Mind: A Good Therapist is Hard to Find," *Ms* (October 1972), 1(4):34.

38. Barbara Ehrenreich and Deirdre English, *Witches, Midwives and Nurses: A History of Women Healers* (Old Westbury, N.Y.: Feminist Press, 1973).

39. Williams, *Notes*.

40. For transactional analysis, see Hogie Wyckoff, "Women's Scripts and the Stroke Economy," in Steiner, ed., *Readings in Radical Psychiatry*, p. 48.

41. Williams, *Notes*.

42. Based on analysis of fifty self-help groups in ten states: see "The Women and Mental Health Project: Women-to-Women Services," *Social Policy* (September–October 1976), 7(2).

43. The adjective "gay" was first applied to theatrical people, then to prostitutes; they behaved differently from earnest, respectable people and at the same time were supposed to be leading "gay" lives.

44. Louis Landerson, "Psychiatry and Homosexuality: New Cures," *Rough Times* (July 1972), 2(8):15.

45. L. J. Hatterer, *Changing Homosexuality* (New York: Delta, 1970).

46. Don Clark, *Loving Someone Gay* (Milbrae, Calif.: Celestial Arts, 1977).

47. C. A. Tripp, *The Homosexual Matrix* (New York: McGraw-Hill, 1975), p. 232.

48. Clark, *Loving Someone Gay*.

49. *Ibid.*, p. 36.

50. Raymond M. Berger, "An Advocate Model for Interventions with Homosexuals," *Social Work* (June 1977), 22(4).

51. Clark, *Loving Someone Gay*, p. 107.

52. *Ibid.*, p. 165.

53. Claude Steiner, "Comment: Principles of Radical Psychiatry," reprinted in *The Black Panther* (December 1977), 7(28):2.

54. Leonard S. Ebreo, "Gay Liberation and Change," *The Radical Therapist* (February 1972), 2(5):6.

55. "Gay Counseling in a Free Clinic: A Group Communal Project," *Journal of Social Issues* (1974), 30(1):9.

56. This success appears precarious, however, given the fact that in a subsequent poll, 69 percent of the psychiatrists surveyed answered "yes" to the question, "Do you think that homosexuality is usually a pathological adjustment?" (*Medical Aspects of Human Sexuality* [November].) This result should perhaps be considered in the light of the present tendency to limit the civil rights already won by homosexuals in several states.

57. Clark, *Loving Someone Gay*, p. 16.

58. *Souder* v. *McGuire*, U.S. District Court for Middle District of Pennsylvania, December 9, 1976 (423 F. Supp. 830–31).

59. Cited by Susan Abrams, "Do Mental Patients Have Rights?" *In These Times* (January 18–24, 1978), p. 5.

60. Cited in *The New York Times*, June 27, 1975, p. 1.

61. Kenneth Donalson has published a book about his experiences, *Insanity Inside Out* (New York: Crown, 1976).

62. Steve Horowitz, "Court-Legislated Reform: Viable Approach or Paper Victory" (n.d.). Mimeo.

63. "I got involved in the suit for a right to treatment in Alabama because we had information that the judge in charge of the case had stated that there was no such thing as an abstract 'right to treatment,' and that he wanted to set conditions that the state of Alabama would have been unable to meet." (Leonard R. Frank, "Interview with Bruce Ennis," *Madness Network News*, [February 2, 1974], p. 10.) Bruce Ennis is one of the best-known lawyers in the movement to change psychiatry through the courts, and he took a particularly active role in the Wyatt case, which resulted not in the closing but in the reform of Alabama mental institutions. See chapter 4.

64. Document translated into French and published in "Les droits des psychiatrisés," *Garde-Fous* (Paris, 1978), (11–12):53–64.

65. *Organizing for Health Care: A Tool for Change*, Source Catalogue (Boston, 1974), no. 3, p. 105.

66. *Health Policy Advisory Center Bulletin* January 1972, no. 37.

67. *Fourth Annual North American Conference on Human Rights and Psychiatric*

Oppression (May 1976). Mimeo. (This quotation is a retranslation from the French.)

68. David Ferleger, "The Vanishing Welcome Mat: Mental Patients Rights." Mimeo.

69. Cited in "Les droits des psychiatrisés," p. 51.

CHAPTER 8: PSY SERVICES AND THEIR NEW CONSUMERS

1. These figures are approximate. We have tried to correct the data by collating the results of several different investigations, which do not always agree among themselves. See especially Judd Marmor, *Psychiatrists and their Patients: A National Study of Private Office Practice* (Washington, D.C.: The Joint Information Service of the American Psychiatric Association and the National Association for Mental Health, 1975); Task Force Report, No. 6, *The Present and Future Importance of Private Psychiatric Practice in the Delivery of Mental Health Service* (Washington, D.C.: American Psychiatric Association, June, 1973); Steven Sharestein, Carl A. Taub, and Irving D. Goldberg, "The Private Psychiatry and Accountability: A Response to the A.P.A. Task Force Report on Private Practice," *American Journal of Psychiatry* (January 1975), 132(1).

2. Marmor, *Psychiatrists and their Patients*, p. 41.

3. Martin L. Gross, *The Psychological Society* (New York: Random House, 1978).

4. Arnold A. Rogow, *The Psychiatrists* (New York: Putnam, 1970).

5. Marmor, *Psychiatrists and their Patients*.

6. On the internal logic of psychoanalysm and its social and political functions, see Robert Castel, *Le Psychanalysme* (Paris: François Maspero, 1973).

7. Peter L. Berger, "Towards a Sociological Understanding of Psychoanalysis," *Social Research* (Spring 1965), 32(1).

8. Charles Kadushin, *Why People Go to Psychiatrists* (New York: Atherton Press, 1969).

9. *Ibid.*, p. 81.

10. We shall mention here only the techniques that are most important, in the sense that they contribute to breaking down the concept of "mental illness." For a more complete treatment, see Robert A. Harper, *Psychoanalysis and Psychotherapy: 36 Systems* (New York: J. Aronson, 1974); and, by the same author, *The New Psychotherapies* (Englewood Cliffs, N.J.: Prentice-Hall, 1975).

11. For the first therapeutic applications of the fundamental work of Wolpe and Skinner, see J. Wolpe, *Psychotherapy by Reciprocal Inhibition* (Stanford, Calif.: Stanford University Press, 1958); O. R. Lindsley and B. F. Skinner, "A Method for the Experimental Analysis of Psychotic Patients," *American Psychologist* (1954), vol. 9. The philosophical, political, and social assumptions behind behavior modification are made clear in B. F. Skinner, *Beyond Freedom and Dignity* (New York: Knopf, 1971).

12. One sign among others, because the number of subjects being treated by behavioral therapy is practically impossible to determine precisely: between 1960 and 1970, the number of articles devoted to behavior modification in four of the most important psychiatric journals multiplied tenfold (Task Force Report, *Behavior Therapy in Psychiatry* (Washington, D.C.: American Psychiatric Association, 1973). Growth of behavior modification in nonpsychiatric applications is even more spectacular.

13. *Ibid.*

14. For a detailed consideration of the methods of behavioral therapy, which space does not permit our giving here, see J. Wolpe, *The Practice of Behavior Therapy* (New York: Pergamon, 1969).

15. Foley, *An Introduction to Family Therapy.*

16. Ross Speck and Carolyn Attenave, *Family Networks* (New York: Pantheon, 1973).

17. Mony El Kaïm, "Broadening the Scope of Family Therapy," *Terapia Familiare* (Rome, 1979).

18. Foley, *An Introduction to Family Therapy,* ch. 6.

19. G. Bateson, D. D. Jackson, D. Haley, J. Weakland, "Towards a Theory of Schizophrenia," in D. D. Jackson, ed., *Communication, Family and Marriage* (Palo Alto, Calif.: Science and Behavior Books, 1968).

20. C. C. Beels and A. Ferbor, "Family Therapy: A View," *Family Process* (September 1969), 8(2).

21. Foley, *An Introduction to Family Therapy.*

22. Cited in *ibid.,* p. 65.

23. William H. Masters and Virginia E. Johnson, *Human Sexual Response* (Boston: Little, Brown, 1966); *idem, Human Sexual Inadequacy* (Boston: Little, Brown, 1969).

24. Cited in Harper, *The New Psychotherapies,* p. 45.

25. Cited in Eugene Kennedy, *Sexual Counseling* (New York: Seabury Press, 1977), p. 192.

26. Helen Singer Kaplan, *The New Sex Therapy* (New York: Brunner-Mazel, 1974).

27. William H. Masters and Virginia E. Johnson, Principles of the New Sex Therapy," *American Journal of Psychiatry* (May 1976), 133(5).

28. Alexander Lowen, *Bioenergetics* (Baltimore, Md.: Penguin, 1975). See also *Depression and the Body* (Baltimore, Md.: Penguin, 1972); and *The Betrayal of the Body* (London: Collier, 1969).

29. Jean-Marie Delacroix, "Les Psychothérapies de groupes corporels avec les psychotiques," *Information psychiatrique* (April 1978), 54(4).

30. Lowen, *Bioenergetics.*

31. Frederick S. Perls, *Gestalt Therapy Verbatim* (Lafayette, Calif.: Real People Press, 1969), p. 44; see also Frederick S. Perls, Ralph F. Hefferline, and Paul Goodman, *Gestalt Therapy* (New York: Julian Messner, 1951).

32. Perls, *Gestalt Therapy Verbatim,* p. 4.

33. Joel Latner, *The Gestalt Therapy Book* (New York: Julian Press, 1973), p. 40.

34. Arthur Janov, *The Primal Scream* (New York: Dell, 1970), p. 9.

35. Arthur Janov, *The Anatomy of Mental Illness: The Scientific Basis of Primal Therapy* (New York: G. P. Putnam's Sons, 1970).

36. Janov, *The Primal Scream*, pp. 206ff.

37. E. Fuller Torrey, "The Primal Therapy Trip: Medicine or Religion?" *Psychology Today* (December 1976), vol. 10.

38. David Freudenlich, "A Historical Perspective on Primal Therapy" (May 1975). Mimeo.

39. William Swartley, "Primal Integration," (n.d.). Mimeo.

40. Transactional analysis is set forth in a number of very popular works by Eric Berne: *Transactional Analysis in Psychotherapy* (New York: Grove Press, 1961); *Games People Play* (New York: Grove Press, 1964); *What Do You Say after You Say Hello* (New York: Grove Press, 1972).

41. Thomas A. Harris, *I'm O.K.—You're O.K.: A Guide to Transactional Analysis* (New York: Harper & Row, 1969).

42. *Ibid.*, p. 197.

43. Berne, *Games People Play*, part 2: "A Thesaurus of Games."

44. Harris, *I'm O.K.—You're O.K.*, p. xv.

45. Muriel James, *The O.K. Boss* (Reading, Mass.: Addison-Wesley, 1975). The basic claim is that everybody wants to be a "boss." Furthermore, "at one time or another, almost everybody is a boss," if only with wife, children, or dog. So everybody may as well be an "O.K. boss."

46. See, for example, Frantz Alexander, "The Dynamic of Therapy in the Light of Learning Theory," *American Journal of Psychiatry* (1963), vol. 120; Judd Marmor, "The Future of Psychoanalytic Therapy," *American Journal of Psychiatry* (1973), vol. 130; Lee Birk and Ann W. Brinkley-Birk, "Psychoanalysis and Behavior Therapy," *American Journal of Psychiatry* (1974), vol. 131.

47. Mimeographed advertising distributed by the Associates.

48. Joel Kovel, *A Complete Guide to Therapy: From Psychoanalysis to Behavior Modification* (New York: Pantheon, 1976), p. 145.

49. Samuel Koch, "The Image of Man in Encounter Group Theory," *Journal of Humanistic Psychology* (Fall 1971), 11:112.

50. Harvey Jackins, *The Human Side of Human Beings: The Theory of Reevaluation Counseling* (Seattle, Wa.: Rational Island, 1965).

51. Thomas Scheff, "Reevaluation Counseling: Social Implications," *Journal of Humanistic Psychology* (Spring 1972), 12:69.

52. Jackins, *The Human Side*.

53. For a more detailed treatment, see Kurt W. Back, *Beyond Words* (New York: Russel Sager, 1972), which is undoubtedly the best general treatment of the question. Even the terminology is not always firmly established. Back suggests calling the whole range of methods treated here "sensitivity training." The "Training group" or "T group" is the most academic and technocratic version,

revolving around the "management science" that was developed at the National Training Laboratory in continuation of Kurt Lewin's research. The term "encounter group" refers primarily to experiments inspired by the Esalen Institute, sometimes known as the "humanist" tendency and strongly influenced by Carl Rogers.

54. Jacob L. Moreno has written the history of his own work in *Who Shall Survive?* 2d ed., (New York: Beacon House, 1953). Concerning the "social" applications of Moreno's work, see C. Loomis, "Sociometries and the Study of New Rural Communities," *Sociometry* (1939), vol. 2.

55. The most comprehensive treatment of these methods may be found in Kenneth D. Benne et al., *The Laboratory Method of Changing and Learning: Theory and Applications* (Palo Alto, 1975).

56. Carl Rogers, *Client-centered Therapy in Current Practice: Implication and Theory* (Boston: Houghton-Mifflin, 1951); and *On Encounter Groups* (Baltimore, Md.: Penguin, 1970).

57. Nathan Hurvitz, "The Origin of the Peer-Help Psychotherapy Movement," *Journal of Applied Behavioral Science* (1976), 12(3).

58. Michael Murphy, "Esalen," *Readings in Social Psychology Today* (Del Mar, Calif.: CRM Books, 1970), p. 149.

59. *Ibid.*

60. Carl R. Rogers, "A Plan for Self Directed Change in an Educational System," *Educational Leadership* (1967), 24(8):717.

61. Arthur Burton, "Encounter, Existence, and Psychotherapy," in Arthur Burton, ed., *Encounter* (San Francisco: Jossey-Bass, 1969), pp. 8–9.

62. *Ibid.*, p. 9.

63. Back, *Beyond Words*, p. 33.

64. Alvin Toffler, *Future Shock* (New York: Random House, 1970), p. 200.

65. Concerning the degradation of labor in the twentieth century owing to technological changes introduced by monopoly capitalism, see Harry Braverman, *Labor and Monopoly Capital* (New York: Monthly Review Press, 1975).

66. Morton A. Leiberman and Jill R. Gardener, "Institutional Alternatives to Psychotherapy: A Study of Growth Center Uses," *Archives of General Psychiatry* (February 1976), 33(4).

67. Morton A. Leiberman, I. D. Yalom, and M. B. Miles, *Encounter Groups: First Facts* (New York: Basic Books, 1973), p. 452.

68. American Psychiatric Association, Task Force Report, *Encounter Groups and Psychiatry* (Washington, D.C., 1970).

69. Gross, *The Psychological Society*, p. 8.

70. "Chewing for Dollars," *Time*, November 28, 1977.

71. Adelaide Bry, *est: 60 Hours that Transform your Life* (New York: Harper & Row, 1976). See also S. Fenwick, *Getting It: The Psychology of est* (Philadelphia, Pa.: J. P. Lippincott, 1976); and R. A. Hargrove, *est: Making Life Work* (New York: Delacorte Press, 1976).

72. Werner Erhard, cited in Bry, est, p. 66.

73. Eva Hoffman, "est: The Magic of Brutality," *Dissent* (Spring 1977), p. 211.

74. Earl Babbie, "est in Prison: General Overview," *American Journal of Corrections* (November–December 1977), p. 23.

75. R. C. Winnett and R. A. Winkler, "Current Behavior Modification in the Classroom: Be Still, Be Quiet, Be Docile," *Journal of Applied Behavior Analysis* (1972), 5:500.

76. George I. Brown, *Human Teaching for Human Learning* (New York: Viking, 1971).

77. Ted Bartel, "The Human Relations Ideology: An Analysis of the Social Origins of a Belief System," *Human Relations* (1976), 29(8).

78. Back, *Beyond Words*, p. 170.

79. Rogers, *On Encounter Groups*, ch. 8.

80. Jane Howard, *Please Touch* (New York: McGraw-Hill, 1970).

81. D. C. Klein, "Sensitivity Training and Community Development," in E. H. Schein and W. G. Bennis, eds., *Personal and Organizational Change Through Group Methods: The Laboratory Approach* (New York: John Wiley, 1965).

82. R. E. Walton, "A Problem-Solving Workshop on Border Conflicts in Eastern Africa," *Journal of Applied Behavioral Science* (1970),6(4). See also L. W. Doob, *Resolving Conflict in Africa* (New Haven, Conn.: Yale University Press, 1970).

83. Back, *Beyond Words*, ch. 11.

84. B. E. Calane, "The Truth Hurts: Some Companies See More Harm than Good in Sensitivity Training," *The Wall Street Journal*, July 14, 1969.

85. These acceptable union strategies and this officially imposed welfare policy of course went hand in hand with systematic repression of the radical demands of exploited groups. This complementary aspect of the issue is beyond the scope of the present study, however.

CONCLUSION: THE PSY WORLD

1. In particular, experiments in England (Maxwell Jones) and the Netherlands (Querido in Amsterdam) served as models. The French *politique de secteur* is sometimes even described in the American psychiatric literature as an example of successful deinstitutionalization. See Martin Gittelmann, "Sectorization: The Quiet Revolution in European Mental Health Care," *American Journal of Orthopsychiatry* (January 1972), 42(1).

2. Richard A. Shartz, "Psychiatry Drifts away from Medicine," *American Journal of Psychiatry* (February 1974), vol. 131, a good example of the school of thought currently dominating the psychiatric profession.

3. For a recent evaluation of research and applications in the area of control policy, see Vance Packard, *The People Shapers* (Boston: Little, Brown, 1977).

4. Nicholas Kittrie, *The Right to Be Different* (Baltimore, Md.: Johns Hopkins University Press, 1971).

5. More than in most other countries, psychiatry in the Soviet Union revolves around prevention and distribution of services in the areas where the users live. This is true to such a degree that, when it came time to set up community mental health facilities in the United States, top American officials from both the government and the psychiatric profession visited the USSR and acknowledged the superiority of Soviet organization in a number of respects. (See U.S. Department of Health, Education and Welfare, *The First U.S. Mission on Mental Health in the USSR*, Washington, D.C., 1969.) As a result, confinement in mental hospitals is only of limited usefulness in the suppression of dissidence (which makes it nonetheless outrageous): "patients," whether dissident or not, must be "severe" cases in order to be committed, which means there can only be relatively few such cases. It is more common to charge dissidents with crimes, the labor camps taking precedence over the mental hospitals.

6. In twenty-five years, the CIA spent more than 25 million dollars through private medical research foundations to perfect drugs and other techniques for controlling human behavior. It also tested LSD on the inpatients of institutions as official as the U.S. Public Health Service Hospital at Lexington, Kentucky, and several federal prisons over a period of eleven years. "In 1954 the CIA hoped to use the knowledge it had acquired about LSD and similar drugs to find effective ways of causing lapses of memory and unusual behavior to discredit their victims, as well as sexual difficulties, decreased awareness, and states of emotional dependence." (*New York Times*, August 2, 1977). The same article reported that the CIA also enlisted the services of such academics as the director of the department of psychiatry and neurology at Tulane University, who was assigned to do research on the pain centers in the brain.

Index